Lange Review

The Fundamentals of Pediatric Sonography: A Registry Review and Protocol Guide

LANGE REVIEW

The Fundamentals of Pediatric Sonography: A Registry Review and Protocol Guide

Jenna N. Laquerre,
RT(R), RDMS (AB, OB/GYN, PS, BR), RVT
Diagnostic Medical Sonography
Adjunct Faculty
Palm Beach State College
Palm Beach Gardens, Florida

Mc
Graw
Hill

New York   Chicago   San Francisco   Athens   London   Madrid   Mexico City
New Delhi   Milan   Singapore   Sydney   Toronto

The Fundamentals of Pediatric Sonography: A Registry Review and Protocol Guide

1 2 3 4 5 6 7 8 9   DSS   27 26 25 24 23 22

ISBN 978-1-264-82789-3
MHID 1-264-82789-X

This book was set in Minion Pro by MPS Limited.
The editors were Sydney Keen Vitale and Kim J. Davis.
The production supervisor was Catherine Saggese.
Project management was provided by Anupam Bose, MPS Limited.

This book is printed on acid-free paper.

Library of Congress Cataloging-in-Publication Data

Names: Laquerre, Jenna N., author.
Title: Lange review. The fundamentals of pediatric sonography : a registry
    review and protocol guide / Jenna N Laquerre.
Other titles: Fundamentals of pediatric sonography
Description: New York : McGraw Hill, [2023] | Includes index. | Summary:
    "This book provides ultrasound educational material and is a registry
    review guide geared towards increased sonographer understanding of
    pediatric-specialized examinations and procedures"—Provided by publisher.
Identifiers: LCCN 2022031907 (print) | LCCN 2022031908 (ebook) |
    ISBN 9781264827893 (paperback; alk. paper) | ISBN 126482789X (paperback;
    alk. paper) | ISBN 9781264827947 (ebook) | ISBN 1264827946 (ebook)
Subjects: MESH: Ultrasonography—methods | Child | Infant | Outline
Classification: LCC RJ51.U45 (print) | LCC RJ51.U45 (ebook) | NLM WN 18.2 |
    DDC 618.92/007543—dc23/eng/20221110
LC record available at https://lccn.loc.gov/2022031907
LC ebook record available at https://lccn.loc.gov/2022031908

McGraw Hill books are available at special quantity discounts to use as premiums and sales promotions or for use in corporate training programs. To contact a representative, please visit the Contact Us pages at www.mhprofessional.com.

Contents

Contributors

Jenna Laquerre, BS, RT(R), RDMS (PS, ABD, OB/GYN, BR), RVT

Jenna is a professor of Sonography at Palm Beach State College and a graduate student at the University of North Florida. She is an alumna of Palm Beach State College in Radiography and Sonography and a Bachelor of Health Sciences graduate from Seminole State College in Healthcare Management and Professional Services. She is American Registry for Diagnostic Medical Sonography (ARDMS) registered in Abdomen, Obstetrics and Gynecology, Pediatric Sonography, Breast, and Vascular Technology, and American Registry of Radiologic Technologists (ARRT) registered in Radiologic Technology. Professor Laquerre is a member of the Lambda Nu National Honor Society for Radiologic and Imaging Sciences, American Society of Radiologic Technologists (ASRT), and Society of Diagnostic Medical Sonography (SDMS). She is a manuscript peer reviewer for the journal Radiologic Technology, published author, educational speaker, and has clinical experience from national institutions including Nemours Children's Hospital and AdventHealth.

Tara K. Cielma, BS, RT(S), RDMS, RDCS, RVT

Tara is a lead sonographer and clinical instructor at Children's National Hospital in Washington, D.C. She is credentialed by the ARDMS in Abdomen, OB/GYN, Neurosonography, Vascular Technology, and Fetal Echocardiography; she also holds credentials from the ARRT in Sonography. Tara is passionate about volunteering and contributing to the sonography community; she serves on the SDMS Conference Management Committee, CME Review Team, and Micro-Volunteer Team. She is a manuscript reviewer for the *Journal of Diagnostic Medical Sonography*, and item writer for the ARDMS. Tara also serves on the Society for Pediatric Radiology Education Committee to advance pediatric sonography. Lastly, Tara has several published chapters ranging from pediatric abdomen, urinary tract, neurosonography, to renal duplex imaging.

M. Robert DeJong, RDMS, RDCS, RVT, FAIUM, FSDMS
Bob DeJong, LLC

Robert is an Ultrasound Technical Manager with a demonstrated history of working in the hospital and healthcare industry since 1976. He is a strong healthcare services professional skilled in clinical research, medical education, healthcare information technology, medical ultrasound, and radiology. He spent the last 28 years gaining experience providing quality ultrasound related education in areas of ultrasound including but not limited to: abdominal, abdominal Doppler including renal arteries and liver Doppler, male reproductive organs, carotid, lower and upper extremity venous Doppler, and pediatrics including TCD on sickle cell children. Recently, he became the new primary author of *Craig's Essentials of Sonography and Patient Care*.

Patty M. Braga, MS, RDMS, RVT, RDCS, RT(R)

Patty is an associate professor and department chair of Palm Beach State College's Diagnostic Medical Sonography program. Professor Braga has served on the SDMS Board of Directors as both Director and Secretary. She is a chairperson on the SDMS Education Committee, which sets national curriculum standards for sonography programs. She serves on the SDMS Ethics Committee, is a Board Liaison for the SDMS Membership Awards and Recognition Committee, and site visitor for the Joint Review Committee on Education in Diagnostic Medical Sonography (JRC-DMS) for schools seeking accreditation through the Commission on Accreditation of Allied Health Education Programs (CAAHEP). In the state of Florida, Professor Braga serves as a Discipline Coordinator for the Florida Department of Education (DOE). She has also presented in both local and national conferences in OB/GYN, vascular, and educational topics.

Diana Mishler, MBA-HM, RT(R)(S), RDMS (ABD, OB/GYN), RDCS (FE)
Western Governor's University

Diana holds an Associate of Science in Radiography and Bachelor of Science in Medical Imaging Technology from Indiana University Kokomo. She is ARRT registered in radiography and sonography, and ARDMS registered in Abdomen, OB/GYN, and Fetal Echocardiography. Diana has been active in the field of diagnostic medical sonography for 14 years, specializing in gynecologic procedure guidance and imaging, standard and high-risk obstetrics, and limited fertility practice. Diana is currently employed with Marion General Hospital. She has served as a Senior Clinical Sales Specialist with Siemens and Program Director at Indiana University Kokomo's Medical Imaging Technology program. Diana is a nationally appointed sonography representative on the ASRT Practice Standards Council as well as 1 of 4 nationally elected sonography chapter delegates to the ASRT House of Delegates. Diana has published several articles and collaborated for a textbook chapter in *Radiology in Global Health*, 2nd edition. She has also contributed to the World Health Organization's (WHO) global sonography guidelines including COVID-19 protocols. Additionally, she has formally reviewed multiple chapters published in various textbooks.

Marjorie Quevedo, BS, RDMS, RDCS, RVT
AdventHealth University—Orlando Campus
Marjorie is a faculty member in the department of Diagnostic Medical Sonography at AdventHealth University. She graduated from the Cardiovascular Sonography program from Florida Hospital College of Health Sciences in 2006 and then from the General Sonography program at Florida Hospital College in 2007. She also graduated from Adventist University of Health Sciences in 2015 with her bachelor's degree in Diagnostic Medical Sonography. Marjorie holds credentials as a Registered Diagnostic Medical Sonographer (RDMS) in Abdomen and Obstetrics/Gynecology, Registered Diagnostic Cardiac Sonographer (RDCS) in Adult Echocardiography, and Vascular Technology (RVT). She has worked for the Adventist Health hospital system in California as a Lead Sonographer and has worked for several years at varying private physician offices. Marjorie currently is a member of the SDMS and American Institute of Ultrasound in Medicine (AIUM), and volunteers for both organizations. She has been published in the *Journal of Diagnostic Medical Sonography*.

Reviewer

David Dinan, MD
Nemours Children's Health System

Dr. Dinan is a board-certified Radiologist with an added Certificate of Qualification in Pediatric Radiology from the American Board of Radiology. He attended medical school at the University of Pennsylvania, completing a residency in Diagnostic Radiology at Beaumont Hospital in Royal Oak, Michigan before completing a fellowship in Pediatric Radiology at the Children's Hospital of Philadelphia. He has been practicing Pediatric Radiology exclusively for the last 12 years and currently serves as an Emergency Radiologist for Nemours Children's Health System. He has a strong interest in quality and patient safety with a focus on peer review. He holds an appointment as Assistant Professor at both the University of Central Florida and Florida State University.

Preface

Lange Review: The Fundamentals of Pediatric Sonography: A Registry Review and Protocol Guide provides ultrasound educational material and is a registry review guide geared toward increased sonographer understanding of pediatric-specialized examinations and procedures.

The Image Gently Alliance's mission statement is to improve safe and effective imaging care of children worldwide. Through this alliance, Image Gently advocates for use of sonographic imaging as an opportunity to decrease radiation dose exposure to a radiosensitive population. In recent years, pediatric sonography has gained recognition as a dedicated specialty. Beginning in 2015, the ARDMS created the Pediatric Sonography (PS) registry examination, providing specialized credentials to sonographers routinely providing care for a pediatric population.

The intent of this material is to enlighten sonographers in the practice of pediatric-specific exams. This comprehensive review guide covers topics outlined by the ARDMS for the PS registry exam, as well as supporting sonographic and radiologic images, schematics, questions, and correlating answers. Unique to this review is the inclusion of scan protocols for various pediatric-specific exams, including but not limited to imaging of the appendix, bowel (i.e., intussusception), dynamic hip, transcranial Doppler studies, and more.

The development of this review was made possible with numerous image contributions from Tara K. Cielma, BS, RT(S), RDMS, RDCS, RVT, text and review question contributions by M. Robert DeJong, LLC, RDMS, RDCS, RVT, FSDMS, FAIUM, Patty M. Braga, MS, RDMS, RVT, RDCS, RT (R), Diana Mishler, MBA-HM, RT(R)(S), RDMS, RDCS (FE), Marjorie Quevedo, BS, RDMS, RDCS, RVT, a dedicated material review performed by pediatric radiologist Dr. David Dinan, and medical illustration contributions by Isaiah Forestier, graphic designer. This review was produced by sonographers with experience in pediatric imaging from accredited institutions including Nemours Children's Hospital, Children's National Hospital, Children's Hospital of Philadelphia, and AdventHealth for Children.

We would like to graciously thank our family, friends, and colleagues for their steadfast support throughout the extensive period of research that went into the creation of this material. We are thankful to McGraw Hill for the opportunity to publish this material and would like to acknowledge their kindness and support throughout the publication process. To the sonographer with a passion for pediatrics, we wish you the very best in the future success of your career. Your gaining of knowledge will be of service to many children and patient families, and we hope you find this material useful!

Jenna N. Laquerre, BS, RT (R), RDMS
(AB, OB/GYN, PS, BR), RVT
Diagnostic Medical Sonography
Adjunct Faculty
Palm Beach State College

1

Sonographic Anatomy of the Skull and Brain

Anatomy of interest to sonographers in the pediatric skull and brain includes the calvarium and skull base, meninges, fissures, supratentorial brain, gyri, sulci, choroid plexus, ventricles, cavum septum pellucidi, thalamus, basal ganglia, cerebellum and cerebrospinal fluid (CSF).

Sutures, which are initially fibrous joints, allow for some mobility overlapping in young infants during birth and are located between the cranial bones. The major sutures of the calvarium are the sagittal, coronal, lambdoid, metopic, parieto-mastoid, and squamosal sutures.

From childhood into adulthood, the sutures fuse to protect the brain. The major cranial bones of interest are the frontal, parietal, temporal, occipital, sphenoid, and ethmoid bones. Cranial bones appear hyperechoic on sonography and demonstrate posterior shadowing.

Sonography of the neonatal brain is performed through the fontanelles (anterior, posterior, mastoid, and sphenoid) of the pediatric skull. The fontanelles allow for an acoustic window throughout the first year of life and begin to close near 9 months of age. However, the acoustic windows via these fontanelles may become limited even within the first 3 to 6 months of life. The anterior fontanelle is the main acoustic window, although the brain can be visualized through the posterior and mastoid fontanelles for axial views.

The anterior (bregma, frontal) fontanelle closes around 2 years of age. The posterior fontanelle is used to visualize infratentorial structures including the occipital horn of the lateral ventricles. The mastoid fontanelle is most commonly used to evaluate the posterior fossa, although it can enable evaluation of other structures (i.e., circle of Willis, posterior ventricles). The sphenoid fontanelle is infrequently used; however, it is an option to visualize the frontal lobes and anterior horns of the lateral ventricles.

Fissures of the brain are hypoechoic infoldings (i.e., because they fill with fluid), dividing the cerebrum into anatomical sections. Fissures include the longitudinal (interhemispheric), parietooccipital, transverse, lateral (Sylvian), and central fissures. The longitudinal fissure measures <6 millimeters and separates the cerebrum into right and left hemispheres. The lateral (Sylvian) fissure separates the temporal lobe from the anterior and parietal lobes, containing the middle cerebral artery.

In premature infants, the gyri and sulci of the brain are undeveloped giving it a smooth appearance (Fig. 1-1), compared to the mature sulcation pattern in the full-term infant (Fig. 1-2). Sulci are superficial depressions (grooves) in the gray matter and gyri are elevations between the sulci. Sulci appear hyperechoic on ultrasound and gyri appear hypoechoic.

The meninges are membranous coverings of the spinal cord and brain (central nervous system [CNS]) that protect these structures and provide nutrients. Meninges include the inner pia mater, arachnoid layer, and external dura mater. The arachnoid layer lets CSF exit the brain and flow into the venous system by way of the subdural and subarachnoid spaces.

CSF is a clear fluid present in the intracranial ventricular system, subarachnoid space, and spinal cord. The fluid is created by epithelial cells within the choroid plexus. It helps to transport waste products from the brain and spinal cord for filtration by the bloodstream. CSF flows from the choroid plexus of the lateral ventricle, foramen of Monro, third ventricle,

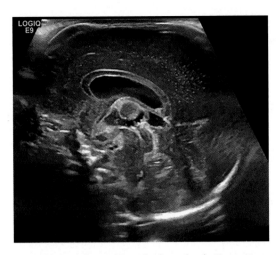

FIGURE 1-1. Preterm infant at 23 weeks. Smooth sulcation pattern with cavum vergae and interpositi present.

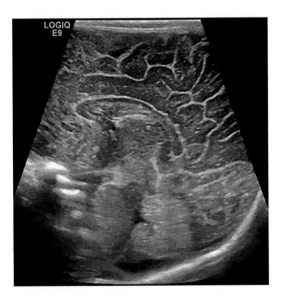

FIGURE 1-2. Full-term infant with mature sulcation pattern and closure of CSP.

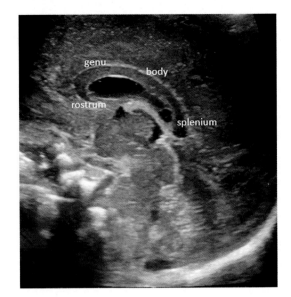

FIGURE 1-3. The four segments of the corpus callosum on a 26-week neonate.

cerebral aqueduct, fourth ventricle, foramen of Magendie, and over the brain and spinal cord, before being resorbed into the bloodstream. Alternative to the foramen of Magendie, CSF may also exit the foramen of Luschka (lateral apertures), also termed the foramina of Luschka.

The communicating third, fourth, and lateral ventricles make up the ventricular system, containing CSF. Ventricular components include frontal, occipital, and temporal horns, as well as the body and atrium (i.e., trigone region). The lateral ventricles are the largest cavity of the ventricular system. The third ventricle is narrow, and the fourth ventricle is positioned posterior to the medulla oblongata and anterior to the cerebellum. Approximately 90% of neonates are seen with asymmetric lateral ventricles with the left being larger than the right, and frontal horns appearing smaller than the ventricular atrium (trigone).

The choroid plexus is located within the third, fourth, and lateral ventricles, attached to the third ventricle's tela choroidea. The choroid plexus creates CSF and is formed by pia mater folds.

The corpus callosum (Figs. 1-3 and 1-4) acts to send information between the cerebral hemispheres and is comprised of a thick band of myelin-coated nerve fibers. The corpus callosum is hypoechoic on ultrasound and is located midline in the brain forming the lateral ventriclar roof.

The cavum septum pellucidum (CSP) is also located midline, between the bodies and frontal horns of the lateral ventricles (Fig. 1-4). Embryonically, the CSP is fashioned from two leaves positioned opposite one another which enclose, forming the anechoic cavity (cave, cavum) of the septi pellucidi. By 6 months gestational age, the leaves of the septi pellucidi come together in a caudal to cranial (rostral) manner. The CSP appears large in early gestation and regresses in size during the gestational period. This cavity most often is completely obliterated by 2 to 3 months postnatal age; however, a residual or small CSP can be seen as a normal variant in 30% of adult patients if the cavity does not fully close.

The thalamus is positioned in the central cerebrum, functioning as a relay station for nerve impulses to the cerebral cortex. This structure forms the upper and posterior walls of the third ventricle and lateral ventricle floor (Fig. 1-4). Sonographically, this structure is hypoechoic and has a round or ovoid appearance.

The germinal matrix (caudothalamic notch) is a delicate vascular rudimentary embryonic structure that regresses throughout the gestational period. It is often nonvisualized after 37 weeks gestational age. The germinal matrix is a common site for subependymal hemorrhage in premature neonates. It forms gray matter of the brain through the production of glial and neural cells.

The cerebellum is located in the posterior fossa (Fig. 1-4). This structure is separated from the cerebrum by the tentorium cerebelli and is connected to the brainstem. The cerebellum, like the supratentorial brain (i.e., cerebrum), consists of gray and white matter. The cerebellum is the largest component of the hindbrain and is made up of two hemispheres, connected

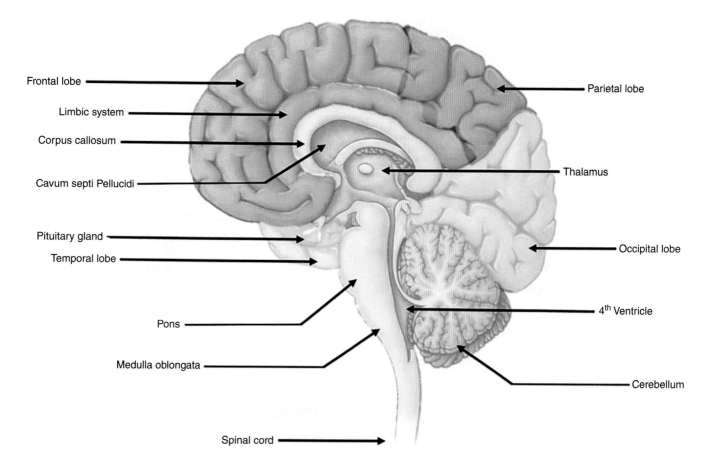

Frontal lobe

Limbic system

Corpus callosum

Cavum septi Pellucidi

Pituitary gland

Temporal lobe

Pons

Medulla oblongata

Spinal cord

Parietal lobe

Thalamus

Occipital lobe

4th Ventricle

Cerebellum

FIGURE 1-4. Anatomic structures of the brain. Courtesy of contributor Tara Cielma.

by the vermis. The cerebellum controls posture, balance, and voluntary movements.

A 7.5-MHz phased or vector array transducer is used for premature infants, and a 5-MHz transducer is needed for larger older infants. Increasing the number of focal zones provides increased lateral resolution by narrowing the acoustic beam. A standoff pad may be required for optimization of superficial structures such as the sagittal sinus.

The patient should be less than 6 months of age (term infants) for this exam for an adequate fontanelle window and optimal penetration. In patients over 6 months of age, the examination may be limited by suboptimal penetration and limited acoustic windows via the fontanelle(s). For neonatal intensive care unit patients the ultrasound unit should be brought portable and sterile gel should be used. If feasible, the sterile gel should be moderately warmed prior to use for reduction of heat loss in the neonate.

Imaging includes coronal anterior to posterior views, followed by sagittal midline to right and midline to left. Using a phased or vector array transducer, coronal and sagittal images of the neonatal brain are standardly performed through the anterior fontanelle. Axial (mastoid) views of the posterior fossa can also be obtained using a phased or vector array transducer demonstrating the cerebellum and fourth ventricle and anatomic side should be labeled. For imaging of the superficial sagittal

sinus, a high-frequency linear transducer is used to evaluate for patency and flow in both the coronal and sagittal planes. Care must be taken to not obliterate flow by applying too much pressure. Copious gel or a standoff pad may be useful. Superficial coronal images can be taken through the open fontanelle(s) to check for extra-axial fluid collections between the cranium and brain parenchyma. Doppler images of the extra-axial spaces should be taken with a high-frequency linear transducer. Doppler is also indicated for abnormalities such as intracranial cystic lesions and vein of Galen malformation.

During coronal imaging, it is important the sonographer image as symmetrically as possible. The sonographer obtains images from anterior to posterior, identifying major anatomic landmarks in each image. In the supine neonate whose head is positioned near the sonographic monitor, the transducer notch is standardly directed toward the patient's right ear.

Still images:

1. To obtain the frontal-most view, the acoustic beam is angled anteriorly toward the patient's face to demonstrate the orbital ridges and frontal lobe. The interhemispheric (longitudinal) fissure can be seen dividing the cerebrum into right and left hemispheres. The ethmoid sinus and orbital ridge can be seen in this view (Fig. 1-5).

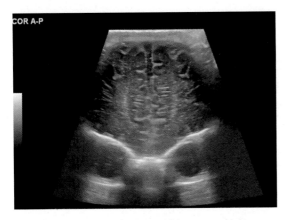

FIGURE 1-5. Anterior-most coronal view of the neonatal brain.

2. Sliding and angling the transducer posteriorly demonstrates the frontal horn of the lateral ventricles and midline CSP (Fig. 1-6). The caudate nucleus, germinal matrix, corpus callosum, and thalamus begin coming into view (Fig. 1-7). The sonographer should observe the echogenicity of the basal ganglia, which are regions of gray matter positioned at the base of the bilateral cerebral hemispheres.

3. Sliding and angling the transducer more posterior demonstrates the temporal lobe and Sylvian fissures. The Sylvian fissure produces a Y-shaped appearance in the coronal plane and separates the frontal and temporal lobes. Posterior to the frontal horns is the body of the lateral ventricle. This view also demonstrates the temporal horn of the lateral ventricle, thalamus, and choroidal fissure.

4. Sliding and angling the transducer posteriorly demonstrates the CSP, thalamus, third ventricle, and foramen of Monro. Just prior to visualization of the occipital lobes, the quadrigeminal plate, cisterna magna, tentorium cerebelli, thalamus, and body and temporal horn of the lateral ventricle are visualized.

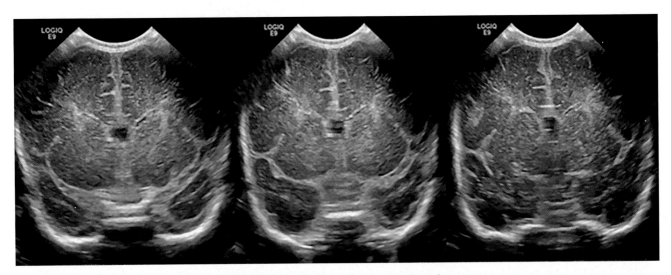

FIGURE 1-6. Coronal anterior brain in a preterm infant.

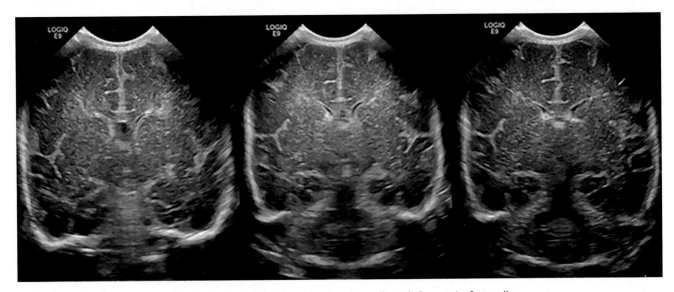

FIGURE 1-7. Imaging the above noted structures through the anterior fontanelle.

5. Sliding and angling the transducer posteriorly, the occipital lobes and choroid plexus comes into view (Fig. 1-8), extending along the body of the lateral ventricles into the atria (trigone) of the lateral ventricles (Fig. 1-9). The sonographer should observe the echogenicity of the periventricular white matter as it relates to the choroid plexus. Echogenicity of the white matter should not surpass echogenicity of the choroid plexus.

6. The final posterior coronal image obtained is of the occipital lobes (Fig. 1-10), with demonstration of the interhemispheric fissure. This is achieved by directing the acoustic beam posteriorly towards the base of the skull.

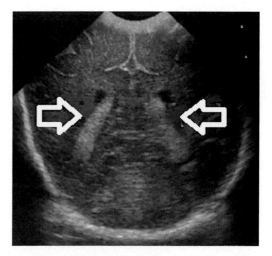

FIGURE 1-8. Choroid plexus (bilateral hyperechoic areas demonstrated with arrows).

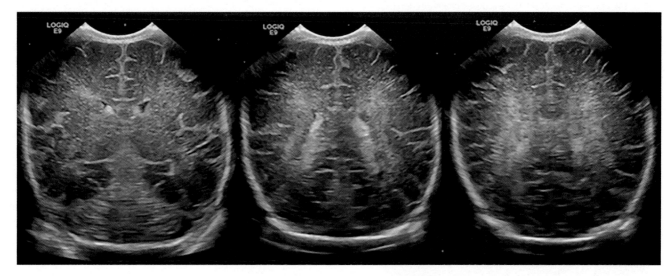

FIGURE 1-9. Occipital lobe and choroid plexus.

Cine-clip: 1. It may also be helpful for radiologist evaluation for the sonographer to obtain an anterior to posterior cine-loop of cranial structures.

Note: It should be noted that protocol may vary based upon institution and/or radiologist or interpreting physician imaging preference. There should be a minimum of six coronal images (Fig. 1-11) and five sagittal images (inclusive of sagittal midline and two lateral images which are obtained bilaterally) (Fig. 1-12). Providing additional images and/or cine-clip documentation aims at documenting an adequate representation and greater detail of the various neonatal intracranial structures.

Following coronal evaluation, the sonographer begins sagittal imaging for evaluation of ventricular size and configuration and structural appearance of the cerebellum, cerebellar vermis, cerebrum, fourth ventricle, and caudothalamic groove. This is

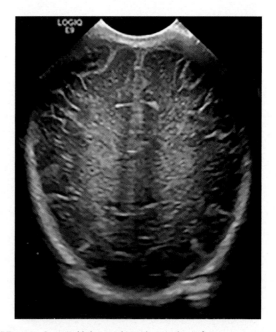

FIGURE 1-10. Occipital lobes and interhemispheric fissure.

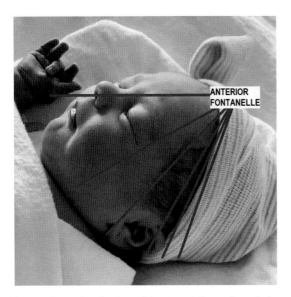

FIGURE 1-11. Coronal projections of the acoustic beam through the anterior fontanelle.

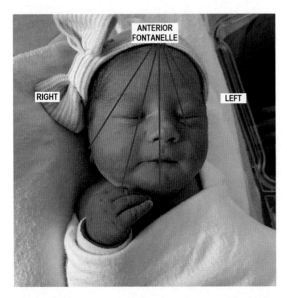

FIGURE 1-12. Sagittal projections of the acoustic beam through the anterior fontanelle.

achieved by rotating the transducer 90-degrees from coronal plane. In the supine neonate whose head is positioned near the sonographic monitor, the transducer notch is standardly directed toward the patient's face.

Still images:

1. The initial sagittal image obtained is sagittal midline (Fig. 1-13(a) and (b)), identifying major landmarks including the corpus callosum, CSP, frontal and occipital lobes, third ventricle, cerebellar vermis, and massa intermedia.

> **Note:** When this view is properly produced, it has been referred to in other sources as creating the "lady in the dress" sign, where the thalamus creates the head, the third ventricle creates the face, the corpus callosum appears to create an eccentric hat, and the vermis of the cerebellum creates a flared ballgown-style dress.

From the sagittal midline view, the sonographer will begin to slide and angle the transducer laterally (Fig. 1-14). The transducer is angled midline to right and midline to left, to perform a bilateral evaluation.

2. The angled right parasagittal view involves the sonographer angling from midline laterally. The landmark for this image is the "C"-shaped lateral ventricle. The sonographer should identify the germinal matrix (caudothalamic notch, see Fig. 1-15(a) and (b)), evaluating for the presence of a discrete hemorrhage. The caudate nucleus, thalamus, and cerebellum can also be identified in this image.

3. The angle right tangential parasagittal view involves further lateral angulation of the transducer. In this view the Sylvian fissure and temporal lobe is demonstrated (Fig. 1-16).

4. The angled left parasagittal view involves the sonographer angling from midline laterally. The landmark for this image is the "C"-shaped lateral ventricle. The sonographer

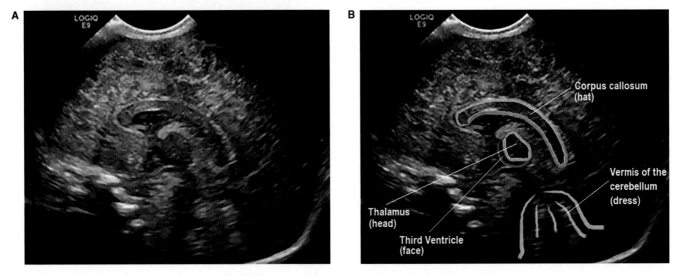

FIGURE 1-13. Sagittal midline structures of the brain.

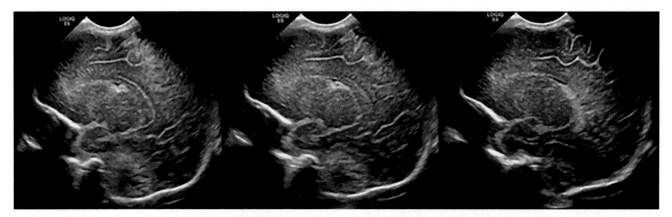

FIGURE 1-14. Sagittal brain, lateral to midline.

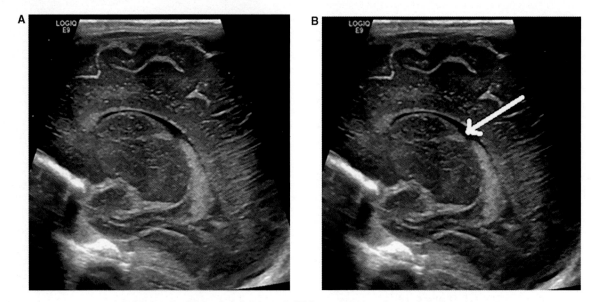

FIGURE 1-15. (A) Caudothalamic notch. **(B)** Arrow depiction of caudothalamic notch.

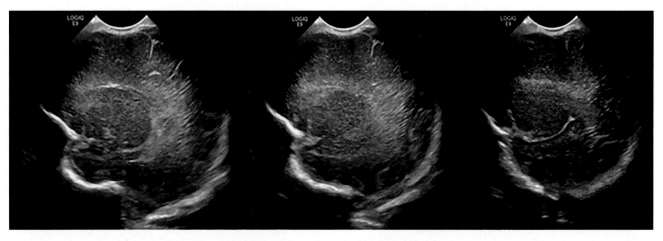

FIGURE 1-16. Sagittal temporal lobe (lateral brain).

should identify the germinal matrix (caudothalamic notch) evaluating for the presence of a discrete hemorrhage. The caudate nucleus, thalamus, and cerebellum can also be identified in this image.

5. The angle left tangential parasagittal view involves further lateral angulation of the transducer. In this view the Sylvian fissure and temporal lobe is demonstrated.

Cine-clip:

1. It is also beneficial for the sonographer to obtain midline to lateral right, and midline to lateral left cine-loops for radiologist evaluation.

> **Note:** Sliding and angling the transducer involves miniscule movements for direction of the acoustic beam, creating various slices of the neonatal brain.

To achieve imaging of vasculature, the sonographer should switch from a phased or vector array to a high-frequency linear array transducer. In sagittal plane, the anterior cerebral artery can be readily visualized. It is here the sonographer should assess velocity of flow and resistive indices utilizing color and spectral Doppler when indicated. In coronal plane, the sagittal sinus and superficial structures can be identified. The sonographer should ensure minimal pressure is used for optimal demonstration of this anatomic region.

Axial views of the posterior fossa are obtained through the mastoid fontanelles which are located posterior to the ears.

Still images:

1. To obtain the right mastoid fontanelle view, place the transducer behind the right ear with the transducer notch directed toward the patient's face. Demonstrate the pons, cerebellum (Fig. 1-17), and interpeduncular fossa. Sonographically the cerebellum is hypoechoic. The fourth ventricle, which is anechoic to hypoechoic with hyperechoic walls, is seen posterior to the pons and medulla and anterior to the cerebellum (Figs. 1-18 and 1-19).

2. To obtain the left mastoid fontanelle view, place the transducer behind the left ear with the transducer notch directed toward the patient's face.

> **Note:** For optimal patient cooperation, mastoid images should be obtained following necessary coronal and sagittal views. It is speculated that neonates may exhibit minimal discomfort because of aural response to acoustic energy pulses emitted by the transducer.

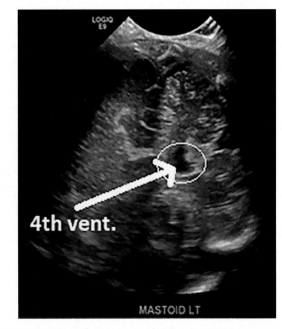

FIGURE 1-18. Mastoid fontanelle view of the cerebellum and fourth ventricle.

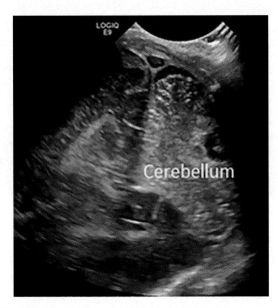

FIGURE 1-17. Mastoid fontanelle view of the cerebellum.

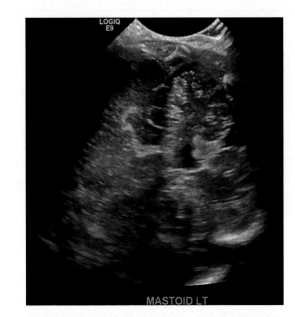

FIGURE 1-19. Mastoid fontanelle view of the cerebellum and fourth ventricle.

2

Sonographic Anatomy of the Spine

While in utero the neural tube begins formation by canalization and retrogressive differentiation of the caudal cell mass, which is known as "secondary neurulation." Within the canal of the neural tube is a layer of cells that generate nerve fibers, nerve cell bodies, and neuroglia.

During secondary neurulation, cell necrosis decreases the size of the caudal neural tube to form the conus medullaris, filum terminale, and ventriculus terminalis.

By 3 weeks gestation, the neural tube is completely formed with the cephalic end of the tube closing before the caudal end. The caudal end of the neural tube forms the spinal cord, while the cranial end forms the brain.

Upon closure of the neural tube, dorsal induction begins at 5 weeks gestation and is the first step in central nervous system maturation. During ventral induction, the neural tube forms the rhombencephalon, mesencephalon, and prosencephalon at 7 to 12 weeks gestational age. Overlapping ventral induction, proliferation, and migration occur at 8 weeks gestation.

During proliferation, glioblasts and neuroblasts begin multiplying. Disruption associated with proliferation may result in brain abnormalities during development, while migration disruption may result in abnormal neuron location. Neuron communication begins to occur around 6 months gestational age.

The final stage of central nervous system maturation includes myelination, in which myelin sheaths develop to insulate axons. This begins at 6 months gestational age and continues throughout life.

For infant spinal cord imaging, a high frequency linear transducer between 5 and 17 MHz should be utilized, placing the transducer midline over the spinous processes. This exam is most successfully performed on infants under 6 months of age. Above 6 months in age, acoustic windows are limited by the underlying spine. The caregiver should be instructed to feed the infant prior to the exam for patient comfort and cooperation. The patient is scanned in prone position with the bed in a slight reverse Trendelenburg position for filling of cerebrospinal fluid in the lower spinal canal. Placing a rolled washcloth or infant blanket under the infant's abdomen will also aid in arching the back for optimal visualization of the interspinous spaces. The lumbar spine is imaged in two planes, sagittal and transverse, and lumbar vertebrae should be labeled by counting both inferiorly from the thoracic spine (i.e., lowest pair of ribs) and superiorly from the sacrum. The sonographer should evaluate cord position within the spinal canal, cord motion, and presence of syrinx (hydromelia), cysts, lipomas, or thickened filum terminale. If abnormal findings are observed, they should be documented in two imaging planes.

In healthy infants, the position of the conus medullaris should be located above the L2-L3 disc space, with the cord ending between T12 and L2. A conus tip below the level of the L2-L3 disc space is suggestive of a tethered cord.

Filar cysts are of no clinical significance and are an anatomic variant of the spinal cord. Additional variants of the spinal cord are discussed in Chapter 14, "Spinal Malformations."

Sonographic imaging of the infant spine is often performed for the assessment of suspected closed neural tube defects. This may be indicated following an abnormal clinical examination. Common reasons for sonographic evaluation include skin dimpling in the sacral region, sacrococcygeal skin defects, posterior masses or cystic lesions, hair tufts overlying the spinal canal, anal stenosis or atresia, skin discoloration or hemangioma overlying the spine, abscess or infectious processes, and post-surgical follow up. Less commonly, spinal ultrasound is used as guidance for spinal interventional procedures (i.e., lumbar puncture).

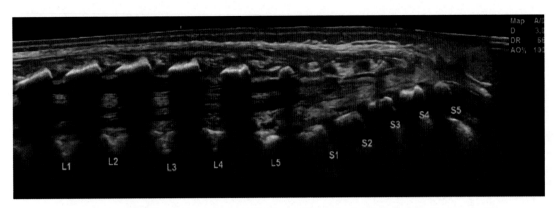

FIGURE 2-1. Normal ultrasound of the pediatric spine in a 2-week-old patient.

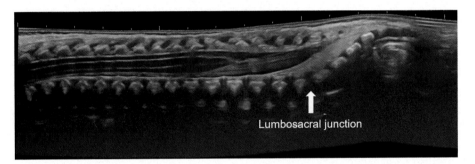

FIGURE 2-2. Lumbosacral junction. Extended field of view with clear conus and visible rectum.

Ultrasound of the spine includes:

1. Sagittal imaging of the lumbar and sacrococcygeal spine:
   a. Document level of each lumbar vertebra (Fig. 2-1); and
   b. Demonstrate relationship to conus (Fig. 2-2).
2. Transverse imaging of the lumbar and sacrococcygeal spine.
   a. Evaluate the conus.
3. In the presence of a dimple, provide dedicated sagittal and transverse images at the level of the dimple with a high-resolution transducer and stand-off pad for visualization of the skin surface to exclude a tract or communication between the skin and spine.
4. Panoramic of conus to coccyx.
5. Cine-clip of sagittal spine demonstrating the conus.

Sonographic Anatomy of the Abdomen

3

The pediatric abdomen is evaluated in its entirety as an abdominal complete, or abdominal limited ultrasound evaluation. An abdominal complete ultrasound entails survey and documentation of the pancreas, aorta, inferior vena cava (IVC), liver, gallbladder, biliary tree, bilateral kidneys, adrenal glands, spleen, and bladder. Adrenal glands become difficult to see as patient age progresses and may not be visualized in older children. An abdominal limited ultrasound is any sonographic examination of the abdomen which is less than what is evaluated in the abdomen complete exam. This may involve evaluation of the right upper abdominal quadrant, including structures evaluated in the abdominal complete excluding the spleen, left kidney, adrenal glands, and bladder. An abdomen limited ultrasound can also include specific evaluation of the appendix, pylorus, bowel for presence of pathologies (i.e., intussusception), survey for ascites, or sole evaluation of the spleen. Transducer selection is based upon patient habitus, ranging from a higher frequency selection for neonates and infants, to a low- to mid-frequency transducer for adolescents. For an abdominal ultrasound, patients should be fasting to reduce bowel gas artifact which obscures anatomy and to improve visualization of abdominal structures. However, fasting may not be feasible in an emergent care setting. Patient preparation of fasting is based upon patient age.

Length of fasting time is based upon the patient's age. This is generally expressed as nil per os (NPO), the Latin abbreviation which translates to "nothing by mouth," describing the length of time by which a patient should go without food or drink prior to a medical examination. General guidelines for patient preparation and fasting include the following: a newborn less than one year of age should fast 2 hours (particularly important in cases of suspected biliary atresia). Patients less than 5 years of age should be NPO 4 hours prior to an abdominal ultrasound. Patients greater than 5 years of age should remain NPO for 6 hours. Adolescents approaching adulthood should be fasting a full 6 to 8 hours prior to abdominal ultrasound exam to reduce bowel gas artifact and fully distend the gallbladder.

All abdominal organs should be scanned in two imaging planes. Bowel loops should be briefly evaluated, documenting images only in the presence of a bowel abnormality, unless a specific bowel exam is ordered (i.e., cross-sectional view of bowel with bowel if wall thickness measurement is abnormal). A sample complete abdomen protocol would include the following:

1. Pancreas
   a. Still images:
      i. Transverse (long-axis view of pancreas) include head, body, and tail anterior to the splenic vein (Figs. 3-1, 3-2, and 3-3)

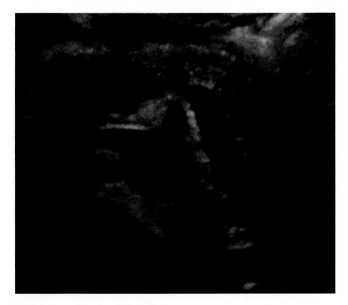

FIGURE 3-1. Transverse pancreas.

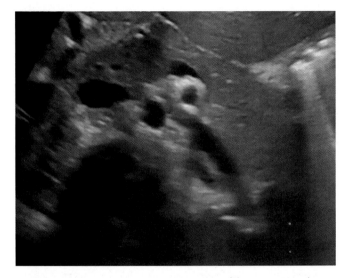

FIGURE 3-2. Transverse pancreas, accentuation of the pancreatic tail.

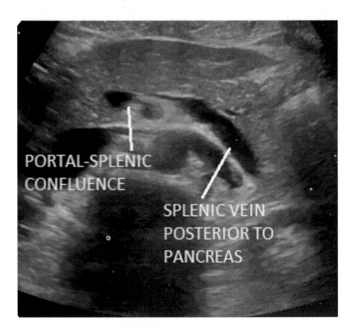

FIGURE 3-3. Vasculature posterior to pancreas.

    ii.   Transverse pancreas head (to include common bile duct [CBD]) (Fig. 3-4)

    iii. Transverse pancreas with color Doppler (Fig. 3-5)

Note: The sonographer should survey the portal-splenic confluence for proper hepatopetal flow direction. In this region, briefly evaluate the relationship of the superior mesenteric artery (SMA) and superior mesenteric vein (SMV). The SMA is positioned anterior to the abdominal aorta and the SMV anterior to the inferior vena cava (IVC).

    iv. Sagittal pancreas (adjacent to aorta)

2. Aorta

  a. Still images:

    i.   With and without color Doppler

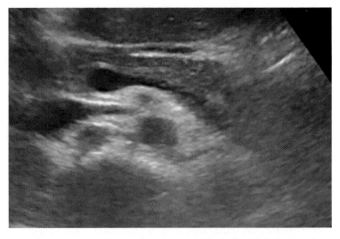

FIGURE 3-4. Transverse pancreas, accentuation of the pancreatic head.

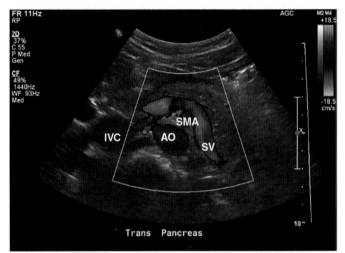

FIGURE 3-5. Transverse pancrease with color Doppler, demonstrating the portal-splenic confluence posterior to pancreatic head and body.

    ii.   Sagittal aorta proximal to include celiac axis and SMA

    iii. Sagittal aorta, mid

    iv. Sagittal aorta, distal

    v.   Sagittal aorta, bifurcation

    vi. Transverse aorta, proximal

    vii. Transverse aorta, mid

    viii. Transverse aorta, distal

    ix. Transverse aorta, bifurcation

Note: Aortic measurements and spectral Doppler evaluation are generally not required for a standard abdominal evaluation unless pathology is identified or this is a preferred by the clinical institution. When measuring the aorta, an outer-to-outer (OTO) wall measurement is standard. Other measurement methods include leading edge-to-leading edge (LELE) or inner-to-inner (ITI) wall measurement. The leading edge method involves caliper placement at the outer edge of the anterior aortic wall to the inner edge of the posterior aortic wall. It is important in subsequent scans the same measurement method be followed for reproducibility and evaluation of any change in aortic diameter. For a dedicated aortic evaluation, spectral Doppler evaluation is performed in sagittal imaging plane at proximal, mid, and distal segments, including evaluation of the bilateral common iliac arteries. The sonographer should obtain two samples at each location measuring peak systolic velocity (PSV) and end diastolic velocity (EDV).

3. IVC
   a. Still images:
      i. With and without color Doppler
      ii. Sagittal IVC
4. Liver
   a. Still images:
      i. Sagittal, far left hepatic lobe (Fig. 3-6)
      ii. Sagittal, left lobe at aorta (origins of celiac, SMA, and pancreas) (Fig. 3-7)
      iii. Sagittal, left lobe at proximal IVC with middle hepatic vein (Fig. 3-8)
      iv. Sagittal, right lobe at region of main lobar fissure and gallbladder (Fig. 3-9)
      v. Sagittal, right lobe at dome (Fig. 3-10)
      vi. Sagittal, right lobe and diaphragm interface (to exclude presence of right pleural effusion)
      vii. Sagittal, right lobe at mid clavicular line (with measurement of liver length)
      viii. Sagittal, right lobe and kidney interface (to compare organ echogenicities) (Fig. 3-11)

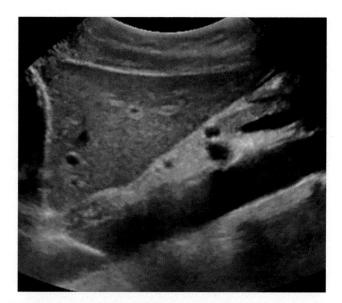

FIGURE 3-7. Sagittal left lobe of the liver at level of aorta.

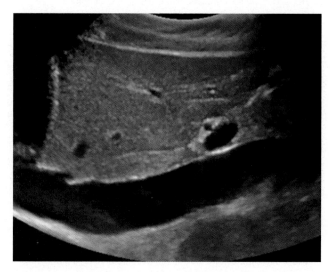

FIGURE 3-8. Sagittal left lobe of the liver at level of the IVC.

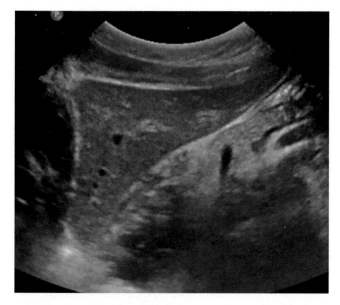

FIGURE 3-6. Sagittal left lobe of the liver.

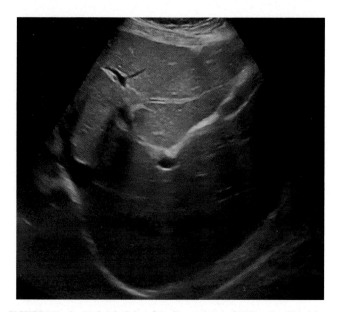

FIGURE 3-9. Sagittal right lobe of the liver at level of MLF and gallbladder.

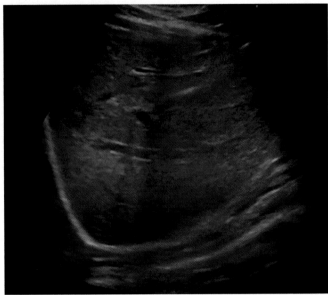

FIGURE 3-10. Sagittal right lobe of the liver at level of dome.

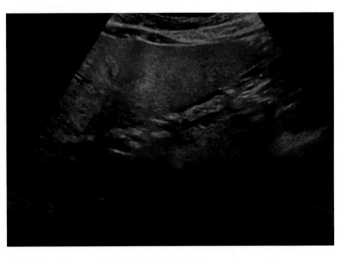

FIGURE 3-12. Transverse left lobe of the liver.

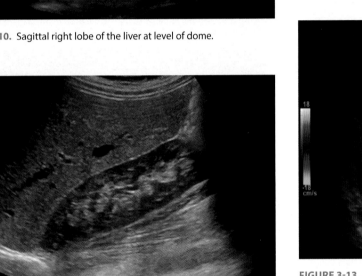

FIGURE 3-11. Sagittal right lobe of the liver at level of right kidney.

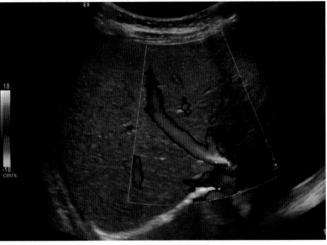

FIGURE 3-13. Transverse right lobe of the liver at level of hepatic veins; use of color Doppler demonstrating patency of the hepatic veins.

ix. Transverse, left lobe and heart (to exclude presence of pericardial effusion) (Fig. 3-12)

- Dependent on clinical institution, cardiology may protest/refrain from excluding pericardial effusion on a standard sonographic abdominal evaluation at some institutions. In this case, provide transverse view of left lobe only.

x. Transverse, junction of right and left lobes at hepatic veins and IVC confluence (Figs. 3-13 and 3-14)

xi. Transverse, right lobe at main portal vein (demonstrating right and left portal vein branches, with and without color Doppler to demonstrate direction of flow) (Figs. 3-15 and 3-16)

xii. Transverse, right lobe and right kidney interface (Fig. 3-17)

b. Cine clip: Transverse liver superior to inferior

Note: Shear wave elastography (SWE) is an imaging technique that measures the shear wave speed in a medium (tissue) to quantify the medium's stiffness. Limitations of SWE include patient motion and patients with increased body habitus. If an abnormality is visualized (i.e., biliary atresia, portal hypertension, cirrhosis, hepatomegaly, hepatitis C, cystic fibrosis, Alpha 1, antitrypsin deficiency, transaminitis, and so forth) and shear-wave module is available, the operator should use shear-wave module providing measurements for radiologist's review. Stiffness measurements are provided in distance divided by time, such as m/s, or in Young's Modulus form of kPa. When using shear wave technology within the liver, samples should be obtained approximately 1 to 2 centimeters from the capsule of the liver, avoiding areas of vasculature.

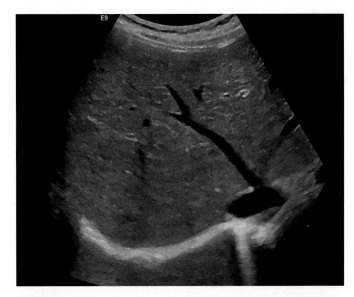

FIGURE 3-14. Transverse right lobe of the liver at level of hepatic veins.

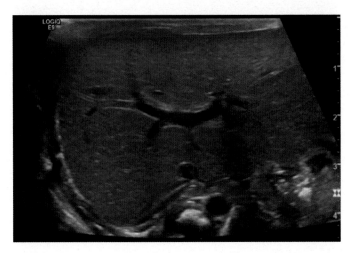

FIGURE 3-15. Transverse right lobe of the liver demonstrating portal vein.

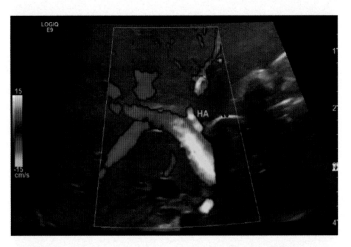

FIGURE 3-16. Transverse right lobe of the liver at level of the portal vein; use of color Doppler demonstrating patency of the portal vein and branches, as well as the adjacent hepatic artery (annotated HA).

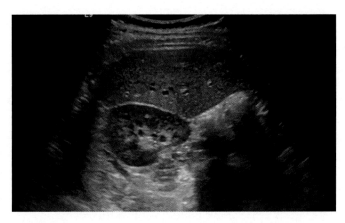

FIGURE 3-17. Transverse right lobe of the liver at level of right kidney.

5. Gallbladder
   a. Still images:
      i.   Sagittal, supine (with and without anterior wall measurement)
      ii. Transverse, supine (with and without anterior wall measurement)
      iii. Sagittal, left lateral decubitus (Fig. 3-18)
      iv. Transverse, left lateral decubitus

Note: Gallbladder images are obtained in two patient positions, most often supine and left lateral decubitus. The sonographer should fully scan through the gallbladder neck, body, and fundus in sagittal (longitudinal) and transverse views. If gallstones are visualized, the sonographer should document mobility and utilize color Doppler to differentiate from alternative etiologies (i.e., gallbladder polyp).

6. CBD
   a. Still images:
      i. Elongated view of CBD (with and without measurement and color Doppler)
      ii. Elongated view of CBD at head of pancreas (include long axis of the mail portal vein)

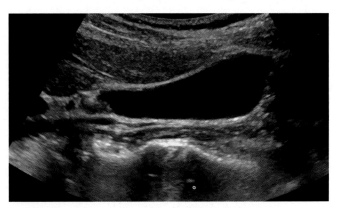

FIGURE 3-18. Sagittal view of the gallbladder with patient in left lateral decubitus position.

7. Right Kidney
   a. Still images:
      i. Sagittal, lateral to medial
      ii. Sagittal, midline (with measurement at parenchymal edge)
      iii. Transverse, superior to inferior
      iv. Transverse, mid (with and without color Doppler and measurement)

Note: Obtain measurement of anteroposterior and transverse diameter of renal pelvis at parenchymal edge in presence of dilation.

   b. Cine clip: Transverse superior to inferior, prone (supine position in larger habitus adolescents)
8. Right Adrenal Gland
   a. Still images:
      i. Coronal view with adjacent liver, right kidney, and IVC
9. Left Kidney
   a. Still images:
      i. Sagittal, lateral to medial
      ii. Sagittal, midline (with measurement at parenchymal edge)
      iii. Transverse, superior to inferior
      iv. Transverse, mid (with and without color Doppler and measurement)

Note: Obtain measurement of anteroposterior and transverse diameter of renal pelvis at parenchymal edge in presence of dilation.

   b. Cine clip: Transverse superior to inferior, prone (supine position in larger habitus adolescents)
10. Left Adrenal Gland
    a. Still images:
       i. Coronal view with adjacent spleen, left kidney, and aorta
11. Spleen
    a. Still images:
       i. Sagittal interface of spleen and left kidney (to compare organ echogenicities)
       ii. Sagittal splenic hilum (with and without color Doppler) (Fig. 3-19)
       iii. Sagittal spleen with measurement, demonstrate diaphragm to exclude the presence of left pleural effusion) (Figs. 3-20 and 3-21)
       iv. Transverse, superior to inferior (with measurement) (Fig. 3-22)

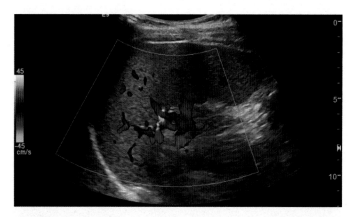

FIGURE 3-19. Sagittal spleen with color Doppler demonstrating patency of splenic artery and vein.

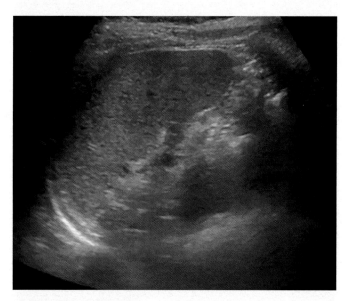

FIGURE 3-20. Sagittal spleen.

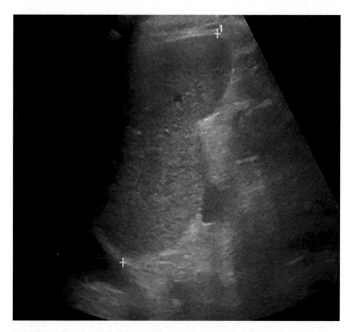

FIGURE 3-21. Sagittal spleen with splenic length measurement.

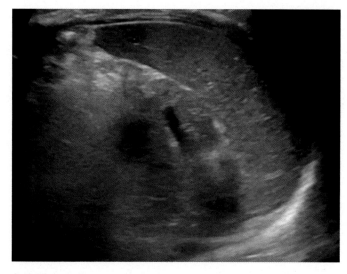

FIGURE 3-22. Transverse spleen.

12. Urinary Bladder
   a. Still images:
      i. Sagittal (with and without measurement)
      ii. Transverse (with and without measurement and color Doppler for demonstration of ureteral jets)
      iii. Obtain bladder volume, L × W × H × 0.52
      iv. Allow patient to empty bladder and obtain post-void measurements

> **Note:** In presence of hydronephrosis with urinary bladder fully distended, re-image bilateral kidneys and urinary bladder post-void. Briefly evaluate female pelvis, only archiving incidental images of uterus and ovaries if abnormality is suspected.

For a limited abdomen exam for evaluation of ascites, a linear 5- to 17-MHz transducer should be used. A curvilinear transducer is appropriate for larger habitus adolescents. Still images should be obtained in two orthogonal planes at each abdominal quadrant. Transverse superior to inferior cine clips should be provided of the right, middle, and left abdomen. The protocols for intussusception and appendix are discussed in pathology section of the review guide.

PANCREAS

The pancreas is an organ composed of accessory digestive exocrine and hormone-secreting endocrine tissues, as well as fibrous stroma parenchyma, vessels, nerves, and lymphatics. The exocrine tissues are comprised of acinar and ductal elements, making up 80% of the pancreas. The endocrine tissues are made of islet cells, which make up 2% of the pancreas. The pancreatic lymphatics, nerves, vessels, and fibrous stroma comprise the remaining 18% of pancreatic tissue. The pancreas regulates carbohydrates by secreting insulin and glucagons

from Islets of Langerhans cells, and pancreatic enzymes play a large role in the process of digestion. Insulin regulates glucose metabolism and blood glucose levels. Without insulin, glucose cannot pass through cell walls. Diabetes mellitus can be caused by lack of insulin or insulin resistance. In patients with diabetes mellitus, not enough insulin is secreted. This causes the body to be unable to utilize glucose, which in turn causes hyperglycemia. Normally, the pancreas is homogeneous and isoechoic to the liver. The head of the pancreas sits in the C-loop of the duodenum which is commonly termed the "romance of the abdomen." The main pancreatic duct is also referred to as the duct of Wirsung, which joins the CBD. Normal variants include an annular pancreas, ectopic pancreatic tissue, and pancreatic divisum. The normal duct of Wirsung measures less than 3 millimeters in the head of the pancreas. The duct of Santorini is an accessory duct and small branch of the main pancreatic duct, located in the head of the pancreas. The size of the pancreas varies with patient age as shown below:

Neonates less than 1 month of age: AP diameter of the head 1.0 cm, body 0.6 cm, tail 1.0 cm

Infants 1 to 12 months of age: AP diameter of the head 1.5 cm, body 0.8 cm, tail 1.2 cm

Children 1 to 5 years of age: AP diameter of the head 1.6 cm, body 1.0 cm, tail 1.8 cm

Children 5 to 10 years of age: AP diameter of the head 1.7 cm, body 1.0 cm, tail 1.8 cm

Adolescents 10 to 19 years of age: AP diameter of the head 2.0 cm, body 1.1 cm, tail 2.0 cm

LIVER

The liver is the body's largest solid organ located in the right upper abdominal quadrant. It receives most of its nutrient-rich blood supply from the hepatic portal vein and a lesser extent of oxygenated blood from the hepatic artery. The right, middle, and left hepatic veins drain filtered blood from the liver into the IVC. The liver is responsible for numerous functions including blood filtration, drug metabolization, regulation of blood chemical levels, plasma protein synthesis, glycogen storage, and bile excretion. Bile is a byproduct of hepatocytes mainly comprised of conjugated bilirubin, cholesterol, bile salts, phospholipids, and water. It is drained from the liver via the right and left hepatic ducts, where it joins the cystic duct for storage in the gallbladder or excretion via the common bile duct into the duodenum. For an optimal sonographic window, the patient should be fasting. Fasting allows for maximum gallbladder distension as a hepatic imaging landmark and minimal bowel gas for best visualization of hepatic structures. Sonographic images are obtained in sagittal and transverse imaging planes of the right and left liver lobes, demonstrating pertinent anatomical landmarks throughout. The caudate lobe can be identified adjacent to the left liver lobe, separated by the ligamentum venosum. The pediatric liver is completed with development by the age of 15, with the right liver lobe growing at a faster rate than the left. The liver parenchyma should appear homogeneous, similar in echogenicity to the right kidney cortex, with fissures and ligaments hyperechoic.

Nomenclature of Couinaud and Bismuth (Fig. 3-23) are most often used for defining segmental anatomy of the hepatic lobes. Claude Couinaud, a French surgeon, described this division of the liver in 1957. The Couinaud classification separates the liver into eight individual wedge-shaped segments. Each wedge apex is directed toward the porta hepatis. From a surgical standpoint, this nomenclature is followed as a guide for extended and subsegmental liver resections. It may be necessary for radiologists to adhere to this nomenclature to provide colleagues (i.e., surgeons) accurate pre-surgical information. These segments are:

1. Segment 1 caudate lobe
2. Segment 2 superolateral segment of left lobe (left of the left hepatic vein [LHV], above portal)
3. Segment 3 inferolateral segment of left lobe (left of the LHV, below portal)
4. Segment 4 medial segment of the left lobe (includes quadrate lobe), divided into (4a and 4b) by the left portal vein:
   4a. Above portal
   4b. Below portal
5. Segment 5 anteroinferior segment of the right lobe (between middle hepatic vein [MHV] and right hepatic vein [RHV], below portal)
6. Segment 6 posteroinferior segment of the right lobe (right of RHV, below portal)

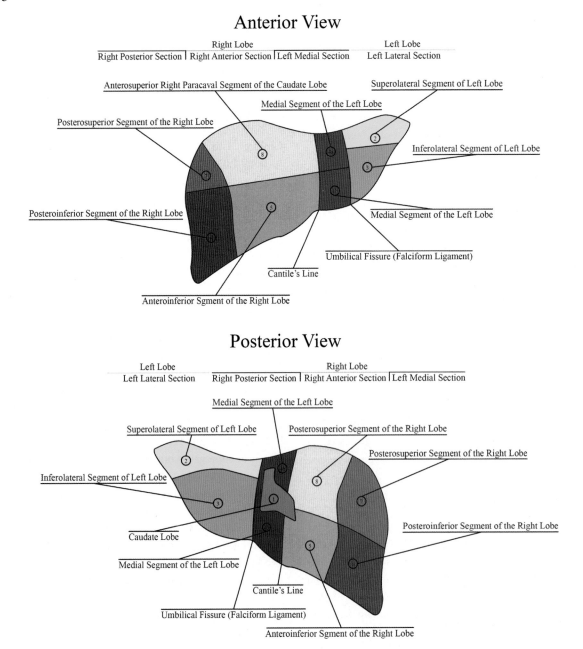

Anterior View

Right Lobe | Left Lobe
Right Posterior Section | Right Anterior Section | Left Medial Section | Left Lateral Section

Anterosuperior Right Paracaval Segment of the Caudate Lobe
Superolateral Segment of Left Lobe
Medial Segment of the Left Lobe
Posterosuperior Segment of the Right Lobe
Inferolateral Segment of Left Lobe
Posteroinferior Segment of the Right Lobe
Medial Segment of the Left Lobe
Umbilical Fissure (Falciform Ligament)
Cantile's Line
Anteroinferior Sgment of the Right Lobe

Posterior View

Left Lobe | Right Lobe
Left Lateral Section | Right Posterior Section | Right Anterior Section | Left Medial Section

Medial Segment of the Left Lobe
Superolateral Segment of Left Lobe
Posterosuperior Segment of the Right Lobe
Posterosuperior Segment of the Right Lobe
Inferolateral Segment of Left Lobe
Posteroinferior Segment of the Right Lobe
Caudate Lobe
Medial Segment of the Left Lobe
Cantile's Line
Umbilical Fissure (Falciform Ligament)
Anteroinferior Sgment of the Right Lobe

FIGURE 3-23. Nomenclature of Couinaud and Bismuth. (Illustration created by and used with permission from Isaiah Forestier.)

7. Segment 7 posterosuperior segment of the right lobe (right of RHV, above portal)

8. Segment 8 anterosuperior right paracaval segment of the caudate lobe (between MHV and RHV, above portal)

Hepatic ligaments and fissures include the falciform ligament, ligamentum teres, ligamentum venosum, and main lobar fissure (Fig. 3-24, Table 3-1). The falciform ligament separates the right and left lobes of the liver. The ligamentum teres is a remnant of the fetal umbilical vein which is also known as the round ligament of the liver. This ligament runs along the free edge of the falciform ligament from the umbilicus into the left lobe. The ligamentum venosum separates the left lobe from the caudate lobe. The ligamentum venosum is the obliterated ductus venosus. In fetal life, the ligamentum venosum shunts blood between the umbilical vein and IVC to bypass the liver. The main lobar fissure passes through the middle hepatic vein and gallbladder fossa, separating the right and left hepatic lobes. The main lobar fissure appears to connect the portal vein to the gallbladder, serving as a useful anatomic marker.

Liver size will vary dependent on the pediatric patient's age, height, weight, and gender. Based on age alone, liver length in the neonatal patient ranges from 4 to 5 centimeters. Adolescent's liver length is between 6 and 10 centimeters. Approaching adulthood liver length ranges between 15 and 17 centimeters. In the infant, the liver can normally extend up to 3.5 centimeters below the costal margin. In children, the liver can normally extend 2 centimeters below the costal margin.

Flow within the portal vein is normally hepatopetal, providing the liver with important nutrients needed to function along with the hepatic artery. The hepatic artery feeds the liver with 25 to 30% of its overall blood supply. The portal vein supplies the remaining 70 to 75%. The hepatic veins drain blood from the liver. The middle hepatic vein divides the liver into right and left lobes. Riedel's lobe is a congenital variant more common in females projecting (tongue-like projection) from the anterior right lobe of the liver to the iliac crest.

TABLE 3-1 • Helpful Hints—Ligaments of the Liver
Falciform ligament separates the right and left lobes.
Main lobar fissure passes through the middle hepatic vein and gallbladder fossa, separating the right and left lobes.
Ligamentum teres runs along the free edge of the falciform ligament, separating the right and left lobes.
Ligamentum venosum separates the left lobe and caudate lobes.

GALLBLADDER AND BILIARY SYSTEM

The gallbladder is a small tear drop shaped organ (may vary) that stores bile and appears anechoic when distended on ultrasound. The gallbladder remains distended while the patient is fasting. Postprandially, the hormone cholecystokinin (CCK) triggers the gallbladder to contract, releasing the stored bile to aid in digestion. The gallbladder is positioned on the liver's visceral surface, and is divided into four sections: neck, infundibulum, body, and fundus. When gallstones obstruct the cystic duct, they are commonly positioned within the infundibulum of the gallbladder. Normal variants include Phrygian cap, junctional fold, septations, and Hartman's pouch. Hartman's pouch is a bulge of the inferior infundibulum. Junctional fold is a variant in which the gallbladder folds at the neck region. Phrygian cap is the most common congenital anatomic variant of the gallbladder. Phrygian cap is a fold at the fundal region of the gallbladder. This variant resembles a head garment (cap) worn in television series *The Smurfs* and originally worn by citizens in Phrygia between 1200 and 1700 BCE (modern day Turkey). The normal thickness of the gallbladder wall is less than 3 millimeters. In infants, the gallbladder should measure less than 1.5 to 3 centimeters in length. In patient's greater than 1 year of age, the gallbladder should measure between 3 and 7 centimeters. The cystic duct connects the gallbladder neck to the common hepatic duct (CHD). The biliary system stores and transports

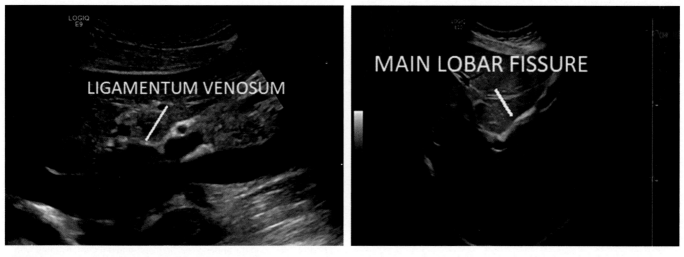

FIGURE 3-24. Two commonly visualized ligaments of the liver.

bile between the liver, gallbladder, and duodenum. The CBD is the junction of the CHD and cystic duct. The CBD traverses the liver, passing through the pancreatic head region, and adjoins the main pancreatic duct at the ampulla of Vater. The CBD then empties into the duodenum of the small intestine at the sphincter of Oddi. Internal lumen diameter of the CHB and CBD varies dependent on patient age.

- In infants 0 to 1 year of age, the CHD should average 1.3 millimeters, falling in a range of 1.0 to 2.0 millimeters.
- In children between 2 and 5 years of age, the CHD should average 1.7 millimeters, measuring between 1.0 and 3.0 millimeters.
- In children between 6 and 8 years of age, the CHD should average 2.0 millimeters.
- In children between 9 and 11 years of age, the CHD should average 1.8 millimeters, measuring between 1.0 and 3.0 millimeters.
- The internal lumen diameter of the CHD in adolescents between 12 and 16 years of age should average 2.2 millimeters, measuring between 1.0 and 4.0 millimeters.

The CHD is not routinely measured on a general abdominal evaluation. The CBD is positioned next to the hepatic artery and portal vein, making up the portal triad.

- In infants 0 to 1 years of age, the CBD should average 1.2 millimeters.
- In children 1 to 10 years of age, the CBD should average 2.0 millimeters.
- In children and adolescents greater than 10 years of age, the CBD should average 3.0 millimeters.

CBD diameter amongst the pediatric population is narrower than that of an adult patient. In adulthood, a general guideline for CBD diameter is an increase of 0.1 to 0.2 millimeter(s) per decade of life until age 60, in which the CBD may increase up to 1 millimeter per decade. It is normal for the CBD to exhibit an increase in diameter up to 1-millimeter post-cholecystectomy.

SPLEEN

The spleen is an intraperitoneal organ composed of lymphoid tissue, red blood cells, and reticuloendothelial cells. The purpose of this organ is to filter blood and participate in immune response. This organ is best visualized in right lateral decubitus position with a 3.0- to 7.5-MHz transducer, depending on the child's age and habitus. A high-resolution linear transducer is best indicated for superficial lesion evaluation.

The spleen is a homogeneous organ, more echogenic than the kidney and equal to or more echogenic than the liver. The spleen is held in place by the gastrosplenic and splenorenal ligaments and may be enlarged if it is seen extending below the inferior margin of the left kidney.

The spleen is a secondary site of disease due to infection, inflammatory, and neoplastic conditions. Splenic pulp is divided into red and white pulp. Red pulp is comprised of blood-filled sinusoids and mononuclear phagocytic cells, while white pulp is comprised of lymphatic tissue sheaths surrounding vessels and cells. In utero the spleen's importance is to aid in production of red blood cells, but this organ is haematopoietically inactive in child and adulthood. Postnatally, hematopoiesis of the spleen can resume with disorders such as osteopetrosis and thalassemia major.

SMALL AND LARGE BOWEL

In utero the gastrointestinal (GI) tract develops from the primary yolk sac as a pouch-like extension and within 6 weeks gestational age divides into the foregut, midgut, and hindgut. Arterial supply to the foregut is via the celiac artery, to the midgut is via the SMA, and hindgut via the inferior mesenteric artery. Gut rotation occurs when the gut herniates into the base of the umbilical cord before returning to the fetal abdomen between 12 and 14 weeks gestational age. Anatomy of the GI tract is comprised of the esophagus, stomach, small bowel (duodenum, jejunum, ileum), and large bowel (colon). The duodenum is in the upper central abdomen. The jejunum is located in the left upper quadrant and courses down to the ileum in the right lower quadrant of the abdomen. The colon (large intestine) originates at the cecum which is the proximal-most part of the ascending colon. Subsequential parts of the large intestine from the ascending colon include the transverse colon, descending colon, sigmoid colon, and rectum, which continues into the anal canal. The appendix is a blind-ending (Fig. 3-25) tubular extension of the cecum, located in the right lower quadrant of the abdomen. Normal bowel wall thickness is 3 to 4 millimeters. Congenital anomalies of the GI system include Meckel's diverticulum and macrogastria. Meckel's diverticulum is the most common pediatric congenital anomaly of the GI tract.

The four abdominal quadrants should be scanned with graded compression when evaluating small bowel. A linear or

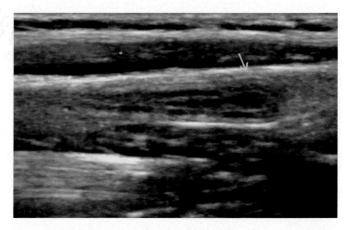

FIGURE 3-25. Sagittal appendiceal tip (blind-ending) demonstrated with arrow.

curvilinear 5.0- to 7.0-MHz transducer is best implemented to displace interposing gas and increase conspicuity of abnormal bowel loops. The small bowel is located centrally and large bowel peripherally within the abdomen. The average thickness of the small bowel wall is between 2 and 3 millimeters. Wall thickening greater than 3 millimeters may indicate bowel disease along with increased color Doppler suggesting intestinal inflammation.

The large bowel, or colon, is not best visualized with sonography due to fecal contents and gas producing strong acoustic reflection and posterior shadowing artifact. When the colonic lumen is fluid-filled, discrete hypoechoic and hyperechoic bowel layers can be visualized. From innermost to outermost the layers of the bowel ("gut signature") include the echogenic superficial mucosa, hypoechoic muscularis mucosa, echogenic submucosa, hypoechoic muscularis propria, and outer hyperechoic serosal layer (Fig. 3-26). The submucosal layer is the thickest layer. The large intestine has haustra which distinguishes it from the small bowel. The ascending colon extends from the cecum to the hepatic flexure and is located on the right side of the abdomen. The transverse colon lies midline in the upper abdomen and extends from the hepatic flexure to the splenic flexure. The descending colon extends from the splenic flexure to the sigmoid colon and is located on the left side of the abdomen. The descending colon empties into the rectum. Colonic wall thickening can be caused by inflammatory, infectious, ischemic, or neoplastic disease. The large bowel (colon) is considered thickened when greater than 4 millimeters.

Key differences between the large and small bowel:

- The small bowel lumen contains valvulae conniventes (these are folds that slow food passage for nutrient absorption).
- The small bowel is the primary site of nutrient absorption and assists in the breakdown of food.
- The large bowel (colon) is shorter in length, but wider in diameter than the small bowel.
- The large bowel does not produce digestive enzymes and does not contain villi.

- The large bowel is primarily responsible for water absorption which dries and stores stool until evacuation.
- The large bowel contains haustra.

The appendix is a compressible, blind-ending (Figs. 3-25, 3-27, and 3-28) structure which normally measures less than 6 millimeters in maximum diameter (Fig. 3-29). The location of the appendix is at the lower end of the cecum, a portion of the

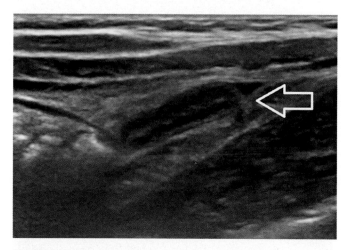

FIGURE 3-27. Appendiceal tip.

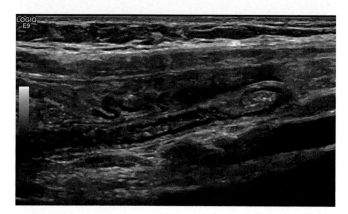

FIGURE 3-28. Blind-ending.

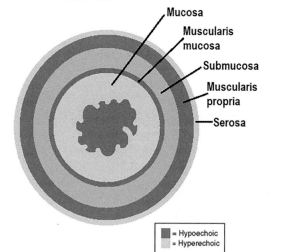

FIGURE 3-26. Layers of the bowel.

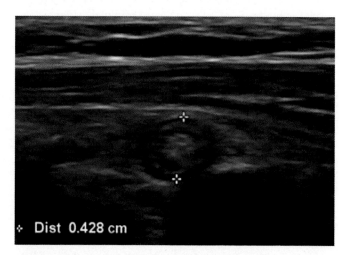

FIGURE 3-29. Transverse appendix with AP measurement.

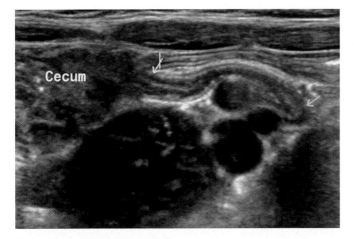

FIGURE 3-30. Relationship to cecum.

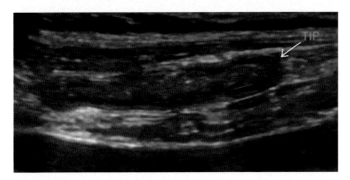

FIGURE 3-31. Sagittal appendix.

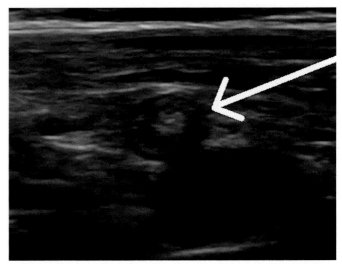

FIGURE 3-32. Transverse appendix.

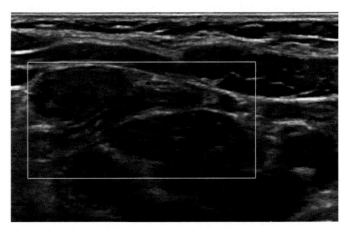

FIGURE 3-33. Non-hyperemic.

large intestine (Fig. 3-30). The appendix has a tubular appearance in long axis (Fig. 3-31) and target appearance in the axial plane (Fig. 3-32), although not all layers of the appendix are always easily appreciated. The normal appendix consists of five distinct layers, comprising the "gut signature" visualized within the small and large intestine. These layers include the innermost echogenic layer which represents the interface of mucosa and lumen, thy hypoechoic mucosal layer, the echogenic submucosal layer, the hypoechoic muscularis propria later, and the outermost echogenic serosal layer. On color Doppler imaging, the normal appendix usually has no flow or minimal scattered color signal (Fig. 3-33). The normal appendix should compress when pressure is applied (Fig. 3-34).

URINARY SYSTEM

The urinary system can be evaluated as part of a complete abdominal scan or on its own as part of a retroperitoneal scan, including the bilateral kidneys, adrenal glands if indicated, and urinary bladder. Transducer selection and frequency is like that of an abdominal scan, and the patient is not required to be

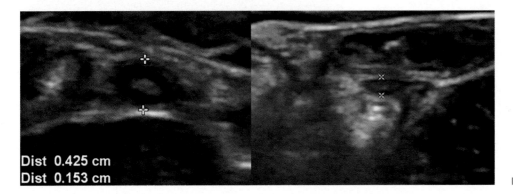

Dist 0.425 cm
Dist 0.153 cm

FIGURE 3-34. Compressible.

fasting unless a renal artery or vein Doppler is requested. The patient's bladder should be distended for optimal visualization, and urinary jets should be documented when possible.

The complete urinary system includes two kidneys, two ureters, one urinary bladder, and the urethra. These structures are located within the retroperitoneum. The urinary system functions to filter waste, conserve water and metabolites, and regulate blood composition. It is also responsible for regulating blood pressure, acid-base balance, and produces erythropoietin, a substance that controls red blood cell production within bone marrow. The kidneys regulate blood volume by the resorption or excretion of sodium and potassium. Waste products are excreted through blood filtration. Waste byproducts include metabolites, such as urea and creatinine. Nephrons are the functional unit of the kidneys and are comprised of renal corpuscles and tubules. The nephrons filter blood to excrete wastes and some water, forming urine.

KIDNEYS

The bilateral kidneys are located within the retroperitoneal cavity in the mid-back. These organs are protected by the rib cage and are part of the upper urinary tract. The right kidney lies slightly lower than the left because of the right liver lobe. Morison's pouch is the space between the right kidney and right liver lobe.

In young children, kidneys are located caudal in comparison to adults and older children. During fetal development, the kidneys begin in the pelvis and migrate to the abdomen. This migration continues until the fifth to sixth year of life.

From outer to inner, the kidneys are comprised of renal fascia, perinephric fat, a fibrous renal capsule, cortex, medulla, and renal pelvis. The medulla consists of renal pyramids. Urine drains from the renal pyramids into the minor and major calyces, before draining into the renal pelvis. Additionally, ureters and the main renal artery and vein enter the renal hilum on the medial aspect of each kidney.

Sonographically, the kidneys are homogeneous with a smooth outer contour. The renal cortex is relatively isoechoic or slightly hypoechoic to the liver, with the renal pyramids more hypoechoic than the cortex. In neonates, the cortex can be slightly hyperechoic to the liver which is considered normal.

In adults, the normal kidney is 9 to 12 centimeters in length. However, in pediatrics, renal size varies greatly depending on the patient's age and weight. In premature infants, normal standards for kidney length are compared alongside patient body weight (Table 3-2). In term infants through adolescence, kidney length is compared to patient's age (Tables 3-3 and 3-4). Normal renal variants include extrarenal pelvis, column of Bertin, fetal lobulation, and dromedary hump.

TABLE 3-2 • Normal Kidney Length in the Premature Infant, According to Body Weight		
Body Weight in Grams	**Lower Limit Kidney Length (mm)**	**Upper Limit Kidney Length (mm)**
Body Weight 600g	26.4	35.7
Body Weight 700g	27.2	36.5
Body Weight 800g	27.9	37.2
Body Weight 900g	28.7	38.0
Body Weight 1,000g	29.4	38.7
Body Weight 1,100g	30.1	39.5
Body Weight 1,200g	30.9	40.2
Body Weight 1,300g	31.6	41.0
Body Weight 1,400g	32.4	41.7
Body Weight 1,500g	33.1	42.5
Body Weight 1,600g	33.9	43.2
Body Weight 1,700g	34.6	43.9
Body Weight 1,800g	35.4	44.7
Body Weight 1,900g	36.1	45.4
Body Weight 2,000g	36.9	46.2
Body Weight 2,100g	37.6	46.9
Body Weight 2,200g	38.4	47.7
Body Weight 2,300g	39.1	48.4
Body Weight 2,400g	39.9	49.2
Body Weight 2,500g	40.6	49.9
Body Weight 2,600g	41.3	50.7
Body Weight 2,700g	42.1	51.4
Body Weight 2,800g	42.8	52.2
Body Weight 2,900g	43.6	52.9
Body Weight 3,000g	44.3	53.7

Source: Esmaeili M, Keshaki M, Younesi L, Karimani A, Otoukesh H, Esmaeili M. Ultrasound measurement of kidney dimensions in premature neonates. *Int J Pediatr.* 2020;8(10): 12235–12242.

TABLE 3-3 • Normal Kidney Length in the Infant, According to Age		
Age of Infant	**Lower Limit Kidney Length (cm)**	**Upper Limit Kidney Length (cm)**
Full Term Newborn to 2 Weeks	3.6	6.0
1 Month	4.0	6.1
6 Weeks	4.1	6.2
2 Months	4.2	6.3
2 ½ Months	4.3	6.4
3–3 ½ Month	4.4	6.5
4 Month	4.5	6.6
4 ½ Months	4.6	6.7
5–5 ½ Months	4.7	6.8
6–6 ½ Months	4.8	6.9
7 Months	4.9	7.0
7 ½ Months	5.0	7.1
8 Months	5.1	7.2
8 ½–9 Months	5.2	7.3
9 ½ Months	5.3	7.4
10–10 ½ Months	5.4	7.5
11 Months	5.5	7.7
11 ½ Months	5.6	7.8

Sources: Obrycki Ł, Sarnecki J, Lichosik M, et al. Kidney length normative values in children aged 0–19 years: a multicenter study. *Pediatr Nephrol.* 2022;37(5):1075–1085; Rosenbaum DM, Korngold E, Teele RL. Sonographic assessment of renal length in normal children. *AJR Am J Roentgenol.* 1984;142(3):467–469.

TABLE 3-4 • Normal Kidney Length in the Pediatric Patient, According to Age		
Age of Pediatric Patient	**Lower Limit Kidney Length (cm)**	**Upper Limit Kidney Length (cm)**
1 Year	5.2	8.0
1 ½ Years	5.4	8.1
2 Years	5.5	8.3
2 ½ Years	5.6	8.4
3 Years	5.7	8.6
3 ½ Years	5.9	8.7
4–4 ½ Years	6.0	8.8
5 Years	6.4	9.2
5 ½ Years	6.5	9.3
6 Years	6.7	9.4
6 ½ Years	6.8	9.5
7 Years	7.0	9.8
7 ½ Years	7.0	9.8
8 Years	7.2	9.9
8 ½ Years	7.3	10.1
9 Years	7.4	10.2
9 ½ Years	7.5	10.3
10 Years	7.7	10.3
10 ½ Years	7.8	10.5
11 Years	7.9	10.6
11 ½ Years	8.1	10.8
12 Years	8.2	11.0
12 ½ Years	8.3	11.1
13 Years	8.5	11.2
13 ½ Years	8.6	11.3
14 Years	8.7	11.4
14 ½ Years	8.9	11.0
15 Years	9.0	11.7

URETERS AND BLADDER

The ureters are tube-like structures which begin in the ureteropelvic junction of the renal hilum and empty into the ureterovesical junction of the posterolateral bladder. Due to presence of overlying bowel gas artifact and their small diameter, unless dilated, the ureters are not visualized sonographically. The ureters lie posterior to the renal vessels and are comprised of

TABLE 3-4 • (Continued)		
Age of Pediatric Patient	Lower Limit Kidney Length (cm)	Upper Limit Kidney Length (cm)
15 ½ Years	9.1	11.8
16 Years	9.2	11.9
16 ½ Years	9.2	11.9
17 Years	9.5	12.2
18 Years	9.8	12.7

Sources: Obrycki Ł, Sarnecki J, Lichosik M, et al. Kidney length normative values in children aged 0–19 years: a multicenter study. *Pediatr Nephrol.* 2022;37(5):1075–1085; Rosenbaum DM, Korngold E, Teele RL. Sonographic assessment of renal length in normal children. *AJR Am J Roentgenol.* 1984;142(3):467–469.

fibromuscular tissue. Prior to entering the ureterovesical junction of the bladder, the right and left ureters cross anterior to the common iliac bifurcation, enter the bladder wall obliquely, and end at the ureteral orifice.

The urinary bladder, located within the pelvis, is a hollow pouch which acts as a muscular container that accumulates the continuous production of urine. Sonographically, the bladder appears as an anechoic structure when filled. To visualize the bladder on ultrasound, patients should be instructed to drink fluids and avoid emptying their bladder prior to exam. The bladder wall contains transitional epithelium, allowing it to stretch as urine accumulates. On the inferior aspect of the bladder is a urethral opening. Nerve endings signal the brain for the bladder muscles to tighten when the bladder becomes full, and these nerves aid in the excretion of urine. Increased pressure from the bladder triggers the internal and external ureteral sphincters to relax, so urine may be excreted from the body.

A renal and bladder protocol is ideally performed with a full bladder, although a full bladder is not required for evaluation of the kidneys. A 2- to 10-MHz transducer is used, using the highest possible frequency that allows for adequate penetration.

Parents of patients under 1 year of age should be instructed to bring a bottle for the patient to drink during the exam. Patients between 1 and 3 years of age should drink 4 to 6 oz. of water 30 minutes prior to the exam. Patients 3 to 6 years of age should drink 8 to 12 oz. of water 30 minutes prior to the exam. If possible, continent patients should be asked not to void 1 hour prior to their ultrasound. Patients between 6 to 12 years of age should drink 12 to 16 oz. of water 30 minutes prior to the exam. Patients over 12 years of age should drink 18 to 32 oz. of water 1 hour prior to the exam.

The sonographer should evaluate the bladder first, particularly in young incontinent patients. If the bladder is full, it

should be imaged including anterior wall thickness measurement. Normal thickness of the bladder wall is less than 3 millimeters when the bladder is distended. If the bladder is not full at the time the exam begins, the sonographer should begin with the kidneys and image the bladder last to measure an accurate wall thickness. A collapsed bladder may exhibit a greater wall thickness measurement than the distended bladder and it may be challenging to adequately assess a true thickened bladder wall versus fabricated thickening. If indicated, ureteral jets should be documented, and a bladder volume should be obtained using two orthogonal imaging planes. If patients are toilet trained and continent, the kidneys should be imaged while the bladder is full, allowing for more sonographic information in the presence of hydronephrosis. The patient should then be asked to void, and post-void images calculating a residual bladder volume should be obtained. A retroperitoneal protocol of the urinary system includes bilateral renal, adrenal, and bladder images as described in the complete abdominal protocol. Adrenal glands become difficult to see as patient age progresses and may not be visualized in older children.

Note: The sonographer should ensure renal length is accurately measured, providing the longest measurement possible from upper to lower pole. In young patients, a standoff pad or copious gel should be used if necessary.

The sonographer should focus the acoustic beam and use the highest transducer frequency possible to best demonstrate shadow artifact when it is present (i.e., if using a curvilinear C 5-1 transducer, transition to C 9-4 or C 8-5). Use of focusing and decreasing spatial pulse (via increasing transducer frequency) improves spatial resolution (imaging detail). In cases of urolithiasis, sonographers should provide a split-screen image depicting twinkle-artifact (Fig. 3-35) of the stone. A wide acoustic beam may not optimally demonstrate useful acoustic shadowing artifact posterior to a stone. If the acoustic beam is wider than the region of posterior shadowing, acoustic reflections may include surrounding tissue signals which blend with and decrease the concentration of the acoustic shadow. Focusing narrows the acoustic beam and improves lateral resolution. The focus should be positioned at the region of interest. Ureteral jets should also be observed bilaterally, to determine whether there is a blockage of the ureter.

The sonographer should evaluate for a dilated extrarenal pelvis or proximal ureter. This should be observed in the coronal plane as it may be visible from a posterolateral approach when there is obscuring bowel gas from the anterior approach. In the presence of pelviectasis, the sonographer should measure the maximum anteroposterior dimension of the renal pelvis at the parenchymal edge in addition to extraparenchymal location. If ureterectasis is present, this should also be measured. In newborns or infant males with dilated collecting systems, the sonographer should investigate for a dilated posterior urethra.

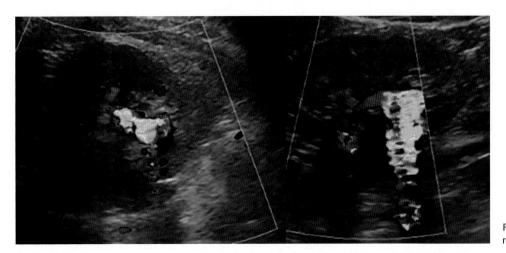

FIGURE 3-35. Color-Doppler twinkle representation of renal calculi.

This may be a sign of posterior urethral valves or lower urinary tract obstruction. Additionally, during evaluation of the bladder, the sonographer should carefully observe for presence of dilated distal ureters or ureterocele. These findings may be visualized intermittently due to peristalsis. When necessary, the sonographer should utilize multiple scanning planes to document findings including adenopathy, perirenal fluid/hematoma, iliopsoas abscess, or vascular abnormality. If the sonographer suspects acute pyelonephritis, color Doppler maps of the entire kidney are performed to document any altered perfusion. Additionally, areas of abnormal echogenicity should be noted (i.e., focal hypoechoic areas).

4

Sonographic Anatomy of the Neck

Imaging of soft tissues in the pediatric neck is well seen on ultrasound with a high frequency linear transducer, between 7 and 20 MHz. Imaging of the neck is performed with the patient in a supine position and the neck hyperextended.

Structures of the neck include the parotid, submandibular, and sublingual salivary glands, major vessels, thyroid gland, parathyroid glands, and lateral neck structures.

The largest salivary gland is the parotid gland. This gland is located inferior to the earlobe and is comprised of two lobes. The larger superficial lobe makes up 80% of the parotid gland, while the smaller deep lobe makes up only 20%. Normally the parotid gland is homogeneous and hyperechoic to the adjacent masseter muscle, surrounded by small lymph nodes.

The submandibular salivary gland is drained by the Wharton duct into the oral cavity and is located in the submental region. Wharton's duct is the main excretory duct of the submandibular gland where sialoliths (calculi) of the salivary glands most commonly form. The submandibular gland is homogeneous and hyperechoic to the adjacent muscles.

The sublingual glands are the smallest salivary glands, lying below the floor of the mouth anterior to the submandibular glands.

The carotid artery perfuses both cerebral circulation and the face and neck. The right carotid artery originates as a branch of the brachiocephalic trunk (formerly termed the *innominate artery*), which is the first branch of the aortic arch. The left carotid artery is a direct branch of the aortic arch. The common carotid arteries continue superiorly and bifurcate into the external and internal carotid arteries. The external carotid artery (ECA) is slightly smaller than the internal carotid artery (ICA). The ECA primarily perfuses the face, neck, and head, while the ICA perfuses intracranial structures. The internal jugular vein returns venous blood from the brain, neck, and upper facial region to the heart. It descends from the neck into the thorax where it joins the subclavian vein to form the brachiocephalic vein (formerly known as the *innominate vein*). The carotid artery and jugular vein are the great vessels of the neck and are seen lateral to the thyroid gland.

CAROTID ARTERIES

For evaluation of the bilateral carotid arteries, a high frequency linear transducer should be used. In very young patients, a linear array hockey stick transducer can be used. This transducer offers high resolution and a small transducer footprint. The patient lies supine with the neck hyperextended and the head turned contralateral to the side being evaluated.

Still images are obtained bilaterally and include:

1. Transverse common carotid artery (CCA)
   a. Proximal
   b. Distal
   c. Bulb
   d. Bifurcation
2. Sagittal CCA
   a. With and without color Doppler
   b. With spectral Doppler evaluation, two samples at each location measuring peak systolic velocity (PSV)
   c. Proximal CCA
   d. Distal CCA
3. Sagittal external carotid artery
   a. With and without color Doppler
   b. With spectral Doppler evaluation, two samples at each location measuring PSV

4. Sagittal internal carotid artery (ICA)
   a. With and without color Doppler
   b. With spectral Doppler evaluation, two samples at each location measuring PSV
   c. Proximal ICA
   d. Mid ICA
   e. Distal ICA
5. Sagittal vertebral arteries
   a. With and without color Doppler
   b. With spectral Doppler evaluation, two samples at each location measuring PSV

Note: Ensure sample gate (Fig. 4-1) is appropriate in size and placed in the center of the vessel. A sample volume angle should be parallel to the vessel wall and equal to or less than 60 degrees. Heel-toe the transducer as necessary to align vessel wall and Doppler angle.

THYROID GLAND

The thyroid gland contains right and left lobes connected by an isthmus and is covered by a fibrous tissue capsule (Fig. 4-2). It is the body's largest endocrine gland. The right and left lobes of the thyroid fuse at the isthmus at approximately 7 weeks gestational age. Thyroid tissue is positioned posterior to the sternohyoid and sternothyroid muscles and anterolateral to the trachea. The thyroid secretes hormones triiodothyronine (T3) and thyroxine (T4), mediated by thyroid stimulating hormone (TSH) from the pituitary gland, all which play a role in our growth, metabolism, development, temperature, and heart rate. Lab values relevant to the thyroid include T3, T4, TSH, and calcitonin. The thyroid obtains its blood supply via the superior and inferior thyroid arteries and is drained by the superior, middle, and inferior thyroid veins.

Sonographically, the normal thyroid appearance is homogeneous. The measurements vary depending on a pediatric patient's age and height. Generally, the length of the bilateral thyroid lobes range between 2 and 3 centimeters, with the connecting isthmus being 2 to 6 millimeters in AP dimension. During imaging of the thyroid gland, notable adjacent sonographic landmarks of the neck include the common carotid arteries, internal jugular veins, strap muscles, and anterior tracheal wall. The strap muscles are made up of sternohyoid, sternothyroid, thyrohyoid, and omohyoid. The thyroid is also surrounded by the sternocleidomastoid and longus colli muscles.

For evaluation of the thyroid gland, a 5 to 17 MHz linear transducer should be used. The patient lies supine with the neck hyperextended; a rolled towel may be placed behind the patient's neck for comfort. The thyroid is evaluated, and surrounding tissues are surveyed for abnormality.

Still images include:

1. Transverse isthmus
   a. With and without measurement
2. Transverse bilateral lobes of the thyroid (Figs. 4-2 and 4-3)
   a. With and without color Doppler
3. Sagittal right lobe (Figs. 4-4 and 4-5)
   a. Medial, mid, lateral
   b. Mid with measurement
   c. Mid with color Doppler

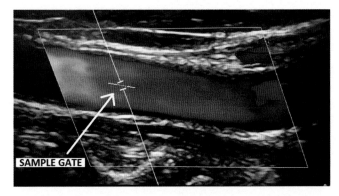

FIGURE 4-1. Sample gate.

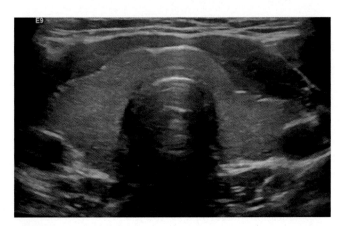

FIGURE 4-2. Transverse thyroid gland.

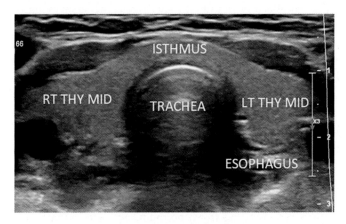

FIGURE 4-3. Transverse thyroid gland with labeling.

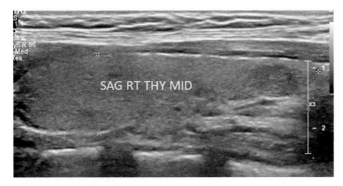

FIGURE 4-4. Normal, sagittal thyroid.

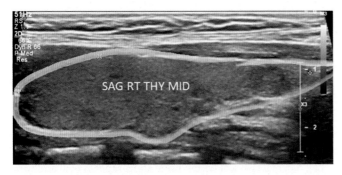

FIGURE 4-5. Normal, sagittal thyroid (parenchyma borders highlighted).

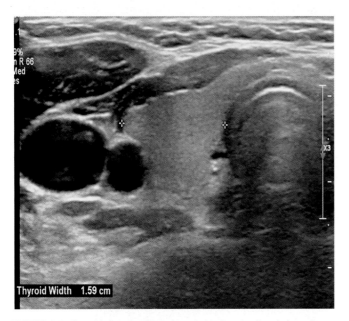

Thyroid Width   1.59 cm

FIGURE 4-6. Carotid artery and jugular vein landmarks directly lateral to transverse right thyroid lobe.

4. Transverse right lobe
   a. Superior, mid, inferior
   b. Mid with measurement (Fig. 4-6)
   c. Mid with color Doppler (Fig. 4-7)
5. Sagittal left lobe
   a. Medial, mid, lateral
   b. Mid with measurement
   c. Mid with color Doppler

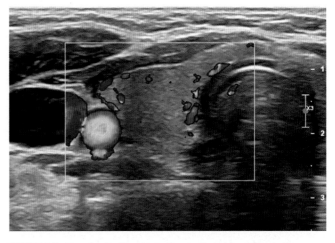

FIGURE 4-7. Use of color Doppler to demonstrate blood flow in the transverse thyroid.

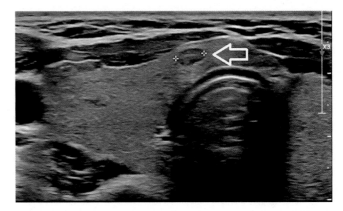

FIGURE 4-8. Thyroid nodule.

6. Transverse left lobe
   a. Superior, mid, inferior
   b. Mid with measurement
   c. Mid with color Doppler
   Cine-clips include (minimum of):

1. Transverse right lobe
2. Transverse left lobe

Note: Any abnormal finding within the thyroid tissue (Fig. 4-8) should be documented with color Doppler and measured (per updated TIRADS guidelines two measurements in transverse plane and single measurement in sagittal plane). Do not mistake the esophagus (left) for a thyroid nodule. In transverse plane, the esophagus has a gut-signature appearing as a circular target sign postero-medial to the left lobe of the thyroid. When in doubt, the sonographer can instruct the patient to swallow.

PARATHYROID

The parathyroid is a set of four endocrine glands that secrete parathyrin, also called *parathyroid hormone* (PTH), maintaining serum calcium in the blood. A fifth parathyroid gland is possible and is referred to as a *supernumerary parathyroid*. There are typically two superior parathyroid glands located posterior to the mid thyroid gland and two inferior parathyroid glands located posterior to the inferior thyroid. The normal parathyroid glands are generally not visualized by ultrasound unless enlarged.

An exam for evaluation of the parathyroid may be ordered if patient presents with history of parathyroidism or prior parathyroid surgery.

A high-frequency (5-17 MHz) linear transducer should be used. Patient preparation and positioning is like that of the thyroid gland.

Expected location of parathyroid glands should be imaged, surveying from the bilateral carotid arteries to midline and from the inferior thoracic inlet to the superior carotid artery bifurcation.

It is possible parathyroid glands may be positioned in the subclavicular region and upper mediastinum. This is the most common ectopic location for parathyroid adenomas, followed by the thyroid gland, carotid sheath, undescended gland, and the retroesophageal space. The patient should be instructed to swallow to visualize this area in real-time. The majority of supernumerary parathyroid glands are located within the thymus.

Additionally, the upper mediastinum can be surveyed by angling the ultrasound transducer beneath the sternum from the sternal notch region. When an exam of the parathyroid is requested, the thyroid tissue should also be evaluated following the above thyroid protocol.

Sonographic appearance includes hypoechoic flattened oval structures that are isoechoic to hypoechoic in comparison to the thyroid gland. Parathyroid glands each measure approximately 4 to 6 millimeters or greater in length.

Still images include:

1. Transverse images of expected right parathyroid gland location
   a. Superior at carotid bifurcation
   b. Common carotid
   c. Inferior thoracic inlet
2. Sagittal images of the expected right parathyroid location
3. Transverse images of expected left parathyroid gland location
   a. Superior at carotid bifurcation
   b. Common carotid
   c. Inferior thoracic inlet

4. Sagittal images of the expected left parathyroid location

Cine-clips include:

1. Transverse right (area of superior-inferior thyroid)
2. Transverse left (area of superior to inferior thyroid)

Note: The normal parathyroid may not be visualized due to the glands' small size and location.

LYMPH NODE SURVEY/SOFT TISSUE NECK

While performing a lymph node survey, zones of the neck (Fig. 4-9) and a body-marker should be labeled on each image. Patient positioning is like that of a thyroid evaluation. A high frequency 5 to 17 MHz linear transducer should be used. The three largest or most abnormal lymph nodes should be measured and interrogated bilaterally, according to individual institution guidelines or radiologist preferences (Figs. 4-10 and 4-11). Normal cervical lymph node appearance is oval and well-defined with a homogeneous hypoechoic cortex and hyperechoic hilum, similar to that of the kidney. Abnormal changes

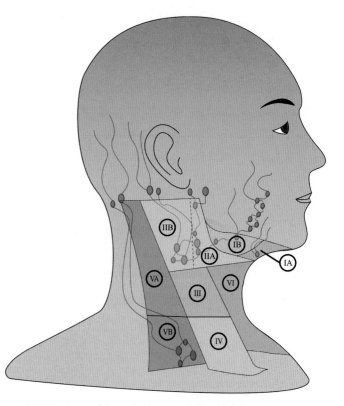

FIGURE 4-9. Zones of the neck: Zone IA—Submental; Zone IB—Submandibular; Zone IIA—Parotid (Ant/Med to Int. Jug.); Zone IIB—Parotid (Post to Int. Jug.); Zone III—Upper/Mid Jugular V; Zone IV—Lower Jugular V; Zone VA—Post. Triangle (Base of Skull to Cricoid); Zone VB—Post. Triangle (Cricoid to Clavicle); Zone VI—Ant. Cervical/Paratracheal; Zone VII—Supraclavicular. (Illustration created by and used with permission from Isaiah Forestier.)

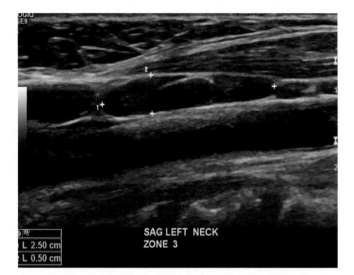

FIGURE 4-10. Sagittal lymph node (largest) at level of the upper/mid jugular vein.

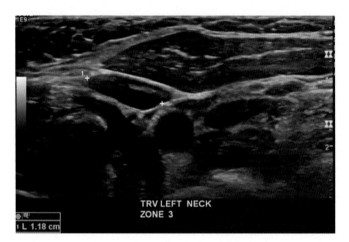

FIGURE 4-11. Transverse lymph node (largest) at level of the upper/mid jugular vein.

include inhomogeneous echotexture, round shape, and markedly hypoechoic appearance with central hyperechogenicity no longer visualized.

The cervical lymph node chain is visualized in the internal and external jugular vein region, with the internal jugular chain consisting of the largest nodes. Within the internal jugular chain, the jugulodigastric node is typically the largest.

Still images include:

1. Right neck, using a body marker demonstrate:
   a. Sagittal and transverse zone IA
   b. Sagittal and transverse zone IB
   c. Sagittal and transverse zone IIA
   d. Sagittal and transverse zone IIB
   e. Sagittal and transverse zone III
   f. Sagittal and transverse zone IV
   g. Sagittal and transverse zone VA
   h. Sagittal and transverse zone VB
   i. Sagittal and transverse zone VI
   j. Sagittal and transverse zone VII
2. Left neck, using a body marker demonstrate:
   a. Sagittal and transverse zone IA
   b. Sagittal and transverse zone IB
   c. Sagittal and transverse zone IIA
   d. Sagittal and transverse zone IIB
   e. Sagittal and transverse zone III
   f. Sagittal and transverse zone IV
   g. Sagittal and transverse zone VA
   h. Sagittal and transverse zone VB
   i. Sagittal and transverse zone VI
   j. Sagittal and transverse zone VII

Note: Image documentation at each zone of the neck ensures a complete survey is performed by the sonographer; however, some institutions may request image documentation of neck zones only in the presence of a finding or pertaining to the patient's area of concern.

If the concern for a palpable soft tissue lump on the neck (Fig. 4-12) exists, still images should be obtained in two imaging planes with documented relationship to anatomical landmarks. Patient positioning is like that of a thyroid evaluation. A high frequency 5 to 17 MHz linear transducer should be used.

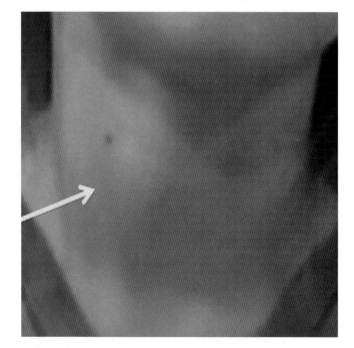

FIGURE 4-12. Right cervical lymphadenopathy.

If a thyroglossal duct cyst is suspected, the sonographer should document the presence or absence of thyroid tissues and mass location in relation to the strap muscles and hyoid bone. A thyroglossal duct cyst is a congenital cyst of the neck that presents as a palpable, visible neck mass. This is typically found in the midline neck as an anechoic or hypoechoic structure, but may be located at, above, or below the hyoid bone.

See soft-tissue imaging protocol listed under "Pathology of Superficial Structures" in Chapter 28.

5

Sonographic Anatomy of the Chest

LUNG

While diagnostic radiographs are the conventional exam for the evaluation of chest pathology, sonography is helpful in identifying and localizing specific anomalies. The lungs are located in the thoracic cavity. Each lung is separated into lobes. The right lung is comprised of three lobes and the left lung is comprised of two lobes. The lungs function to supply oxygen to the body via the bloodstream. The lungs take in oxygen and excrete carbon dioxide from the blood. Oxygen travels from the trachea into bronchi, bronchioles, and alveoli where gas exchange occurs. Sonographically, because the lungs are air-filled structures, certain artifacts may be visualized. A mirror image, reverberation, or comet tail artifact may be seen at echogenic visceral and parietal pleura lines. When pleural effusion is present, the fluid appears anechoic surrounding or overlying the lung parenchyma.

DIAPHRAGM

The diaphragm is a muscle that separates the thoracic and abdominal cavities. The diaphragm is dome-shaped, with the right dome slightly more superior due to the large underlying right hepatic lobe. Diaphragmatic muscle fibers insert on the central tendon, which is an aponeurosis. Sonographically the diaphragm appears as a smooth, slightly curved, echogenic line adjacent to the spleen and liver (Fig. 5-1). The diaphragm expands and contracts, accommodating inhalation and exhalation of the lungs.

> **Note:** Because many organs lie close to the diaphragm, to reduce organ motion often we ask the patient to suspend respiration. As the lungs fill with air, the diaphragm moves downward thus pushing abdominal organs downward. Therefore, we ask our patients to take in a deep breath and hold during abdominal exams—the diaphragm pushes our kidneys inferior helping us avoid rib shadowing!

Imaging of the diaphragm may be requested to rule out diaphragmatic paralysis, paresis, or paradoxical motion. No patient preparation is required for this exam. A 2-10 MHz sector transducer should be used. This procedure entails a survey of diaphragmatic excursion while the patient breathes spontaneously, and diaphragmatic thickness may be measured. The diaphragm should move superior with expiration and inferior with inspiration. Sonography is the modality of choice due to capability for real-time imaging and portability. It should be documented on the technologist worksheet whether the patient is on ventilator support. If the patient is on ventilator support, the doctor, nurse or respiratory therapist should be present to suspend support as needed during the exam. Quantitative imaging may be accomplished by utilizing M-mode. This can be done by evaluating one hemidiaphragm at a time in a lateral subcostal approach, or a transverse subxiphoid angle. The first cursor is placed at the end of expiration and the second cursor at peak inspiration (Fig. 5-2).

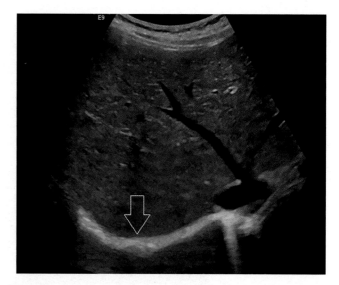

FIGURE 5-1. Diaphragm adjacent to the right liver lobe and aerated lung.

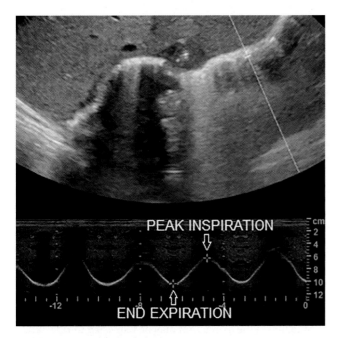

FIGURE 5-2. M-mode caliper placement.

The excursion is measured by calculating the difference in centimeters. Diaphragm motion can be normal, diminished, or absent.

Typically, normal excursion occurs when there is >4 centimeters of motion. More precisely, in females excursion is approximately 3.7 centimeters and in males approximately 4.7 centimeters. However, a variance in this measurement may be observed based upon patient age (i.e., preterm infants versus adolescents, see Table 5-1).

As a result, normal diaphragmatic motion can also be described as less than 50% difference between each diaphragm. On M-mode display, normal diaphragmatic motion appears as a horizontal wavy line (Fig. 5-3). An abnormal result occurs when there is less than 4 centimeters of excursion or greater than a 50% difference between hemidiaphragms. M-mode display

TABLE 5-1 • Variance of Diaphragmatic Excursion in Preterm Infants

Diaphragmatic Excursion Variance by Patient Age in Preterm Infants	
26–28 Weeks GA	5.5 ± 0.2 mm
29–31 Weeks GA	4.8 ± 0.2 mm
32–34 Weeks GA	4.6 ± 0.2 mm
35–37 Weeks GA	4.4 ± 0.3 mm

Source: From Bahgat E, El-Halaby H, Abdelrahman A, Nasef N, Abdel-Hady H. Sonographic evaluation of diaphragmatic thickness and excursion as a predictor for successful extubation in mechanically ventilated preterm infants. *Eur J Pediatr*. 2021;180(3):899–908. doi: 10.1007/s00431-020-03805-2.

with absent or decreased diaphragmatic excursion will appear as a primarily or entirely flat line (Fig. 5-4).

Thickness of the diaphragmatic muscle can also indicate normality versus a weakened diaphragm. During inspiration, the diaphragm contracts. During contraction of the diaphragmatic muscle, the diaphragm is 20% thicker than it is during expiration. The exact measurement among a pediatric population for diaphragmatic thickness can vary greatly based on patient age. Typically, diaphragmatic thickness increase of less than 20% with inspiration is indicative of a weakened diaphragm. Additionally, patients on mechanical ventilation will exhibit a decrease in diaphragmatic thickness due to acquired diaphragmatic atrophy.

For imaging of the diaphragm, still images include:

1. Sagittal right liver with cursor crossing the right hemidiaphragm
2. Sagittal measurement of right inspiration curve height (with and without ventilator support)
3. Sagittal spleen with cursor crossing the left hemidiaphragm

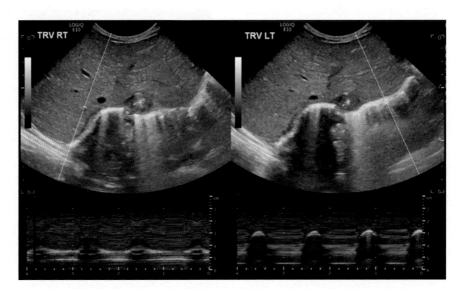

FIGURE 5-3. Normal motion of each hemidiaphragm with M-mode quantification.

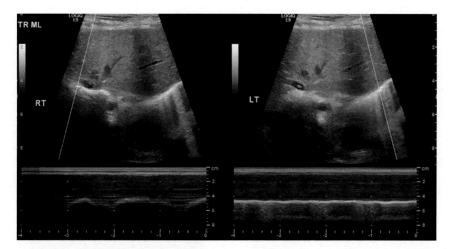

FIGURE 5-4. Abnormal motion on left. M-mode tracing shows diminished excursion on left (note absence of undulation), compared to robust movement on the right.

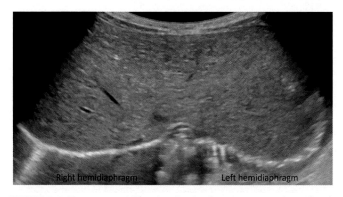

FIGURE 5-5. Transverse midline view for simultaneous comparison of each hemidiaphragm.

4. Sagittal measurement of left inspiration curve height (with and without ventilator support)

5. Transverse subcostal bilateral hemidiaphragms (angle up toward the chest, if possible, obtain bilateral diaphragms in single image) (Fig. 5-5)

Cine-clips include:

1. Coronal right hemidiaphragm during respiration

2. Coronal left hemidiaphragm during respiration

3. Transverse subcostal view of bilateral hemidiaphragms during respiration, demonstrate bilateral hemidiaphragms in single cine-clip to compare diaphragmatic excursion

> **Note:** To best view structures of the pediatric chest, imaging approaches may include supraclavicular, suprasternal, parasternal, trans-sternal, intercostal, sub-xiphoid, sub-diaphragmatic, and posterior paraspinal acoustic windows. Suprasternal views help to best evaluate apices of the lungs, upper mediastinum, and great vessels. In neonatal patients, trans-sternal views with the transducer placed directly over the sternum is useful for imaging the thymus, which lies anterior to the great vessels.

THYMUS

The thymus changes in appearance as the patient ages, being largest in neonatal patients and young infants. The thymus begins developing between 6 and 8 weeks gestational age and is located anterior to the great vessels and posterior to the sternum. The thymus is a bi-lobed, triangular lymphoid organ that functions to secrete hormones, including thymosin, thymopoietin and thymulin. These hormones aid in the creation of T cells in utero and early childhood, assisting in boosting the immune system. Intercostal sonographic windows help to image the pleural space and lung parenchyma. The thymus may be located through a suprasternal, parasternal, subxiphoid, or transcostal approach. The sonographer should demonstrate presence of the thymus in relation to the heart and great vessels. Lastly, subdiaphragmatic views best visualize the deep lower lung and pleura, or sulcal, space. Sonographically, the thymus is a smooth, hypoechoic organ with internal echogenic strands—giving it a "starry sky" appearance. The thymus has also been described as having a liver-like appearance (Fig. 5-6).

If the ordering provider requests examination of the thymus, a 2-10 MHz sector or 5-17 MHz linear transducer should be used. No patient preparation is required for this exam.

When imaging the thymus, a measurement in three dimensions should be obtained. The size of the thymus varies with age, with mean length of the left lobe being approximately 2.9 centimeters and the right lobe approximately 2.5 centimeters. It should be noted that cervical extension of the thymus is a normal variant. In cases of a neck mass, the sonographer may be able to show that it extends into the mediastinum and is connected to the mediastinal thymus. Cervical extension of the thymus is rare but may mimic other neck masses.

> **Note:** The thymus may be difficult to visualize as patients age. During puberty, it atrophies and undergoes fatty replacement.

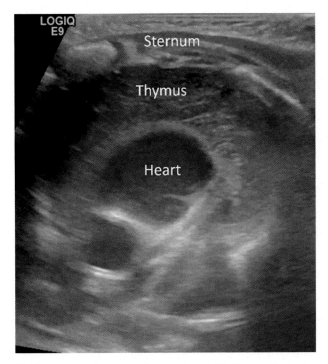

FIGURE 5-6. Normal sonographic appearance of the thymus, located in the anterior mediastinum.

IMAGING OF THE PLEURAL SPACE

Ultrasound of the chest is often performed to assess for suspected pleural effusion (Figs. 5-7 and 5-8). A 2-10 MHz sector, 5-8 MHz sector, or 5-17 MHz linear transducer is used for this examination. The unilateral or bilateral hemithoraces should be evaluated to determine the presence of and complexity of a pleural effusion (Fig. 5-9). It is preferred that the patient is sitting for this examination, however it may be performed supine when necessary. It is also preferred that the patient has a documented radiograph of the chest, prior to performing an ultrasound of the chest.

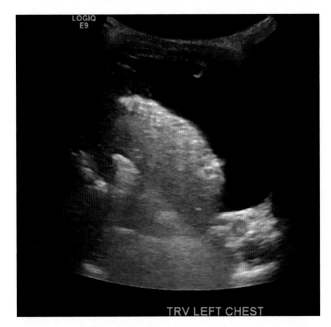

FIGURE 5-7. Transverse left chest with moderate left pleural effusion.

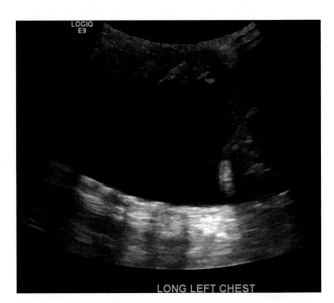

FIGURE 5-8. Sagittal left chest with moderate left pleural effusion.

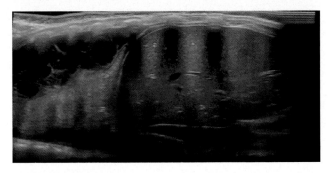

FIGURE 5-9. Coronal panoramic image of right lung consolidation with a complex effusion.

Still images include:

1. Transverse superior, mid, inferior hemithorax (with and without fluid pocket measurement in largest plane, if present)
2. Sagittal image for volume calculation of fluid pocket

Cine clips include:

1. Sagittal cine clip of effusion, demonstrate presence or absence of septations
2. Transverse cine clip of effusion, demonstrate presence or absence of septations

MEDIASTINUM

If the ordering provider is concerned for a mediastinal mass, a 2-10 MHz sector or 5-17 MHz linear transducer should be used. No patient preparation is required for this exam. For evaluation of these areas, the sonographer scans the suprasternal notch or intercostal spaces in two imaging planes, demonstrating relationship of the mediastinal mass of interest in relation to the heart and great vessels. A cine-clip should be obtained, documenting motion of any visualized mass in relation to the chest wall during respiration.

Sonographic Anatomy of the Breast

6

A palpable mass or skin change may be indications for an ultrasound of the pediatric breast. The patient's area of concern should be scanned using a high-frequency linear transducer. The most common benign breast mass in young women is fibroadenoma (Fig. 6-1).

The location of the scan should be documented to include a clock-face body marker (Fig. 6-2), with radial or antiradial orientation labeled in lieu of sagittal and transverse (Fig. 6-3), and the anatomical side. The sonographer should indicate the distance from the nipple in centimeters.

If a lesion is visualized, standard color Doppler should be performed to document presence or absence of flow. Using color or power Doppler with vocal fremitus technique involves the patient speaking or humming to produce a vibration of the chest wall. This allows for demonstration of color artifact remaining at the periphery of a lesion versus central extension. Color flow artifact which remains peripheral while the patient hums most often correlates to a benign lesion, while color flow artifact which enters a lesion's center correlates with a potential invasive malignancy. Strain-elastography (SR) should also be used when available in the presence of a finding. SR is known as *static* or *compression elastography*, with strain being the manual compression of a lesion (like manual palpation). Decreased strain values correlate to greater elasticity and harder lesions, indicated by a color map. Lesions which have greater elasticity are more likely to be benign.

See soft-tissue imaging protocol listed under "Pathology of Superficial Structures" in Chapter 28.

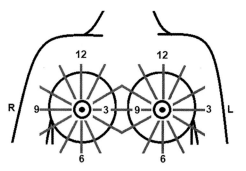

FIGURE 6-2. Clock stations of the anatomical right and left breast.

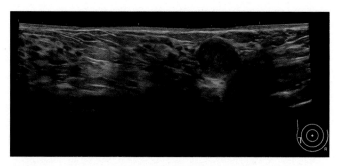

FIGURE 6-1. Panoramic view of the right breast with region-of-interest body marker. A well-circumscribed, hypoechoic, wider-than-tall structure is visualized, consistent with fibroadenoma.

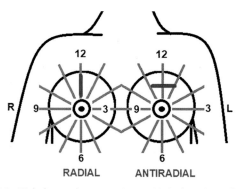

FIGURE 6-3. Right breast demonstrating 12:00 clock station radial positioning of transducer and left breast demonstrating 12:00 clock station antiradial positioning of transducer.

7

Sonographic Anatomy of the Musculoskeletal System

JOINTS

Major joint spaces in the body that can be visualized with ultrasound include the knee, ankle, shoulder, wrist, hip, elbow, foot, and hand.

KNEE

The pediatric knee is evaluated while in slight flexion for visualization of the distal femur and proximal tibial cartilage, with the transducer directed into the intercondylar notch.

Cartilaginous structures have well-defined echogenic margins with hypoechoic echotexture in relation to muscle and bone. Cartilage thickness in a mature knee should measure between 1 and 3 millimeters, with the lateral femoral condyle cartilage thicker than the medial femoral condyle. In younger, skeletally immature patients, the cartilage may be significantly thicker as the ossification centers may be predominantly unossified. In this case, the hypoechoic cartilage may have speckled echoes related to blood vessels. Examples include unossified femoral and humeral heads.

ANKLE

The Achilles tendon of the ankle and foot is most often scanned, particularly in pediatric athletes for tear or rupture, and inserts on the posterior aspect of the calcaneus. The normal Achilles tendon in adolescents is 4 millimeters thick and 5 centimeters long; in adults it is 6 millimeters thick and 6 centimeters long.

SHOULDER

The shoulder joint in neonates and young infants appears as a round hypoechoic cartilaginous structure with bright internal echoes within the glenoid fossa. The shoulder joint is not frequently scanned in pediatric patients, although sonography can be useful to evaluate the shoulder for excluding dislocation of the humeral head from the glenoid cavity. Sonography of the shoulder can also be used to determine if there has been avulsion of the humeral head from the humeral shaft, which can be seen in non-accidental trauma.

WRIST

The four components of the wrist that can be visualized with sonography include the radial, ulnar, volar, and dorsal compartments. Ultrasound is capable of depicting dynamic motion for a more accurate assessment of soft tissue, tendons, ligaments, vessels, muscles, and nerve bundles in patients with swelling, pain, or trauma. Focused sonography may encompass the major joints of the dorsal wrist, including the distal radio-ulnar joint, midcarpal joint, dorsal radiocarpal ligament, and carpometacarpal joint. In examining the dorsal wrist, the hand is pronated. For assessment of the ventral wrist, the hand is supinated. Pathology encountered may include fractures, carpal tunnel syndrome, ganglion cysts, neuromas, and tenosynovitis.

HIPS

The femoral head is the superior-most portion of the femur. At birth, the femoral head is cartilaginous and hypoechoic

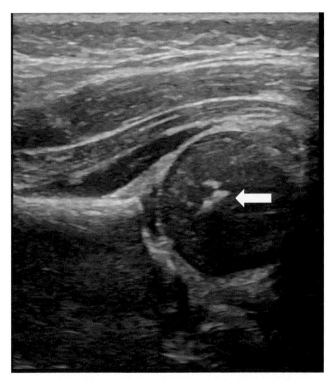

FIGURE 7-1. Normal ossification center seen on a 5-month-old patient.

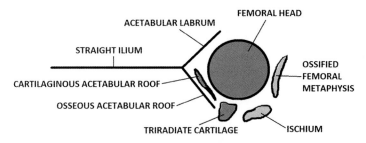

FIGURE 7-2. Diagram of anatomic structures of the hip.

to bone. The femoral head ossification center (Fig. 7-1) develops between the second and eighth months of life. For this reason, examination of the hip is most successfully performed in patients under 6 months of age.

The hip may be evaluated following abnormal findings during a pediatrician's clinical hip exam, history of breech position in utero, presence of asymmetry in thigh skin folds, or for hip clicks. Common clinical hip exams include the Barlow and Ortolani maneuvers or the Galeazzi test (Allis sign), which evaluates for presence of instability (i.e., dislocation and relocation of hips) and leg length asymmetry. With the Barlow maneuver the thigh is adducted and a gentle posterolateral pressure is applied. With this maneuver, a palpable "clunk" may be felt as the femoral head pops out of the acetabulum in the event of a dislocated hip joint. With the Ortolani maneuver, the thigh is abducted and a gentle anteromedial pressure is applied. If the hip is dislocated, a palpable "clunk" is felt as the femoral head is reduced back into the acetabulum. These tests are most sensitive in the neonatal to early infantile period. As the infant ages, hip capsule laxity decreases and contractures develop, limiting accuracy of Barlow and Ortolani maneuvers for DDH evaluation. The Galeazzi test (Allis sign) is performed with the patient lying supine with 90° knee flexion and 45° hip flexion. This test is not limited to the infantile period and can be performed throughout childhood. With this test, the clinician observes for asymmetry of the thigh folds and compares the femur length at knee level to assess for a discrepancy in leg length. It is important to note, in the scenario of bilateral dislocation, a positive Galeazzi sign would not be visualized. Other causes of positive Galeazzi sign include fracture or congenital conditions such as femoral shortening.

The two sonographic methods of evaluating the hip include the dynamic stress technique and the static Graf technique, with both approaches based on identification of the femoral and acetabular landmarks (Fig. 7-2).

Sonographically, the femoral head is rounded and hypoechoic. The acetabulum, which articulates with the femoral head, contains hyperechoic bony and hypoechoic cartilaginous portions. The labrum is a hypoechoic fibrocartilage that is visualized superolateral to the femoral head and adjacent to the ilium. The hypoechoic Y-shaped triradiate cartilage is located posterior to the femoral head (Fig. 7-3).

Please refer to hip protocol information in Chapter 27, section "Developmental Dysplasia of the Hip (DDH)."

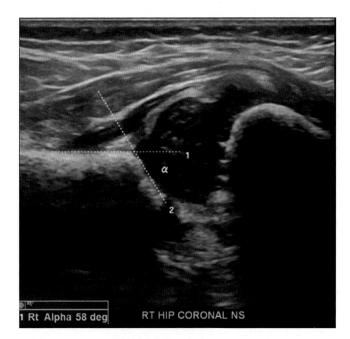

FIGURE 7-3. Coronal hip with alpha angle.

8

Sonographic Peripheral Vasculature

For peripheral vascular exams, sonographers should choose a linear transducer with the highest frequency that allows for adequate penetration, typically between 9 and 14 MHz. Smallest habitus patients (i.e., infants) may require use of a linear array hockey stick transducer. This transducer offers high resolution and a small transducer footprint. Larger habitus patients (i.e., athletic, or obese adolescents) may require lower frequencies of 5 to 8 MHz.

LOWER EXTREMITY VENOUS SYSTEM

In the lower extremity, venous drainage is divided into deep and superficial systems. Both deep and superficial systems drain into the common femoral vein (CFV) of the leg (Fig. 8-1). The lumen of a normal vein is anechoic, and the walls are thinner than those of the adjacent artery. The lower extremity veins should be entirely compressible when pressure is applied with the transducer in transverse imaging plane (Fig. 8-2). Complete compression of the lower extremity veins confirms there is no clot material (thrombus) within the interior vessel lumen on B-mode imaging.

During color and spectral Doppler evaluation, expiration causes spontaneous venous flow to increase in the lower extremity, and inspiration causes spontaneous venous flow to decrease in the lower extremity. This is because venous flow fluctuates with respiration. During inspiration, the diaphragm moves downward, compressing the abdomen and increasing abdominal pressure, which decreases venous blood flow in the bilateral lower extremities. During expiration, the abdominal cavity decompresses, and in turn increases venous blood flow in the lower extremities.

Clinical indications for a venous exam include extremity discomfort, pain, edema, and erythema. Risk of untreated venous thrombosis includes life-threatening pulmonary embolism (PE) and superior vena cava syndrome.

Sonographic appearance of venous thrombosis varies according to age of thrombus. In the acute setting, thrombus can be nearly anechoic and difficult to visualize. Color and spectral Doppler imaging will demonstrate absence of flow, providing additional information pertaining to vessel obstruction. Once thrombus material is ruled out via compression technique, the sonographer may squeeze the distal extremity or have the patient plantar flex their foot. These techniques push blood proximally, demonstrating increased flow throughout the lower extremity on color (Fig. 8-3) and spectral Doppler imaging display during evaluation in sagittal imaging plane. This increase in flow is termed *augmentation*, confirming vessel patency (Fig. 8-4). This is a beneficial diagnostic component in negative deep vein thrombosis (DVT) cases for improved clinical confidence.

Note: With a positive venous thrombosis, augmentation technique using manual compression may cause minor patient discomfort and poses the risk of mobilizing loose clot material as blood surges proximally through the vein. Therefore, in the presence of DVT identified using vessel compression technique with the imaging transducer, clinical benefit of augmentation may not outweigh the risk combined with patient discomfort. In lieu of augmentation, sagittal evaluation with color or power Doppler modalities may be utilized to confirm lack of spontaneous venous flow. Augmentation in the scenario of complete venous thrombosis appears as lack of flow on Doppler modalities. A blunted, minimized augmentation is demonstrated with partial thrombus obstruction.

Hint: For the lower extremity venous protocol, the examination table should be placed in reverse Trendelenburg position with head of table elevated 30 to 45 degrees.

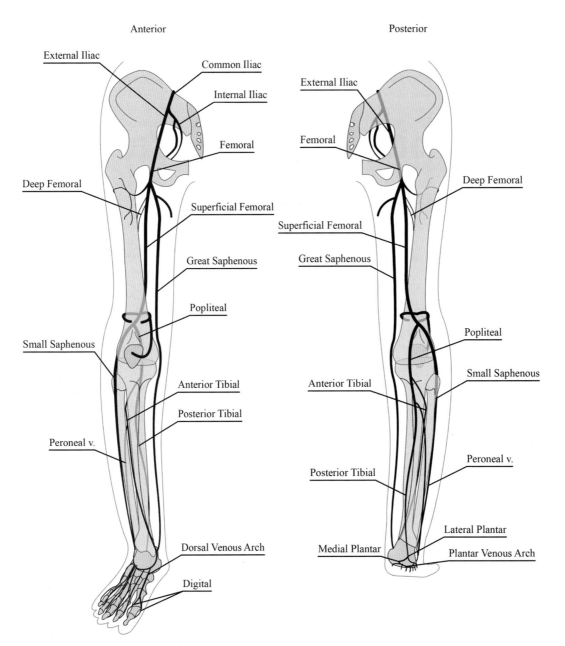

FIGURE 8-1. Lower extremity venous system. (Illustration created by and used with permission from Isaiah Forestier.)

The deep veins of the lower extremity from distal to proximal extremity consist of:

1. The deep digital veins which merge into plantar metatarsal veins
   a. Metatarsal veins which merge with dorsal veins, forming the deep plantar arch
2. Veins of the calf including the posterior tibial veins (PTV), anterior tibial veins (ATV), peroneal veins, gastrocnemius (sural) veins, and soleal veins (sinuses)
   a. PTV course posterior to the tibia
   b. ATV course lateral to the tibia
   c. Peroneal veins course lateral to the fibula

   d. Soleal veins empty into the PTV and peroneal veins
   e. Gastrocnemius ends at the popliteal vein
3. The popliteal vein resides in the popliteal fossa, posterior to the knee
   a. Confluence of the ATV, PTV, and peroneal veins
4. Veins in the thigh consist of the femoral vein (FV), deep femoral vein (DFV), and CFV
   a. The FV courses the medial thigh, and merges with the DFV
   b. The DFV (profunda femoris) and FV merge into the CFV
   c. The CFV continues superior to become the external iliac vein

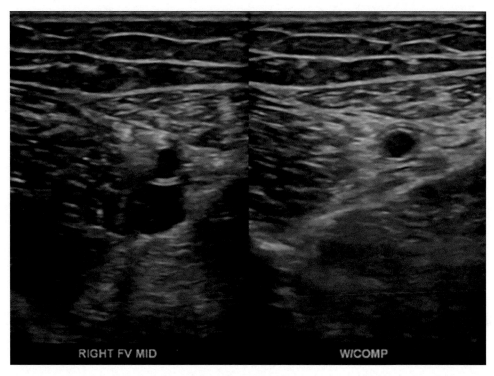

FIGURE 8-2. Demonstration of femoral vein compression; the deep venous system should be evaluated with compression in its entirety to ensure there is no acute thrombus, as acute thrombus may present with an anechoic appearance.

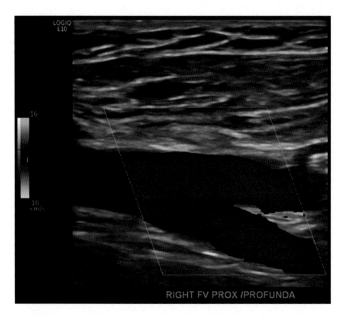

FIGURE 8-3. Color Doppler evaluation demonstrating patency of the femoral vein.

Common clinical protocols include evaluation of the CFV at groin-level to the PTV, ATV, and peroneal veins at ankle level. Should a sonographer scan superior (central) to the CFV, they would encounter the external iliac vein and internal iliac vein, which merge to form the common iliac vein (CIV) and continue proximally to the bifurcation of the inferior vena cava.

The superficial veins of the lower extremity from distal extremity to proximal consist of:

1. Greater saphenous vein (GSV)
   a. The GSV is the body's longest vein.
2. Lesser saphenous vein (LSV)
   a. The LSV ends at the popliteal vein.
3. Superficial veins
   a. Perforating veins of the lower extremity.
   b. Venous stasis may occur as a result of flow reversal and pressure increase in the superficial venous system.

UPPER EXTREMITY VENOUS SYSTEM

The veins of the upper extremity are also divided into deep and superficial systems. The deep veins of the upper extremity drain the palm of the hand to form the radial and ulnar veins. These veins continue merging with other veins located proximally in the arm until blood reaches the superior vena cava (Fig. 8-5). There is more variability in the upper extremity veins compared to the lower extremities. Therefore, it is possible to have duplicate venous systems (i.e., two cephalic veins, two basilic veins, and so forth). During color and spectral Doppler evaluation, expiration causes venous flow to decrease in the upper extremity, and inspiration causes venous flow to increase in the upper extremity. This is because venous flow fluctuates with

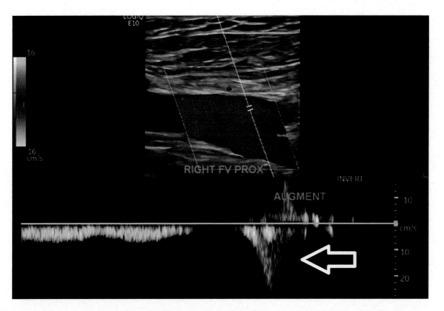

FIGURE 8-4. Patent, compressible, proximal right femoral vein with no suggestion of thrombosis. Augmentation demonstrated and indicated by the white arrow.

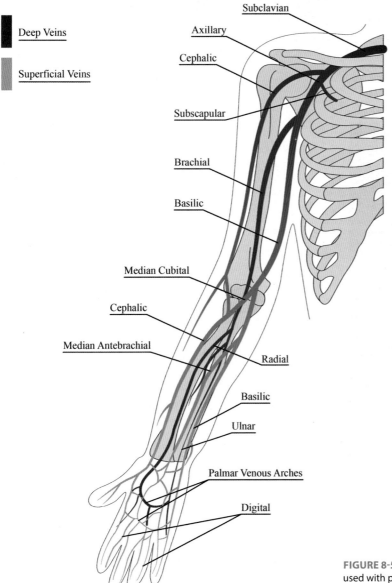

FIGURE 8-5. Upper extremity venous system. (Illustration created by and used with permission from Isaiah Forestier.)

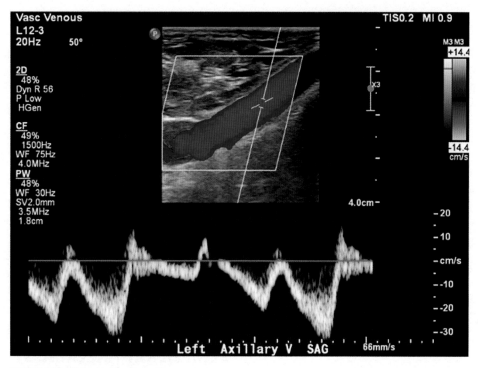

FIGURE 8-6. Patent left axillary vein.

respiration (Fig. 8-6). During inspiration, the diaphragm moves downward, compressing the abdomen and increasing abdominal pressure. In turn, negative pressure in the thoracic cavity creates suction, increasing venous return from the arms, head, and vena cava.

The deep veins of the upper extremity consist of:

1. The deep digital and deep palmar veins, which empty into the radial vein

2. Veins of the distal arm including the radial and ulnar veins

   a. Paired radial veins course the lateral forearm (radial bone)

   b. Paired ulnar veins course the medial forearm (ulnar bone)

> **Note:** The distal veins may not be imaged in evaluation for DVT due to variability and clinical impact, dependent on institution protocol preference

3. Veins of the proximal arm including the brachial and axillary veins

   a. Paired brachial veins, product of radial and ulnar vein junction at antecubital fossa

   b. Axillary vein at level of axilla, product of paired brachial veins and basilic veins

      i. Continues into the subclavian vein

4. Subclavian vein merges with the internal jugular vein (IJV) and becomes the brachiocephalic (formerly termed *innominate*) vein

   a. Courses under the clavicle

5. Veins of the neck which include the internal and external jugular veins, merge into the subclavian vein

The superficial veins of the upper extremity consist of:

1. The superficial digital veins drain into the deep veins

2. Basilic vein (large) courses the medial arm and merges with brachial vein

3. Cephalic vein courses the lateral (radial) arm and merges with the axillary vein

4. Medial cubital vein is at the junction of the basilic and cephalic veins, an area commonly used for venipuncture

Common clinical protocols include evaluation of the jugular vein at neck-level to radial and ulnar veins at wrist level, including the jugular, subclavian, axillary, brachial, basilic, cephalic, radial, and ulnar veins.

VENOUS ACCESS SURVEY

A venous access survey may also be requested. This is generally performed as a preoperative evaluation for transplant patients or in patients requiring complex cardiothoracic surgical intervention. The purpose of a venous access survey is to ensure there will be adequate access for large bore catheters, or to evaluate patients with prior histories of dialysis, multiple catheterizations, or multiple surgeries. A venous access survey is performed using a 5 to 7 MHz linear transducer. However, if the patient has a small anatomical neck area, a 7-MHz vector transducer may be used. When a venous access study is requested, bilateral imaging of the internal jugular veins, subclavian veins, brachiocephalic veins, superior vena cava, CFVs, external iliac veins, and common iliac veins should be obtained.

Additional veins throughout the body can be surveyed (i.e., IV-line access, inclusion of inferior vena cava in renal Doppler or lower extremity exams) when necessary.

Images include:

1. Imaging in two planes from the right atrium of the heart to the common iliac vein confluence should be obtained
   a. Use color Doppler and obtain spectral Doppler waveforms to demonstrate blood flow
   b. Limitations of the distal infrarenal inferior vena cava may be caused by obscuring bowel gas, in which case coronal imaging can be utilized
2. The common and external iliac veins should be surveyed
   a. Caudad to the inguinal ligament, the CFV should be surveyed in two imaging planes
3. The IJV should be surveyed in the anterolateral neck, lateral to the thyroid gland in 2 imaging planes
   a. Respiratory variation is normally seen in this vessel
   b. This vein should be followed to the subclavian vein confluence to ensure it is not a collateral
4. Long-axis view of the subclavian vein is obtained by positioning the transducer in transverse imaging plane inferior to the clavicle
5. The axillary vein should be traced to the IJV confluence
   a. Because of close proximity between the axillary artery and vein, spectral Doppler should be performed
6. Long-axis view of the brachiocephalic vein is surveyed by positioning the transducer medial and oblique to the confluence of the subclavian vein and IJV
   a. Color and spectral Doppler should be utilized to demonstrate flow and presence of an existing line or thrombus
   b. This vein should be followed to the superior vena cava to exclude collateralization
7. The superior vena cava is surveyed when the transducer is placed in a transverse fashion just superior to the sternal notch
   a. Images should be obtained in grayscale, color, and spectral Doppler
   b. It may be required to have the patient hyperextend and laterally rotate (toward the right) their neck for image optimization
   c. If the sonographer faces difficulty, the left brachiocephalic vein can be followed to its confluence with the right brachiocephalic vein
   d. Note that in infants, better imaging may be obtained by taking a right parasternal image of the superior vena cava using the thymus as a window compared to the suprasternal approach

PERIPHERAL ARTERIAL SYSTEM

Arteries can easily be differentiated from veins because the walls are thicker than that of the adjacent veins. Additionally, arteries will not collapse when pressure is applied to them with the imaging transducer. The lumen of a normal artery is anechoic. A triphasic waveform is seen in peripheral arteries of the upper and lower extremities. The peripheral arteries show a triphasic flow pattern with forward flow acceleration in systole, reversal of flow in early diastole, and low amplitude antegrade flow during late diastole. With exercise and warmth, antegrade diastolic flow will increase and will decrease with vasoconstriction. Arterial occlusion is noted when there is absence of Doppler signal or color flow.

LOWER EXTREMITY ARTERIAL SYSTEM

The arteries of the lower extremity (Fig. 8-7) consist of:

1. Iliac arteries
   a. The common iliac arteries arise from the bifurcation of the distal abdominal aorta, further dividing into the internal and external iliac arteries
      i. The left common iliac artery is shorter than the right
      ii. The internal iliac artery is shorter than the external iliac artery
      iii. Multiple collateral branches may be present if there is obstruction of the internal iliac artery

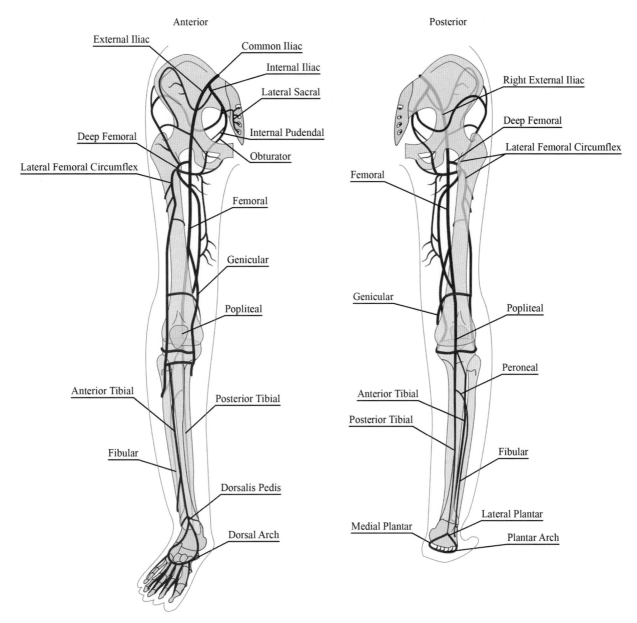

FIGURE 8-7. Lower extremity arterial system. (Illustration created by and used with permission from Isaiah Forestier.)

2. Femoral arteries
   a. The external iliac arteries continue to form the common femoral arteries (CFA)
      i. The CFA divides into the deep femoral artery (DFA, profunda femoris) and superficial femoral artery (SFA)
         • The DFA courses medial to the femur
         • The SFA continues into the popliteal artery, coursing through the adductor (Hunter's) canal

3. Popliteal arteries
   a. Branches into the anterior tibial artery (ATA), posterior tibial artery (PTA), and peroneal artery, bilaterally. The peroneal artery and the PTA come off the tibioperoneal trunk

4. Arteries of the calf
   a. Tibioperoneal trunk
      i. Branches into the PTA and peroneal artery
   b. ATA
      i. Continues into the dorsalis pedis artery of the foot

5. Plantar arch of the foot is a junction of the deep and lateral plantar arteries

UPPER EXTREMITY ARTERIAL SYSTEM

The arteries of the upper extremity (Fig. 8-8):

1. Subclavian artery
   a. Left begins at aortic arch, right begins at brachioce-phalic (formerly termed *innominate*) artery
2. Axillary artery
   a. Level of axilla
3. Brachial artery
4. Ulnar artery
   a. Begins at antecubital fossa
   b. Branches into superficial palmar arch
5. Radial artery
   a. Begins at antecubital fossa
   b. Branches into deep palmar arch
6. Palmar arches
   a. Branches supply digits (fingers) and metacarpals

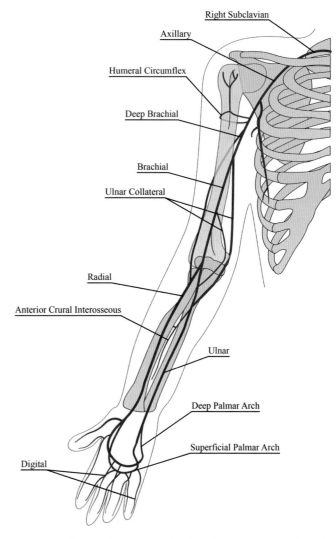

FIGURE 8-8. Upper extremity arterial system. (Illustration created by and used with permission from Isaiah Forestier.)

9

Sonographic Abdominal Vasculature

An artery is a hollow muscular tube enclosed in a sheath, whose purpose is to carry oxygenated blood away from the heart and supply tissues and organs throughout the body. Arteries have three layers, including the tunica intima, tunica media, and tunica adventitia. The endothelial tunica intima is the innermost layer. The muscular tunica media is the middle layer with the capability of handling higher pressures. The adventitial layer is the outermost layer and is comprised of connective tissue.

Unlike the artery, a vein is a hollow collapsible tube. Veins carry deoxygenated blood toward the heart from tissues and organs throughout the body. Veins are aided by muscle contraction and contain venous valves, which are an extension of the intimal layer to prevent backflow of blood. Capillaries are miniscule, one-walled vessels that connect the arterial and venous systems.

The great vessels of the abdomen include the abdominal aorta and inferior vena cava.

The abdominal aorta perfuses the abdomen and lower extremities with oxygenated blood. It has multiple branches including the paired inferior phrenic arteries, celiac axis, paired middle adrenal (suprarenal) arteries, superior mesenteric artery (SMA), paired renal arteries, paired gonadal arteries, inferior mesenteric artery (IMA), paired lumbar arteries, median sacral artery, and bifurcates distally to form the iliac arteries (Figs. 9-1, 9-2). The celiac axis (trunk) is the first branch arising from the anterior proximal abdominal aorta (Fig. 9-3). The three branches that arise from the celiac axis are the common hepatic, left gastric, and splenic arteries. Of these branches, the left gastric artery is the smallest branch and the splenic artery is the largest. The common hepatic artery further bifurcates into the proper hepatic artery and gastroduodenal artery. The SMA is 1 centimeter distal to celiac axis, which supplies the small bowel distal to the duodenum and the first two-thirds of the colon. The gonadal arteries arise from the aorta inferior to the renal arteries. The IMA perfuses the distal one-third of the colon.

An abdominal aorta protocol entails visualization of the proximal, mid, and distal aorta, including distal bifurcation and survey of the bilateral common iliac arteries. The aorta

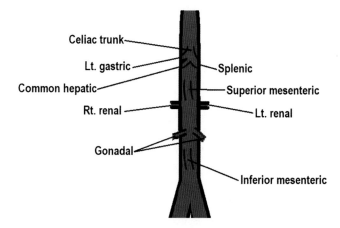

FIGURE 9-1. Main branches of the abdominal aorta.

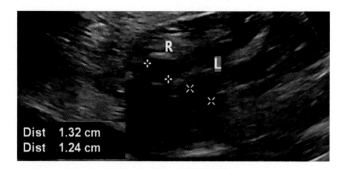

FIGURE 9-2. Common iliac arteries (aorta bifurcation).

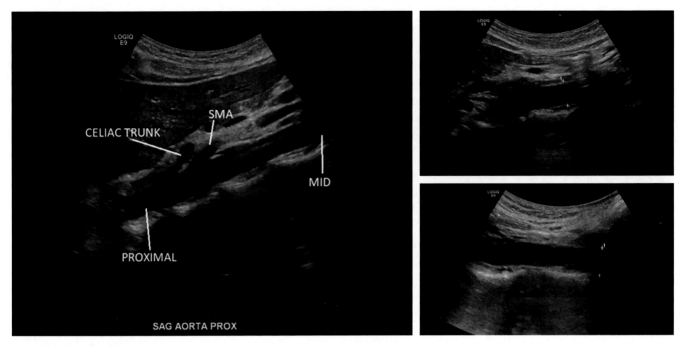

FIGURE 9-3. Sagittal aorta.

TABLE 9-1 • Pediatric mean abdominal aorta diameter by age					
Mean Measurement	**1-3 Years**	**3-7 Years**	**7-11 Years**	**11-15 Years**	**15-17 Years**
Proximal Aorta (cm)	0.9	1.0	1.2	1.5	1.7
Distal Aorta (cm)	0.7	0.8	1.1	1.2	1.4

Source: Akturk Y, Ozbal Gunes S. Normal abdominal aorta diameter in infants, children and adolescents. Pediatr Int. 2018 May;60(5):455-460. doi: 10.1111/ped.13542. PMID: 29498778.

should be evaluated in two imaging planes, providing grayscale, color Doppler, and spectral Doppler images in the long axis and grayscale and color Doppler images in the short axis. In both longitudinal (sagittal or coronal) and short axis (transverse) planes, images with and without wall-to-wall measurement should be obtained. When measuring the aorta, an outer-to-outer (OTO) wall measurement is standard. Other measurement methods include leading edge-to-leading edge (LELE) or inner-to-inner (ITI) wall measurement. The leading edge method involves caliper placement at the outer edge of the anterior aortic wall to the inner edge of the posterior aortic wall. It is important in subsequent scans the same measurement method be followed for reproducibility and evaluation of any change in aortic diameter. The normal anteroposterior and transverse diameter of the abdominal aorta is 3 centimeters or less in adults but varies greatly with age in pediatrics (see Table 9-1). The average proximal aorta measurement for patients between 1 to 3 years of age is 0.9 cm, between 3 to 7 years of age is 1.0 cm, between 7 to 11 years of age is 1.2 cm, between 11 to 15 years of age is 1.5 cm, and between 15 to 17

years of age is 1.7 cm. The average distal aorta measurement for patients between 1 to 3 years of age is 0.7 cm, between 3 to 7 years of age is 0.8 cm, between 7 to 11 years of age is 1.1 cm, between 11 to 15 years of age is 1.2 cm, and between 15 to 17 years of age is 1.4 cm. Normal appearance of the aorta is described as smooth (i.e., without bulging, aneurysm, etc.). For sonographic imaging of the abdominal aorta, a normal patient preparation for abdominal ultrasound is followed using NPO guidelines based upon the patient's age.

IMAGING OF THE ABDOMINAL AORTA

Still images:

1. Proximal abdominal aorta imaged in sagittal and transverse planes, in grayscale (with and without measurement)

Hint: Proximal abdominal aorta is located posterior to the left lobe of the liver, the celiac axis and SMA are identified branching anteriorly at this level.

2. Proximal abdominal aorta imaged in sagittal and transverse planes, with color Doppler

3. Proximal abdominal aorta imaged in sagittal plane, with spectral Doppler waveform obtaining peak systolic velocity (PSV) and end diastolic velocity (EDV) measurements

    a. Asking the cooperative patient to inhale and suspend respiration at this level can aid in image optimization.

    b. For all spectral Doppler samples obtained, ensure angle correction is implemented at 60 degrees or less, heel-toe the transducer so the indicator is positioned parallel to the vessel wall.

4. Mid-abdominal aorta imaged in sagittal and transverse planes, in grayscale (with and without measurement)

5. Mid-abdominal aorta imaged in sagittal and transverse planes, with color Doppler

6. Mid-abdominal aorta imaged in sagittal plane, with spectral Doppler waveform obtaining PSV and EDV measurements

    a. Spectral Doppler sample of the mid-abdominal aorta is obtained inferior to the level of the SMA with sample gate placed in the center of the vessel lumen.

7. Distal abdominal aorta imaged in sagittal and transverse planes, in grayscale (with and without measurement)

8. Distal abdominal aorta imaged in sagittal and transverse planes, with color Doppler

9. Distal abdominal aorta imaged in sagittal plane, with spectral Doppler waveform obtaining PSV and EDV measurements

    a. Spectral Doppler sample of the distal abdominal aorta is obtained at the approximate level of the umbilicus with sample gate placed in the center of the vessel lumen.

10. Distal aortic bifurcation imaged in sagittal and transverse planes, in grayscale

11. Distal aortic bifurcation imaged in sagittal and transverse planes, with color Doppler

12. Right common iliac artery imaged in sagittal and transverse planes, in grayscale (with and without measurement)

13. Right common iliac artery imaged in sagittal and transverse planes, with color Doppler

14. Right common iliac artery imaged in sagittal plane, with spectral Doppler waveform obtaining PSV and EDV measurements

15. Left common iliac artery imaged in sagittal and transverse planes, in grayscale (with and without measurement)

16. Left common iliac artery imaged in sagittal and transverse planes, with color Doppler

17. Left common iliac artery imaged in sagittal plane, with spectral Doppler waveform obtaining PSV and EDV measurements

    a. Spectral Doppler samples of the bilateral common iliac arteries are obtained at or directly below the approximate level of the umbilicus with sample gate placed in the center of the vessel lumen.

The inferior vena cava is a retroperitoneal vascular structure which originates at the confluence of the bilateral common iliac veins. It courses adjacent to the abdominal aorta and lies to the right of the vertebral column. The IVC is thin-walled, anechoic, and unlike other veins throughout the body, lacks valves. Walls of the IVC are collapsible and yield to respiratory changes. The IVC (Figs. 9-4 and 9-5) has multiple branches throughout the abdomen including the lumbar veins, right gonadal vein, bilateral renal veins, right suprarenal vein, hepatic veins, and inferior phrenic veins. The right renal

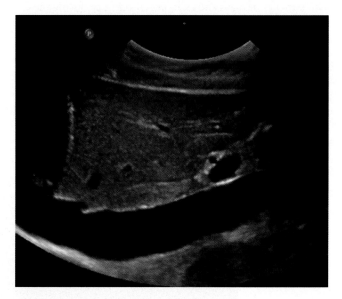

FIGURE 9-4. Inferior vena cava.

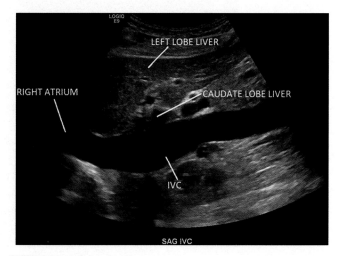

FIGURE 9-5. Inferior vena cava.

vein lies posterior to the inferior vena cava. The left renal vein exits the renal hilum and must pass anterior to the abdominal aorta before reaching the IVC. For this reason, the left renal vein is longer than the right renal vein. The left gonadal vein enters the left renal vein, and then into the IVC. The right gonadal vein enters directly into the IVC. The IVC functions to drain deoxygenated venous blood from the lower extremities, pelvis, abdomen, and lower trunk into the right atrium of the heart.

PORTAL-VENOUS SYSTEM

A confluence of vessels including the splenic vein, gastric vein, cystic vein, superior mesenteric, and inferior mesenteric veins join to form the portal vein, which enters the liver through the hepatoduodenal ligament. The main portal vein supplies 70-75% of blood to the liver. At the liver's hilum, the main portal vein branches into left and right portal veins, perfusing the corresponding lobes of the liver. The proper hepatic artery supplies the additional 25 to 30% of blood to the liver.

When imaging abdominal vasculature in pediatric patients, unlike peripheral vasculature, scan technique more closely resembles technique used to evaluate abdominal structures, and a curvilinear transducer may be used.

Similarly, patient preparation guidelines are like those used for abdominal scans. The patient should be fasting to minimize bowel gas artifact following guidelines according to the patient's age. In very small habitus patients (i.e., neonates and infants) a high frequency linear or sector transducer may be selected for a smaller transducer footprint. In adolescents, a low to mid frequency curvilinear transducer is appropriate. When PSV is measured, Doppler angle correction should be utilized at 60 degrees or less. The indicator is positioned parallel to the vessel wall within the center of the vessel. If a resistive index (RI) is being obtained, angle correction is not a requirement.

An abdominal Doppler protocol entails imaging of the splenic vein at the splenic hilum and posterior to the pancreatic tail, portal-splenic confluence, superior mesenteric vein (Fig. 9-6), main portal vein (Figs. 9-7 and 9-8) including right and left portal vein branches, the hepatic artery (Fig. 9-9) which feeds the liver along with the portal venous system, hepatic veins (Fig. 9-10), inferior vena cava, and proximal aorta (varies by institution) (Figs. 9-11 to 9-13). Imaging of these vascular structures should include grayscale, color Doppler, and spectral Doppler evaluation to determine appropriate direction of flow. Wall measurement of the main portal vein and aorta should be obtained.

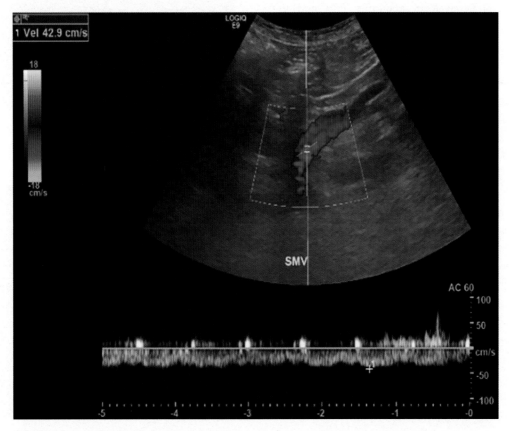

FIGURE 9-6. Superior mesenteric vein.

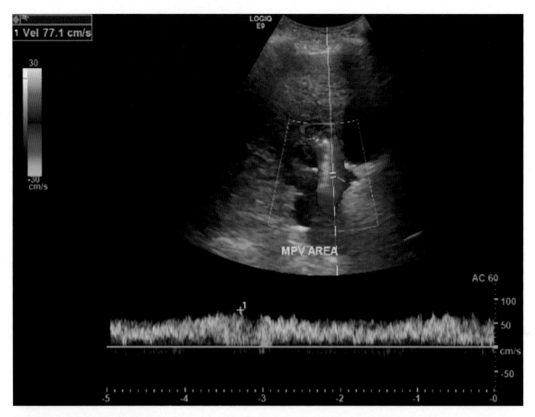

FIGURE 9-7. Main portal vein.

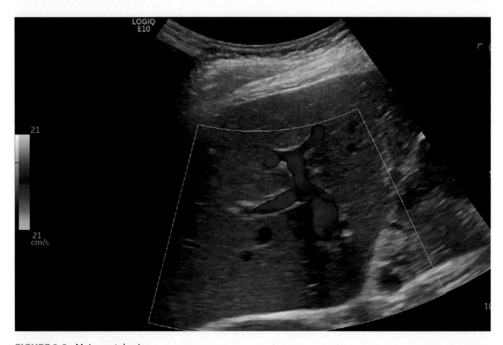

FIGURE 9-8. Main portal vein.

IMAGING AND NORMAL DIRECTION OF FLOW IN THE PORTAL-VENOUS SYSTEM

Normal direction of flow in the portal venous system is hepatopetal, toward the liver (Fig. 9-14). Normal direction of flow in the hepatic veins, which drain the liver, is hepatofugal or away from the liver.

Still images:

1. Coronal images of the splenic vein at the splenic hilum are obtained in grayscale, color, and spectral Doppler, evaluating direction of flow and splenorenal shunting. Normal flow in the splenic vein at the splenic hilum is hepatopetal.

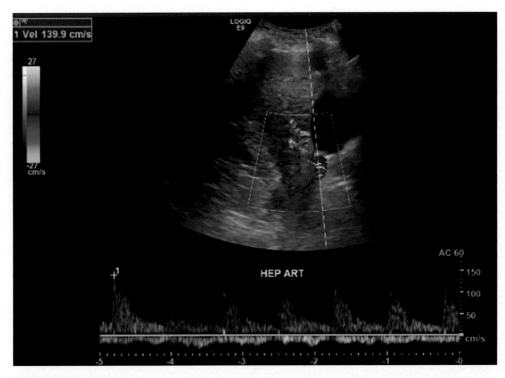

FIGURE 9-9. Hepatic artery.

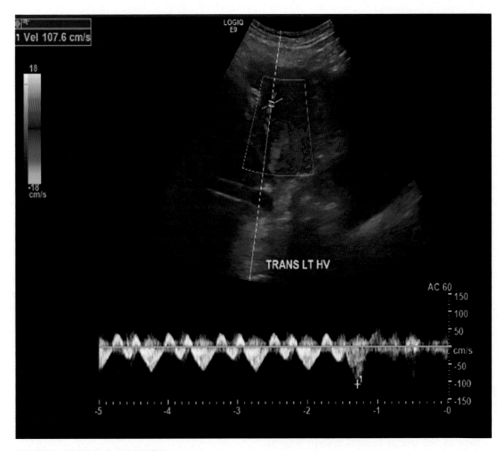

FIGURE 9-10. Hepatic veins (left).

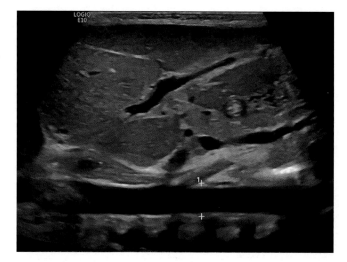

FIGURE 9-11. Aorta.

2. Long-axis images of the splenic vein posterior to pancreatic tail are obtained in grayscale, color, and spectral Doppler. Normal flow in the splenic vein posterior to the pancreatic tail is hepatopetal.

3. Long-axis images of the portal-splenic confluence posterior to the body of the pancreas demonstrate normal hepatopetal flow. Images are obtained in grayscale, color, and spectral Doppler. Spectral display will demonstrate respiratory variation.

4. Long-axis images should be obtained in grayscale, color, and spectral Doppler of the main portal vein at the region of the pancreatic head. The transducer should be slightly obliqued, angling towards the liver until the main portal vein comes into view. Long axis images of the main portal vein at bifurcation may also be imaged (this may vary by institution). Normal flow is hepatopetal.

Note: Flow in the main portal vein should be uniform, with mild changes with respiration and minimal periodicity, or changes in the cardiac cycle. Ensure flow in the main portal vein is higher than the diastolic flow in the hepatic artery. If diastolic flow in the hepatic artery is higher that flow in the main portal vein, the sonographer should notate this on the technologist worksheet and observe the liver parenchyma, providing additional images using a high-resolution linear transducer.

5. Long-axis images should be obtained of the main portal vein in grayscale with measurement. The normal diameter of the portal vein is less than 13 millimeters.

6. Obtain long-axis images in grayscale, color, and spectral Doppler of the right portal vein in the intercostal margin and left portal vein at midline. Normal flow is hepatopetal in these branches. The sonographer should follow the right and left portal veins to their secondary bifurcation.

7. Long-axis images of the hepatic artery are obtained, locating the celiac axis and taking spectral Doppler images of the left celiac axis branch which is the hepatic artery. Normal flow is hepatopetal.

   a. Hepatic artery waveforms should demonstrate a pulsatile, low-resistance waveform and high diastolic flow velocities. The normal resistive index (RI) in a fasting state fluctuates from 0.55 to 0.81 (mean, 0.62-0.74). The RI increases slightly after a meal and with age. RI will be higher at the porta hepatis and lower within the vessel branches closer to the liver periphery. The normal hepatic arterial PSV in a fasting *adult* is approximately 30 to 40 cm/s, and EDV is 10 to 15 cm/s.

Note: There is currently not a widely agreed upon standard hepatic artery PSV in the pediatric population.

8. The sonographer should obtain long-axis images of the right, mid, and left hepatic veins in grayscale, color, and spectral Doppler. Normal flow is hepatofugal and triphasic.

   a. Flow of the hepatic veins has also been referred to as periodic. Pressure changes in the right atrium of the heart (i.e., pressure gradient affecting blood flow) determines appearance of the hepatic vein spectral Doppler waveform. When a Valsalva maneuver is performed, or the patient briefly stops respiration, waveforms may appear blunted in normal patients. Waveforms within the hepatic veins are best evaluated during quiet respiration and when patients briefly stop respiration at end inspiration. Four parts of the typical hepatic vein waveform include a, s, v, and d waves. The a-wave represents atrial contraction, s-wave represents ventricular systole, v-wave represents atrial overfilling, and d-wave represents opening of the tricuspid valve.

9. Images of the inferior vena cava are obtained in the long axis with and without color and spectral Doppler. IVC diameter varies with respiration. Normal flow is hepatofugal. Spectral Doppler waveform will vary based on where the sample gate is placed.

   a. Flow in the proximal inferior vena cava is influenced by activity of the right atrium of the heart and shows

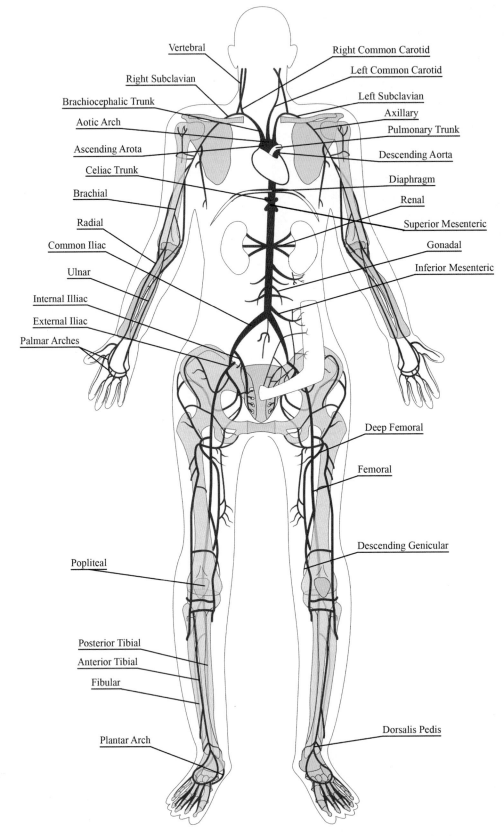

FIGURE 9-12. Arterial system with depiction of abdominal vasculature. (Illustration created by and used with permission from Isaiah Forestier.)

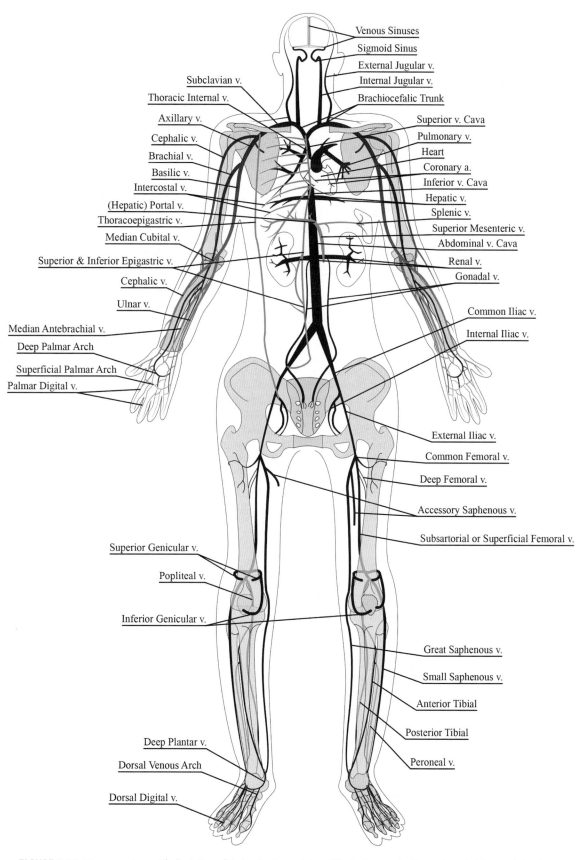

FIGURE 9-13. Venous system with depiction of abdominal vasculature. (Illustration created by and used with permission from Isaiah Forestier.)

Direction of Normal Hepatopeal Flow (Towards the Liver) in the Portal-Venous System

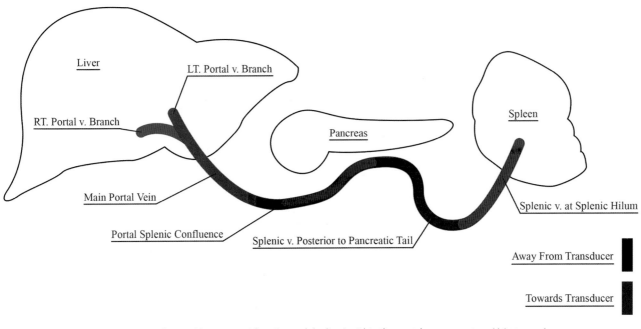

FIGURE 9-14. Diagram of normal hepatopetal flow (toward the liver) within the portal-venous system. Vein traversing anteriorly should depict a positive Doppler shift (toward the transducer). Vein diving posteriorly depicts a negative Doppler shift (away from the transducer). (Illustration created by and used with permission from Isaiah Forestier.)

back-pressure changes similar to those seen with hepatic venous flow. As the sonographer slides the transducer distally from the heart, cardiac activity has a lesser effect on flow velocities, and variations in abdominal or thoracic pressure cause greater variability in forward flow. Waveform appears more monophasic in the common iliac veins, similar to the proximal lower limb veins.

10. Evaluation of the aorta in a portal-venous system evaluation varies by institution. Generally, this evaluation is limited to include grayscale, color, and spectral Doppler imaging of the proximal aorta.

Note: If patent, image and evaluate the umbilical vein and follow this vessel in long axis to the umbilicus. Additionally, the sonographer should survey for porto-systemic collaterals (paraumbilical veins, splenorenal, gastroesophageal junction, coronary vein, mesocaval, etc.).

ABDOMINAL MESENTERIC ARTERIAL VASCULATURE

The postprandial SMA and IMA should demonstrate a low-resistance waveform in the nonfasting patient. In a RadioGraphics study, Chavhan et al. describes normal spectral Doppler

waveforms of the aorta and SMA in pediatrics as having high-resistance patterns. A pre-prandial SMA and IMA in the fasting patient should demonstrate a high-resistance waveform. The normal PSV for a pre-prandial SMA is 110 to 180 cm/s. The normal PSV for a pre-prandial IMA is 93 to 189 cm/s. The normal PSV for the celiac artery is 50 to 160 cm/s. Pre-prandial the normal flow velocity for the portal vein averages 18 cm/s (range 13-23 cm/s). Post-prandial this value rises, and 20 to 40 cm/s is an acceptable range.

Still images:

1. Proximal abdominal aorta imaged in sagittal plane at level of the celiac axis and SMA origin. Evaluate in grayscale, with color Doppler, and spectral Doppler.

2. Elongated celiac artery at origin. Evaluate in grayscale, with color Doppler, and spectral Doppler.

3. Elongated celiac artery at mid. Evaluate in grayscale, with color Doppler, and spectral Doppler.

4. Elongated common hepatic artery. Evaluate in grayscale, with color Doppler, and spectral Doppler.

5. Elongated splenic artery branch of celiac trunk. Evaluate in grayscale, with color Doppler, and spectral Doppler.

6. Elongated SMA at origin (aortic junction). Evaluate in grayscale, with color Doppler, and spectral Doppler.

7. Elongated SMA at proximal. Evaluate in grayscale, with color Doppler, and spectral Doppler.

8. Elongated SMA at mid. Evaluate in grayscale, with color Doppler, and spectral Doppler.

9. Elongated SMA at distal. Evaluate in grayscale, with color Doppler, and spectral Doppler

10. Elongated IMA at origin (aortic junction). Evaluate in grayscale, with color Doppler, and spectral Doppler.

11. Elongated IMA at proximal. Evaluate in grayscale, with color Doppler, and spectral Doppler.

Note: If unable to obtain long-axis images in the sagittal imaging plane, the sonographer should attempt images coronally. Ensure sample gate is appropriate in size and placed in the center of each vessel. A sample volume angle should be parallel to the vessel wall and equal to or less than 60 degrees. Heel-toe the transducer as necessary to align the vessel wall and Doppler angle. If the PSV of the celiac artery is greater than 200 cm/s with normal respiration pattern, or if the patient has or is being evaluated for median arcuate ligament syndrome, obtain a PSV of the celiac artery at origin (aortic junction) with the patient in deep inspiration.

Please note, abdominal renal vasculature is discussed in Chapter 11, Genitourinary System Vasculature.

10

Sonographic Intracranial Vasculature

INTRACRANIAL ANATOMY AND CIRCULATION

Intracranial vessels are well seen through the anterior fontanelle. Most commonly interrogated intracranial arteries include the anterior cerebral (ACA), middle cerebral (MCA), posterior cerebral (PCA), and internal carotid (ICA) arteries. Other important vessels include the sagittal sinus and vein of Galen (Figs. 10-1 and 10-2). Normal arterial blood flow patterns are evaluated with flow velocities and resistive indices (RI). Velocities and RI vary with age. For neonatal intensive care unit patients, spectral Doppler pattern and RI should be demonstrated in the ACA, and color Doppler should be used to demonstrate venous flow in the superior sagittal sinus, internal cerebral vein, vein of Galen, and inferior sagittal sinus. Venous blood flow of the central sagittal sinus veins and vein of Galen include sinusoidal flow (low-amplitude pulsation).

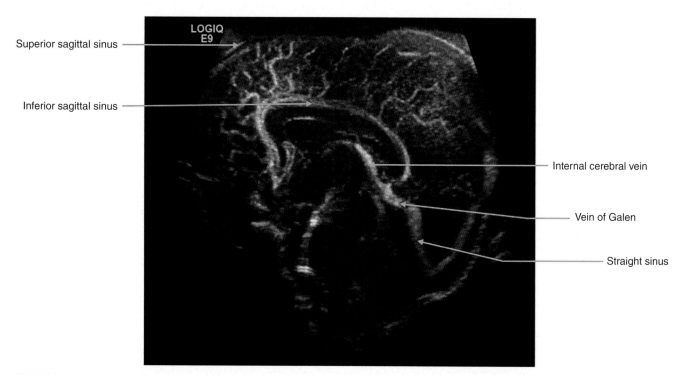

FIGURE 10-1. Intracranial veins.

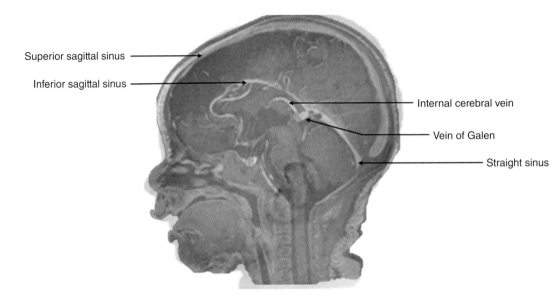

Superior sagittal sinus

Inferior sagittal sinus

Internal cerebral vein

Vein of Galen

Straight sinus

FIGURE 10-2. Intracranial veins.

After blood exits the left ventricle of the heart and travels through the ascending aorta, it enters and is routed through the branches of the aortic arch. These branches listed in order from right to left or proximal to distal are the brachiocephalic artery (formerly called the *innominate*), the left common carotid artery, and the left subclavian artery. The brachiocephalic artery bifurcates to form the right subclavian artery and the right common carotid artery. Both common carotid arteries bifurcate to form the external and internal carotid arteries. The bilateral external carotid arteries (ECAs) route blood to the face and neck structures. It is important to note that while the ECAs do not directly supply blood to the brain, the branches of the ophthalmic arteries, which branch from the cerebral portion of the ICAs, anastomose with the ECAs. This can form collateral blood flow to the brain in the event of ICA occlusion or interruption. The bilateral ICAs become intracranial vessels. These consist of three sections, the petrous, the cavernous, and the cerebral arteries. The cerebral segment of the ICAs branch into the ACA, the MCA, the posterior communicating artery, and the anterior choroidal arteries. These route blood to the anterior portions of the brain.

The vertebral arteries are branches of the right and left subclavian arteries and deliver blood to posterior portions of the brain. They ascend the neck posteriorly and pass through the transverse processes of the sixth cervical vertebrae. They continue superiorly through the transverse processes of the cervical vertebrae before coursing medially to enter through the foramen magnum of the skull. They then converge to form the basilar artery, which joins the posterior circle of Willis.

The circle of Willis (Figs. 10-3 and 10-4) is made up from the branches of the ICAs and basilar artery. This creates the network of vessels that perfuse brain tissue. Anteriorly, the circle of Willis is formed by the right and left ACAs which communicate via the anterior communicating artery. The posterior circle of Willis is formed by the right and left PCAs which communicate via the posterior communicating arteries. The basilar artery is formed by the junction of the bilateral vertebral arteries at the medullo-pontine junction and terminates at the posterior circle of Willis where it branches to join the right and left PCA.

The intracranial venous system forms a complex set of sinuses. Unlike other veins, the veins in this system have no valves. The intracranial venous system is divided into two sets, superficial veins and deep veins; however, it is important to note that the venous systems can present with variable and asymmetrical configurations, frequently including collateral vessels unlike the arterial system. The flow in the intracranial venous system can be quite difficult to visualize with ultrasound and often requires a great deal of adjusting imaging parameters. It is helpful to keep in mind that most of the intracranial venous system drains the blood in a centrifugal radial fashion with most being returned to the sagittal sinuses. The deep system is the exception to this. In the deep venous system, the blood is collected and eventually travels to the straight sinus, which courses in a horizontal fashion posteriorly, or toward the outer posterior area of the brain.

To simplify the process, the flow identification in Table 10-1 includes only the main intracranial veins, as there are many smaller intracranial veins that are unnamed due to multiple variations and collaterals.

The deep system includes the internal cerebral veins, which are comprised of three veins converging just behind the foramen of Monro. These drain into the vein of Galen, along with the basal vein of Rosenthal, which then drain into

Circle of Willis

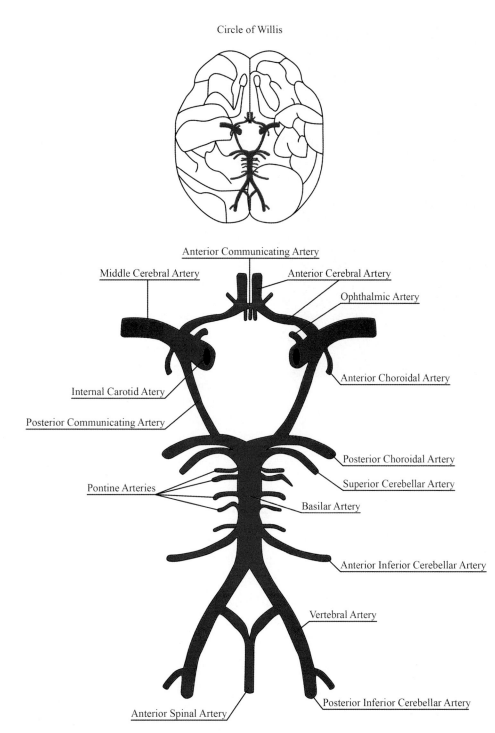

FIGURE 10-3. Circle of Willis. (Illustration created by and used with permission from Isaiah Forestier.)

the straight sinus at the uniting site with the inferior sagittal sinus. The straight sinus is the main site of collection from the deep system. From here, the blood flows to the transverse sinus.

The venous drainage of the head and neck occurs via the internal jugular veins, external jugular veins, and vertebral veins. The external jugular veins drain blood from the face, neck, and portions of the scapular region. The external jugular veins drain into the subclavian vein. The internal jugular veins collect blood from the brain and some superficial areas of the face and neck. These unite with the subclavian veins to become the brachiocephalic (innominate) veins. Note that there are brachiocephalic veins located bilaterally, whereas the brachiocephalic artery is only located on the right. There is a dense plexus of veins around the vertebral arteries. These are formed by small veins draining the neck muscles, joining with the veins

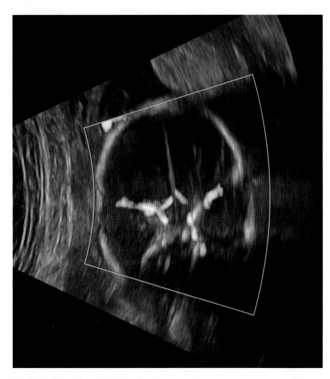

FIGURE 10-4. Circle of Willis in a 21-week fetus.

TABLE 10-1 • The Superficial System Flow
Superior
Superior cerebral veins drain parts of the superior cerebral cortex.
Includes Vein of Trolard, also known as the *superior anastomotic vein*.
Middle
The superficial middle cerebral vein drains the perisylvian area (around the Sylvian fissure).
Connected to the superior sagittal sinus via the anastomotic vein of Trolard.
Connected to the transverse sinus via the anastomotic vein of Labbé.
Inferior
Inferior cerebral veins.
Mostly anastomosed with deep venous system.
Basal vein of Rosenthal, paired, closely related to posterior cerebral arteries and drains into the vein of Galen.

associated with the internal vertebral plexuses. These descend through the transverse foramen of the cervical vertebrae until eventually converging into the vertebral vein and exiting the transverse foramen of the sixth vertebrae bilaterally. The vertebral veins drain into the brachiocephalic veins. These drain into the superior vena cava which returns the blood to the right atrium of the heart.

IMAGING APPROACH FOR EVALUATION OF INTRACRANIAL VASCULATURE

The major intracranial arteries include the ACA, MCA, PCA, and ICAs. Central intracranial veins include the vein of Galen and straight sinus. The midline sagittal image of the neonatal brain through the anterior fontanelle (Figs. 10-5 and 10-6) should demonstrate the vertebral, basilar, internal carotid, ACA, and pericallosal arteries, vein of Galen, and straight and superior sagittal sinuses. The smaller thalamostriate arteries (Fig. 10-7) are seen in sagittal images angling laterally throughout the brain.

Coronal images through the anterior and midbrain show the internal carotid arteries, MCAs, thalamostriate arteries, ACAs, and terminal cerebral veins. From a transtemporal approach (Fig. 10-5), the MCA, A1 segment of ACA, posterior communicating artery, and PCA can be seen (Fig. 10-8).

Normal intracranial arterial blood flow patterns are assessed with RI and flow velocity. RI and flow velocity are dependent on prematurity and vary by age in full-term neonates. In premature infants less than 30 weeks gestational age, diastolic flow in the intracranial arteries may be absent (important to note, other factors can affect this in infants, i.e., patent ductus arteriosus). In full-term infants, antegrade flow is present throughout systole and diastole. Normal venous blood flow pattern of the larger central veins of the sagittal sinus and vein of Galen include sinusoidal flow which has low-amplitude pulsation. The smaller intracerebral and terminal veins should have a continuous monophasic flow pattern (Fig. 10-9).

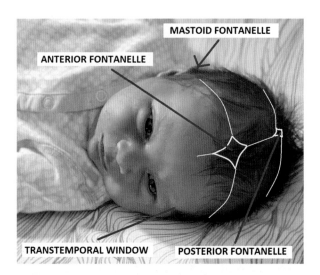

FIGURE 10-5. Common imaging windows used to evaluate intracranial structures and vasculature.

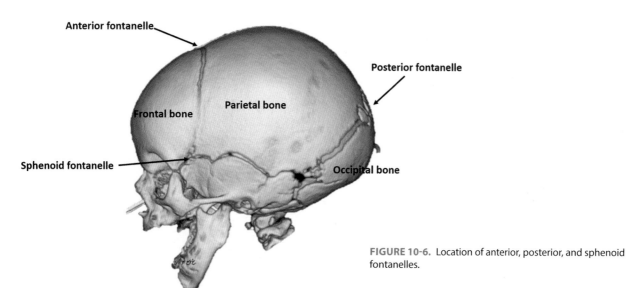

FIGURE 10-6. Location of anterior, posterior, and sphenoid fontanelles.

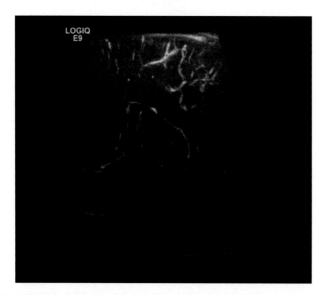

FIGURE 10-7. Thalamostriate vessels in a 28-week neonate.

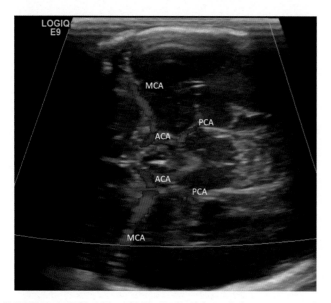

FIGURE 10-8. MCA, ACA, and PCA visualized through the transtemporal imaging window.

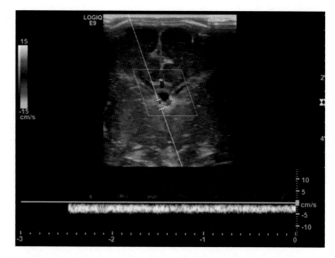

FIGURE 10-9. Continuous monophasic flow pattern in the terminal vein. The common terminal vein is formed by the confluence of the thalamostriate, anterior septal, superior choroidal, and medullary veins, which drain the deep white matter of the brain. The terminal veins course beneath the stria terminalis, posterior to the foramen of Monro. They continue as the internal cerebral veins, which drain over the third ventricle into the vein of Galen.

11

Vasculature of the Urinary System

PEDIATRIC RENAL VASCULATURE

The main renal arteries (MRA) can be seen branching off of the abdominal aorta and course posterior to the main renal veins (MRV). Branches of the MRA include the parenchymal, intrarenal, segmental, interlobar, and outermost arcuate arteries. The MRV lie anterior to the MRA and can be seen emptying into the inferior vena cava (IVC). The right renal vein is shorter than the left, and courses directly into the IVC from the renal hilum. The left renal vein courses past the abdominal aorta prior to reaching the IVC, thus being longer than the right renal vein.

In the MRA and within the renal parenchyma, arterial flow demonstrates a rapid systolic upstroke with antegrade diastolic flow noted throughout the cardiac cycle. During diastole, a continuous gradual drop-off is present, remaining above baseline. The renal arteries should demonstrate a low-resistance waveform (Fig. 11-1). The normal peak systolic velocity (PSV) for the renal arteries is less than 200 cm/s.

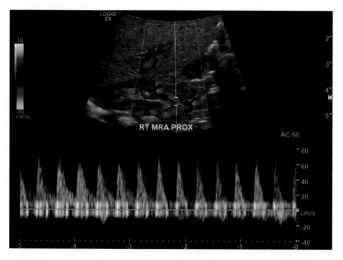

FIGURE 11-1. Normal main renal artery waveform in a 4-week-old patient.

In *adults*, the normal PSV ranges between 100 and 180 cm/s. The normal EDV is 25 to 50 cm/s. The MRA PSV varies with age of the pediatric patient. The PSV of the MRA ranges from 30 to 52 cm/s in neonatal patients to 100 to 110 cm/s in older children. The PSV decreases the further the artery branches into the renal parenchyma. Systolic acceleration time is usually equal to or less than 0.07 seconds throughout the start of systolic upstroke to early systolic peak. For the renal arteries, a renal to aortic ratio (RAR) and resistive index (RI) calculation may be required. RAR is calculated using the following: The highest renal artery PSV is divided by the PSV of the aorta at a level distal to superior mesenteric artery and proximal to renal artery origin.

$$RAR = \frac{\text{HIGHEST RENAL ARTERY PSV}}{\text{AORTIC PSV}}$$

A normal RAR is less than or equal to 3.5 and is valid when the PSV is within certain limits. The RI is calculated using the following:

$$\text{RESISTIVE INDEX (RI)} = \frac{\text{PSV} - \text{EDV}}{\text{PSV}}$$

For evaluation of renal disease processes, intraparenchymal RI may be helpful. Doppler waveforms should be obtained from the interlobar arteries (adjacent to the medullary pyramids) or arcuate arteries (at the corticomedullary junction). A normal RI for the renal arteries is less than or equal to 0.7; however, this value may vary slightly with age—particularly in the first year of life. These differences occur as a result of the physiologic and anatomic immaturity of the neonatal kidney. Renal arterial RI for preterm infants may be as high as 0.9. Infants less than 1 year of age have an RI ranging between 0.6 and 0.8. Adult levels are reached after the first 6 months to 1 year of life. Children

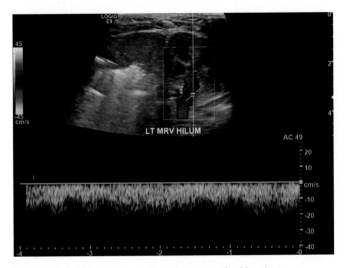

FIGURE 11-2. Patent main renal vein in a 2-month-old patient.

greater than 1 year of age have a RI ranging between 0.5 and 0.7. A normal flow velocity in a renal transplant is 80 to 118 cm/s with intraparenchymal RI of 0.4 to 0.8.

The MRV and intrarenal veins should have continuous flow throughout the cardiac cycle with the direction of flow opposite to that of the MRA (Fig. 11-2). Venous waveforms can show fluctuations in velocity related to cardiac (right atrial contractions) and respiratory motions.

Renal artery Doppler protocol entails a full bilateral renal evaluation and evaluation of arterial renal vasculature. The sonographer should provide grayscale, color Doppler, and spectral Doppler imaging of the MRA at origin, mid, and at the renal hilum (Fig. 11-3). Upper, mid, and lower pole interlobar and arcuate vessels should also be evaluated when indicated. A PSV, EDV, and RI should be obtained. Indication for renal artery Doppler includes renal artery stenosis, renal artery thrombosis and segmental infarction, and pseudoaneurysm or arteriovenous fistula following an interventional study such as renal biopsy.

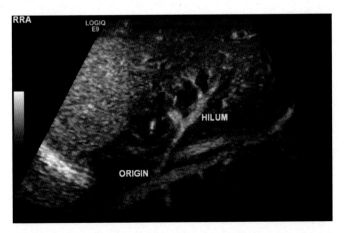

FIGURE 11-3. B-flow depiction of the right renal artery from origin to hilum.

RENAL ARTERY DOPPLER

Still images include:

1. Sagittal grayscale image of the right kidney at lateral
2. Sagittal grayscale image of the right kidney at mid, with and without measurements
3. Sagittal grayscale image of the right kidney at medial
4. Transverse grayscale image of the right kidney at superior
5. Transverse grayscale image of the right kidney at mid, with and without measurement
6. Transverse grayscale image of the right kidney at inferior
7. Long-axis view of right MRA at origin (aortic-end) with color and spectral Doppler
8. Long-axis view of right MRA at mid with color and spectral Doppler
9. Long-axis view of right MRA at renal hilum with color and spectral Doppler (MRA often elongated in transverse renal imaging plane)
10. Superior right renal interlobar and arcuate arteries with color and spectral Doppler
11. Mid right renal interlobar and arcuate arteries with color and spectral Doppler
12. Inferior right renal interlobar and arcuate arteries with color and spectral Doppler
13. Sagittal grayscale image of the left kidney at lateral
14. Sagittal grayscale image of the left kidney at mid, with and without measurements
15. Sagittal grayscale image of the left kidney at medial
16. Transverse grayscale image of the left kidney at superior.
17. Transverse grayscale image of the left kidney at mid, with and without measurement
18. Transverse grayscale image of the left kidney at inferior
19. Long-axis view of left MRA at origin (aortic-end) with color and spectral Doppler
20. Long-axis view of left MRA at mid with color and spectral Doppler
21. Long-axis view of left MRA at renal hilum with color and spectral Doppler (MRA often elongated in transverse renal imaging plane)
22. Superior left renal interlobar and arcuate arteries with color and spectral Doppler
23. Mid left renal interlobar and arcuate arteries with color and spectral Doppler
24. Inferior left renal interlobar and arcuate arteries with color and spectral Doppler

Note: In cases of a renal transplant, the transplanted kidney should be evaluated using the highest frequency transducer that allows visualization of the entire kidney. The sonographer should Doppler the iliac artery proximal to site of anastomosis and provide a cine clip in the kidney's long axis, demonstrating vascular perfusion of the renal transplant. The sonographer should survey for pseudoaneurysms, hematoma, fluid collections, caliectasis, pelviectasis, or ureterectasis. When possible, an attempt should be made to trace the renal artery and vein with color Doppler to the iliac anastomosis.

Renal vein Doppler protocol entails a full bilateral renal evaluation and evaluation of venous renal vasculature, including the grayscale, color Doppler, and spectral Doppler waveforms at IVC, mid, and renal hilum. Doppler of the renal veins may be performed individually or in combination with a renal artery Doppler examination. Indication for renal vein Doppler includes evaluation of vascular patency when there is suspicion for renal vein thrombosis or evaluation of the renal artery and vein following a renal transplant.

RENAL VEIN DOPPLER

Still images include:

1. Sagittal grayscale image of the right kidney at lateral
2. Sagittal grayscale image of the right kidney at mid, with and without measurements
3. Sagittal grayscale image of the right kidney at medial
4. Transverse grayscale image of the right kidney at superior
5. Transverse grayscale image of the right kidney at mid, with and without measurement
6. Transverse grayscale image of the right kidney at inferior
7. Long-axis view of right MRV near IVC junction with color and spectral Doppler
8. Long-axis view of right MRV at mid with color and spectral Doppler
9. Long-axis view of right MRV at renal hilum with color and spectral Doppler (MRV often elongated in transverse renal imaging plane)
10. Sagittal grayscale image of the left kidney at lateral
11. Sagittal grayscale image of the left kidney at mid, with and without measurements
12. Sagittal grayscale image of the left kidney at medial
13. Transverse grayscale image of the left kidney at superior
14. Transverse grayscale image of the left kidney at mid, with and without measurement
15. Transverse grayscale image of the left kidney at inferior
16. Long-axis view of left MRV near IVC junction with color and spectral Doppler
17. Long-axis view of left MRV at mid with color and spectral Doppler
18. Long-axis view of left MRV at renal hilum with color and spectral Doppler (MRV often elongated in transverse renal imaging plane)

12

Vasculature of the Male and Female Reproductive Systems

MALE REPRODUCTIVE SYSTEM

The spermatic cord functions to transport sperm from the testicle. It contains arteries, the pampiniform plexus which is made up of veins, nerves, and lymphatics, and the vas deferens. Pampiniform plexus veins may dilate with the Valsalva maneuver. Sonographic appearance of the spermatic cord appears as hypoechoic tubes with hyperechoic borders in sagittal plane.

The spermatic cord is attached to the testicles (testes), suspending the right testis slightly higher than the left. The bilateral testicles are held in place by the scrotal ligament inside the scrotal sac and covered by the tunica vaginalis. The testes function to produce spermatozoa and hormones. The testes are comprised of 250 to 450 lobules of seminiferous tubules. Between the tubules are Leydig cells, which produce hormones including testosterone and androgen. The size of the Testes varies with patient age; however, before 12 years of age testicular volume should remain less than 5 mL (Table 12-1).

TABLE 12-1 • Testicular Measurements

Age	Length	AP/Width
Neonate	1.5 cm	1.0 cm
1–6 Years	2.0 cm	1.2 cm
Postpubertal	3.0–5.0 cm	2.0–3.0 cm

Source: From Sotos JF, Tokar NJ. Appraisal of testicular volumes: volumes matching ultrasound values referenced to stages of genital development. *Int J Pediatr Endocrinol*. 2017;2017:7. [Published correction appears in *Int J Pediatr Endocrinol*. 2017;2017:10.]

Sonographic appearance of the testes includes bilateral homogeneous, hypoechoic, egg-shaped organs. A hyperechoic linear structure known as the *rete testes* may be seen coursing within the mediastinum. A smooth, hyperechoic capsule known as the *tunica albuginea* surrounds each testis. Lab values associated with the testes include testosterone, hematocrit, white blood cells, and serum placental-like alkaline phosphatase (PLAP). Testosterone and PLAP may increase with malignancy.

The epididymis sits posterolateral to each testis and functions to store and move sperm from each testis into the spermatic cord (vas deferens). The epididymal heads are hypoechoic, hypovascular, and are ovoid to triangular structures that have a continuous body and tail. Anteroposterior measurements of the epididymal heads range between 6 and 12 millimeters.

The testicular artery, also known as the *internal spermatic artery*, is a branch of the abdominal aorta and provides the main blood supply to the testes. The testicular artery enters the spermatic cord at the area of the deep inguinal ring. The capsular arteries give rise to the centripetal arteries, which enter the testes and branch into the transtesticular and transmediastinal arteries. The deferential and cremasteric arteries accompany the testicular artery in the spermatic cord to provide arterial flow to the epididymis, vas deferens, and peritesticular tissues. The pampiniform plexus is the bundle of veins draining from the testes. The right testicular vein empties into the IVC, while the left testicular vein drains into the left renal vein.

Depending on the patient's age, the parent or caregiver may be asked to assist in patient preparation. The patient lies supine and the patient and/or parent or caregiver is instructed to bring the patient's pants and undergarments to knee level, with the legs together for the examination. In the adolescent age group, a folded washcloth or towel should be provided for the patient to place under the scrotum for support, to ensure the bilateral testis are in the same plane. The patient and/or parent or caregiver places the patient's penis on their abdomen and covers it with a towel. For patient comfort and modesty, a sheet or blanket should also be used to cover the patient's legs, so only the area of interest (scrotum) is exposed. The sonographer should use warmed gel for prevention of vasoconstriction and testicular retraction, thickening the scrotal wall. This response (to cold gel) can make the evaluation more difficult.

When imaging superficial structures of the scrotum, a 5 to 17 MHz linear transducer should be used. Equipment settings should be optimized to detect low velocity flow, and Doppler sensitivity should be reduced slightly to decrease motion artifact while increasing detection of difficult-to-detect arterial flow in young children. If demonstration of flow using color Doppler proves difficult, the sonographer may implement power Doppler. Power Doppler is more sensitive to flow in small vessels, but does not provide information pertaining to direction of flow.

The bilateral testis, spermatic cord, pampiniform plexus vessels (Fig. 12-1), epididymis, and inguinal canals should be imaged in addition to evaluation of any pathologies visualized. Ultrasound of the scrotum includes the following.

Still Images

1. Transverse image of bilateral testis side by side, with and without color Doppler (Fig. 12-2), to demonstrate the presence of vascularity, compare echogenicity, and to measure the bilateral scrotal walls

2. Sagittal (Fig. 12-3) and transverse images of the right epididymis, with and without color Doppler and volume measurements

3. Sagittal image of the right testicle, lateral

4. Sagittal image of the right testicle, mid; include images in grayscale, color, and spectral Doppler (Figs. 12-4 and 12-5); and obtain length and anteroposterior measurements

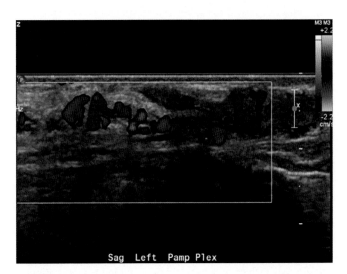

FIGURE 12-1. The pampiniform plexus is a bundle of veins draining from the testes.

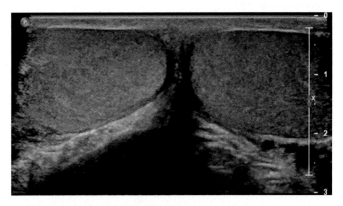

FIGURE 12-2. Transverse bilateral testes.

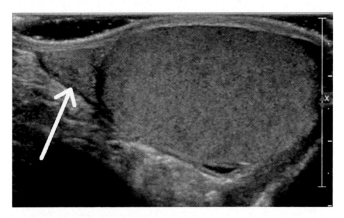

FIGURE 12-3. Sagittal right epididymal head.

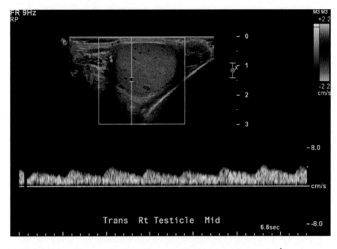

FIGURE 12-4. Demonstration of normal right testicular perfusion.

5. Sagittal image of the right testicle, medial

6. Transverse image of the right testicle, superior

7. Transverse image of the right testicle, mid; include images in grayscale, color, and spectral Doppler; obtain width measurement to calculate volume using the Lambert method for testicular volume measurement, length (cm) × width (cm) × height (cm) × 0.71 = volume (cm^3)

8. Sagittal images of the right spermatic cord and inguinal canal with and without color Doppler; image in cephalic direction from upper pole of each testicle, extending into the inguinal/groin region

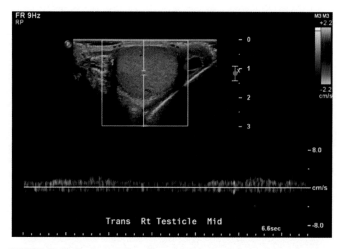

FIGURE 12-5. Demonstration of normal right testicular perfusion on a 14-year-old patient's testicular ultrasound.

9. Sagittal and transverse images of the left epididymis, with and without color Doppler and volume measurements

10. Sagittal image of the left testicle, lateral

11. Sagittal image of the left testicle, mid; include images in grayscale, color, and spectral Doppler; obtain length and anteroposterior measurements

12. Sagittal image of the left testicle, medial

13. Transverse image of the left testicle, superior

14. Transverse image of the left testicle, mid; include images in grayscale, color, and spectral Doppler; obtain width measurement to calculate volume using the Lambert method for testicular volume measurement, length (cm) × width (cm) × height (cm) × 0.71 = volume (cm³)

15. Sagittal images of the left spermatic cord and inguinal canal with and without color Doppler; image in cephalic direction from upper pole of each testicle, extending into the inguinal/groin region

Cine Clips

1. Transverse superior to inferior right testicle

2. Sagittal lateral to medial right testicle

3. Transverse superior to inferior left testicle

4. Sagittal lateral to medial left testicle

Note: If any pathology or dilated pampiniform plexus vessels are visualized, they should be interrogated. If a mass is present within the right testicle, image the area of the inferior vena cava and abdominal aorta for presence of lymphadenopathy or metastasis. If mass is present in the left testicle, image the area medial to the left kidney. If a varicocele is present, the sonographer should obtain an image with and without Valsalva maneuver in both grayscale and color Doppler. Additionally, placing the patient in an upright position may increase varicocele blood flow, optimizing visualization.

FEMALE REPRODUCTIVE SYSTEM

The female reproductive system is comprised of the vaginal canal, cervix, uterus, fallopian tubes, and ovaries.

Sonographically, the bladder is visualized anterior to the uterus and the rectosigmoid colon is positioned posterior to the uterus. When the bladder is filled, posterior enhancement (through-transmission) artifact acts like a "flashlight" to brighten and aid in visualization of structures deep to the bladder, including the vaginal canal, cervix, and uterus. As the bladder fills, the bowel is pushed laterally, also helping in visualization of the female pelvic reproductive structures.

The vaginal canal contains an inner mucosal layer and outer muscular layer, extending to the external cervical os. Sonographically, the vaginal canal is visualized posterior to the bladder and anterior to the rectum.

The cervix begins at the external cervical os where the vaginal canal ends. Sonographically, in transverse view, two acoustic shadow artifacts are visualized, one on each side of the external cervical os, created by the vaginal fornices. The internal os of the cervix meets the junction of the endometrial canal, connecting the vagina and uterus.

The uterus is a muscular, eggplant-shaped organ that is suspended in the female pelvis by the round, broad, and uterosacral ligaments. The endometrium is the inner layer that lines the uterus. It is made up of glandular cells that create secretions. The myometrium is the middle and thickest layer of the uterine wall. It consists primarily of smooth muscle. The perimetrium is the outer serous layer of the uterus.

Uterine positions include retroflexed (posterior), retroverted, anteflexed (anterior), anteverted, levoflexed (left), and dextroflexed (right). Uterine position is determined by position of the uterus in relation to sagittal midline plane. When the bladder is not fully distended, the uterus is commonly anteflexed. Uterine size varies with patient age (Table 12-2).

The lower uterine segment, or isthmus, meets the internal cervical os. The body of the uterus is the largest portion of the

TABLE 12-2 • Uterine Measurements			
Age	Length (cm)	Width (cm)	AP (cm)
Neonate	2.0–4.5	0.8–2.0	0.8–2.0
Infant	3.0–4.0	0.5–1.0	0.1–1.0
Adolescent	3.0–4.0	0.5–1.0	0.1–1.0
Pubertal	5.0–8.0	3.0–5.0	3.0–4.0

Source: From Garel L, Dubois J, Grignon A, Filiatrault D, Van Vliet G. US of the pediatric female pelvis: A clinical perspective. *RadioGraphics*. 2001;21(6): 1393–1407.

TABLE 12-3 • Endometrial Thickness Throughout the Menstrual Cycle

Phase	AP (mm)
Menses	2.0–3.0
Proliferative	4.0–8.0
Secretory	8.0–14.0

Source: From Garel L, Dubois J, Grignon A, Filiatrault D, Van Vliet G. US of the pediatric female pelvis: A clinical perspective. *RadioGraphics*. 2001;21(6): 1393–1407.

TABLE 12-4 • Ovarian Measurements

Menarche Status	Mean Length (cm)	Mean Width (cm)	Mean AP (cm)
Premenarchal	2.5	1.5	0.5
Postmenarche	2.5–5.0	1.5–3.0	0.6–2.2

Source: From Garel L, Dubois J, Grignon A, Filiatrault D, Van Vliet G. US of the pediatric female pelvis: A clinical perspective. *RadioGraphics*. 2001;21(6): 1393–1407.

TABLE 12-5 • Ovarian Follicular Change Throughout the Menstrual Cycle

Day	# Follicles	Size (mm)
5–7	Multiple	1.0–2.0 mm
8–12	1–2 Dominant	14.0 mm
14	1 Dominant	20.0–25.0 mm
15–28	1 Dominant	<20.0–25.0 mm

Source: From Garel L, Dubois J, Grignon A, Filiatrault D, Van Vliet G. US of the pediatric female pelvis: A clinical perspective. *RadioGraphics*. 2001;21(6): 1393–1407.

organ, containing the endometrial cavity. The uterine fundus is the superior portion of the organ.

Thickness of the vascular endometrial layer varies throughout the menstrual cycle; however, it is sonographically difficult to visualize prior to 7 years of age. In pubertal patients, endometrial thickness varies with hormonal status and time of the menstrual cycle (Table 12-3).

The uterus obtains its blood supply from the uterine arteries, which are a branch of the internal iliac arteries. Within the myometrial layer of the uterus, flow then branches into the arcuate, radial, basal (also referred to as *straight*), and spiral arteries. Prepubertal and postmenarchal girls will typically have little to no color flow visualized during Doppler imaging.

The uterus cornua are lateral extensions that meet the bilateral interstitial portion of the fallopian tubes. Sonographically, the normal fallopian tubes are not normally seen. The muscular fallopian tubes transport the ovum via peristalsis from the ovaries to the uterus. They are categorized into four segments: cornual (interstitial, intramural), isthmus, ampullar, infundibular. The distal infundibular portion of the fallopian tubes terminate at the bilateral ovaries. Ovarian location varies within the bilateral adnexal regions. The ovaries function to produce eggs (ova).

Ovarian size and volume varies with age. In infants under 1 year of age ovarian volume should be less than 1.0 cubic centimeters (cc). However, this volume can vary in newborns and breast-fed infants as a result of circulating maternal hormones. In the neonatal period, the mean ovarian volume is ~1.06 cc due to maternal hormonal stimulation response, larger than the ovarian volume observed in the pediatric period. In these groups, it is normal for the ovaries to exhibit follicles. Ovarian volume begins regressing to 1.05 cc +/− 0.67 by age 4 to 12 months of life and decreases to a mean volume of 0.67 cc by 13 to 24 months age. In toddler to adolescent patients less than 13 years of age ovarian volume should range between 0.7 and 4.2 cc (Table 12-4). By the start of menses, ovarian volume is ~9.8 cc +/− 5.8 cc. It is not until the postmenopausal period of life that the ovarian volume will again regress.

In postpubertal patients, cystic follicles may be visualized. Number and appearance of follicles varies throughout the menstrual cycle (Table 12-5).

The ovary receives its blood supply from the main ovarian artery and the adnexal branches of the uterine artery. The main ovarian artery is a branch of the abdominal aorta. Color Doppler on slow flow setting can be visualized in 80% of prepubertal ovaries and 90% of postmenarchal ovaries via transabdominal imaging approach. During the early follicular and late luteal phases, the resistance index (RI) is near 1.0. During the late follicular and early luteal phase, the RI is closer to 0.5. In instances where flow visualization with color Doppler is difficult, power Doppler can be implemented. Power Doppler is sensitive and readily demonstrates flow in small vessels but does not provide information pertaining to direction of flow. The right ovarian vein drains into the IVC, and the left ovarian vein drains into the left renal vein.

Ultrasound of the female pelvis entails demonstration of pelvic anatomical structures including the uterus, ovaries, and adnexal regions ensuring appropriate blood flow is present to organs through use of color and spectral Doppler. For optimal visualization of these structures, it is ideal the patient is prepped with a full bladder.

For patients under 1 year of age, parents should be instructed to bring a bottle for the patient to drink during the exam. This allows for bladder fill (prep) and helps with patient cooperation during the exam. Patients between 1 and 3 years of age should be given 4 to 6 oz of fluids 30 minutes prior to the exam. These patients should be scanned promptly following prep, as they are likely not yet continent. Patients 3 to 6 years of age should be given 8 to 12 oz of fluids 30 minutes prior to the exam. Between 6 and 12 years of age, patients should drink 12 to 16 oz of fluids 30 minutes prior to exam. Patients greater than 12 years of age should drink 18 to 32 oz of fluids 1 hour prior to their examination.

Emergency protocols for ruling out ovarian torsion in the pediatric patient may call for expedited care in the acute care setting. If the provider suspects ovarian torsion and an ultrasound examination is ordered, the emergency department may hydrate the patient via intravenous fluids and oral hydration. The sonographer should check for fullness of the bladder. If not optimally full for diagnostic visualization of the pelvic organs after 45 minutes, the emergency department should begin discussion with the patient's family for option of catheterizing the patient for retrograde filling of the bladder. Once the catheter is placed, the sonographer can determine the amount of necessary retrograde flow by visualizing when adequate fluids have filled the bladder. The bladder of a post-pubertal patient should be full following administration of approximately 400 mL (not to exceed 800 mL). For prepubertal patients, the formula (age in years) $+$ (2) $\times$ (30 mL) $=$ bladder capacity in mL should be used. Once the bladder is appropriately filled, the sonographer should promptly begin the following protocol using a curvilinear or sector 2-10 MHz transducer.

Still Images

1. Sagittal midline uterus
2. Sagittal midline uterus with sagittal and anteroposterior (AP) measurement
3. Sagittal endometrium with AP measurement
4. Sagittal medial uterus
5. Sagittal lateral uterus
6. Sagittal cul-de-sac
7. Transverse vaginal canal
8. Transverse cervix
9. Transverse lower uterine segment
10. Transverse midline uterus
11. Transverse midline uterus with transverse measurement
12. Transverse uterine fundus
13. Transverse right ovary
14. Transverse right ovary with transverse measurement
15. Sagittal right ovary with sagittal and AP measurement
16. Sagittal right ovary with color Doppler
17. Sagittal right ovary with spectral Doppler, identifying arterial and venous flow (Figs. 12-6 to 12-8)

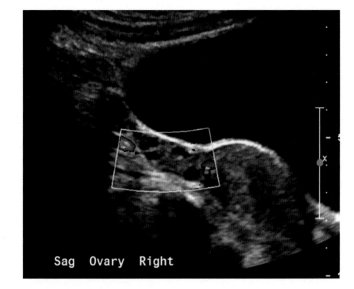

FIGURE 12-6. Sagittal right ovary.

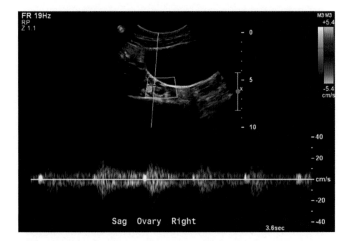

FIGURE 12-7. Normal Doppler evaluation of the ovary in a 16-year-old patient demonstrating arterial waveform.

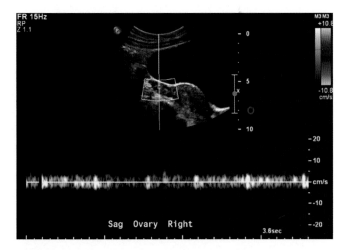

FIGURE 12-8. Normal Doppler evaluation of the ovary in a 16-year-old patient demonstrating venous waveform.

18. Evaluation of the right adnexal region
19. Transverse left ovary
20. Transverse left ovary with transverse measurement
21. Sagittal left ovary with sagittal and AP measurement
22. Sagittal left ovary with color Doppler
23. Sagittal left ovary with spectral Doppler, identifying arterial and venous flow
24. Evaluation of the left adnexal region

Cine Clips

1. Sagittal uterus
2. Transverse uterus
3. Sagittal right ovary
4. Transverse right ovary
5. Sagittal left ovary
6. Transverse left ovary

Note: Pelvic transvaginal ultrasound should be performed in sexually active patients *ONLY*. This exam should be specifically requested by the ordering provider only if there is absence of or poor ovarian visualization transabdominally due to body habitus or technical examination factors. To perform this exam, there should be an agreement amongst the patient, parent or legal guardian, the referring physician, and the radiologist. The patient must fully understand the nature of the procedure, and the patient's parent and a medical staff chaperone (preferably female) must be present during the examination. This exam is not appropriate in a nonsexually active patient. When indicated, a transducer cover is used, covering the endocavitary imaging transducer. Following the exam, the transducer should be cleaned using a high-level disinfectant (i.e., Trophon, Cidex, etc.) (Fig. 12-9).

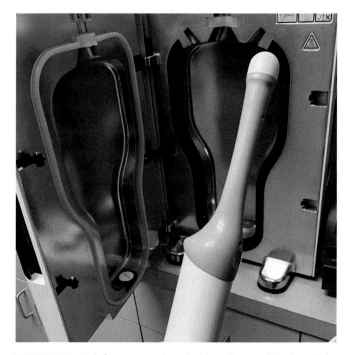

FIGURE 12-9. High-frequency endovaginal transducer and Trophon high-level disinfection unit.

Section I Review: Normal Anatomy and Physiology Normal Perfusion and Function

1. The most common acoustic window used for sonography of the neonatal brain is the
   a. Mastoid fontanelle
   b. Sphenoidal fontanelle
   c. Anterior fontanelle
   d. Posterior fontanelle

2. The neural tube is completely closed by
   a. 3-4 weeks gestation
   b. 2-3 weeks gestation
   c. 9-10 weeks gestation
   d. 5-6 weeks gestation

3. In healthy infants the position of the conus medullaris should be located above
   a. T12 - L1
   b. L1 - L2
   c. L2 - L3
   d. L3 - L4

4. Islet cells make up what percent of the pancreas
   a. 38%
   b. 18%
   c. 9%
   d. 2%

5. The ligamentum teres is a remnant of the
   a. Fetal ductus venous
   b. Fetal umbilical vein
   c. Main lobar fissure
   d. Ligamentum venosum

6. Riedel's lobe is a congenital variant projecting from the
   a. Gallbladder
   b. Lateral left lobe of the liver
   c. Posterior right lobe of the liver
   d. Anterior right lobe of the liver

7. The spleen is a homogenous organ that is
   a. More echogenic than the kidney and the liver
   b. Less echogenic than the kidney and more echogenic than the liver
   c. Less echogenic than the kidney and the liver
   d. More echogenic than the kidney and less echogenic than the liver

8. The appendix is usually located in the
   a. LLQ
   b. LUQ
   c. RLQ
   d. RUQ

9. The average thickness of the small bowel wall is between
   a. 0.5-1 mm
   b. 1-2 cm
   c. 2-3 mm
   d. 4-5 mm

10. The largest salivary gland is the
    a. Parotid
    b. Submandibular
    c. Sublingual
    d. Parathyroid

11. On an ultrasound image, the muscles surrounding the thyroid are
    a. Longus colli, strap and thyroid muscles
    b. Sternocleidomastoid, strap and longus colli muscles
    c. Sternocleidomastoid, strap, and thyroid muscles
    d. Longus colli, sternocleidomastoid and thyroid muscles

12. The view to best image the thymus is
    a. Suprasternal sagittal
    b. Trans-sternal over the sternum
    c. Trans-sternal lateral to the sternum
    d. Parasternal transverse

13. Cartilaginous structures have well-defined _____ margins with _____ echotexture in relation to muscle and bone

    a. Echogenic – anechoic

    b. Hypoechoic – echogenic

    c. Hyperechoic – anechoic

    d. Echogenic – hypoechoic

14. The central arteries of the upper and lower extremities show a

    a. Triphasic flow pattern with forward flow in systole

    b. Biphasic flow pattern with forward flow in systole

    c. Triphasic flow pattern with forward flow in diastole

    d. Biphasic flow pattern with forward flow in diastole

15. The layers of the artery are

    a. Tunica arterial, tunica media, and tunica adventitia

    b. Tunica intima, tunica media, and capillary

    c. Tunica intima, tunica media, and tunica adventitia

    d. Tunica intima, tunica valves, and capillary

16. The common hepatic artery bifurcates into the

    a. Lesser hepatic and greater hepatic artery

    b. Lesser hepatic and gastroduodenal artery

    c. Proper hepatic and pancreatic artery

    d. Proper hepatic and gastroduodenal artery

17. Normal intracranial arterial blood flow patterns will show systolic and diastolic velocities _____and the RI _____ as gestational age increases.

    a. Increasing – increasing

    b. Increasing – decreasing

    c. Decreasing – increasing

    d. No significant changes with age

18. The main renal artery has a _____ waveform

    a. Low impedance

    b. High impedance

    c. Monophasic

    d. Bidirectional

19. The main renal artery peak systolic velocity (PSV) in neonatal patients range from

    a. 10-25 cm/sec

    b. 30-50 cm/sec

    c. 60-75 cm/sec

    d. 100-110 cm/sec

20. The left gonadal vein drains into the

    a. IVC

    b. Aorta

    c. Left renal artery

    d. Left renal vein

21. To best visualize the cerebellum and fourth ventricle, which sonographic window can be used?

    a. Anterior fontanelle

    b. Intercostal window

    c. Mastoid Fontanelle

    d. Suboccipital window

22. The aorta becomes the abdominal aorta after passing through the _____.

    a. Left ventricle

    b. Diaphragm

    c. Rectus abdominis muscle

    d. Peritoneum

23. What is the first branch off the abdominal aorta?

    a. Gonadal artery

    b. Superior mesenteric artery

    c. Celiac trunk

    d. Iliac artery

24. What are the outermost arterial vessels within the bilateral kidneys?

    a. Arcuate arteries

    b. Parenchymal arteries

    c. Intrarenal arteries

    d. Segmental arteries

25. Which ligament separates the left and caudate lobes of the liver?

    a. Ligamentum venosum

    b. Ligamentum teres

    c. Main lobar fissure

    d. Falciform ligament

26. Into which chamber of the heart does the IVC empty?

    a. Left atrium

    b. Left ventricle

    c. Right atrium

    d. Right ventricle

27. **What structure is located directly posterior to the isthmus of the thyroid?**

    a. Esophagus

    b. Trachea

    c. Parathyroid gland

    d. Parotid gland

28. **Which of the following allows for an acoustic window of the neonatal brain in the first year of life?**

    a. Sutures

    b. Meninges

    c. Fissures

    d. Fontanelles

29. **Which fontanelle closes around two years of age?**

    a. Anterior

    b. Posterior

    c. Sphenoid

    d. Mastoid

30. **Which of the following is the largest component of the hindbrain?**

    a. Fourth ventricle

    b. Cerebellum

    c. Cavum septum pellucidum

    d. Choroid plexus

31. **Which structure is visualized in the anterior-most view of the neonatal brain?**

    a. Thalamus

    b. Sylvian fissure

    c. Interhemispheric fissure

    d. Quadrigeminal plate

32. **How long should a newborn less than one year of age remain NPO for an abdominal ultrasound?**

    a. 1 hours

    b. 2 hours

    c. 4 hours

    d. 6 hours

33. **Another name for the main pancreatic duct is the**

    a. Duct of Santorini

    b. Wharton duct

    c. Duct of Wirsung

    d. Langerhans duct

34. **The normal appendix measures less than**

    a. 4 mm

    b. 5 mm

    c. 6 mm

    d. 7 mm

35. **Zone IIA within the neck correlates with which region?**

    a. Submandibular

    b. Supraclavicular

    c. Upper internal jugular

    d. Submental

36. **The muscle that separates the thoracic and abdominal cavities is**

    a. Diaphragm

    b. Mediastinum

    c. Suprasternal

    d. Internal intercostal

37. **When performing an ultrasound of the chest, it is preferred the patient be positioned**

    a. Supine

    b. Upright

    c. Prone

    d. Reverse Trendelenburg

38. **The superior-most part of the femur is the**

    a. Ileum

    b. Labrum

    c. Femoral head

    d. Intercondylar notch

39. **What is being scanned in this image?**

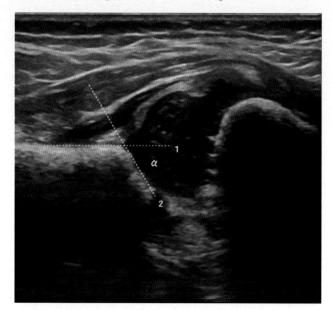

a. Knee joint

b. Ankle joint

c. Shoulder joint

d. Hip joint

40. Which of the following is a superficial vein?

a. Axillary vein

b. Common femoral vein

c. Greater saphenous vein

d. Brachial vein

41. The external iliac artery continues to form the

a. Common femoral artery

b. Profunda femoris

c. Superficial femoral artery

d. Brachial artery

42. The innermost arterial layer is the

a. Tunica adventitia

b. Tunica intima

c. Tunica media

d. Tunica elastica

43. The spinal cord normally ends between which vertebral levels?

a. T11 – L1

b. T12 – L2

c. L1 – L2

d. L2 – L3

44. Which of the following findings would indicate that the sonographer is not evaluating the normal appendix?

a. The structure evaluated is compressible

b. The structure evaluated is continuous

c. The structure evaluated contains five bowel wall layers

d. The structure evaluated is blind-ending

45. The neonatal intracranial region demonstrated in this image is

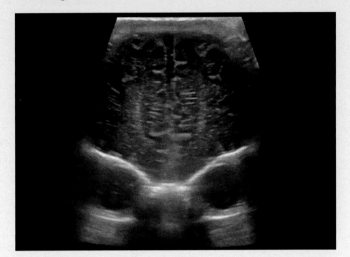

a. Anterior coronal

b. Posterior coronal

c. Midline sagittal

d. Lateral sagittal

46. What structure is being identified in this image?

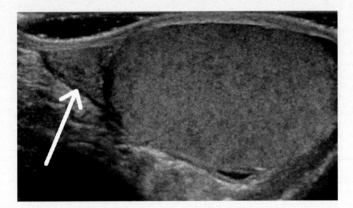

a. Testicle

b. Spermatic cord

c. Epididymis

d. Pampiniform plexus

47. Which of the following is a major intracranial artery?

a. Anterior cerebral

b. Parasellar

c. Thalamostriate

d. Pericallosal

13

Intracranial Processes

INTRAVENTRICULAR HEMORRHAGE

Intraventricular hemorrhage (IVH) and periventricular leuko-malacia are the most common central nervous system (CNS) complications of prematurity. Hemorrhage risk factors include birth at less than 30 weeks gestational age and birth weight of less than 1,500 grams. IVH is a bleed that occurs within the lateral ventricles of the brain. Grade I IVH involves hemorrhage only within the germinal matrix. Grade II IVH involves the germinal matrix and IVH without the presence of hydrocephalus. Grade III IVH involves the germinal matrix and IVH with

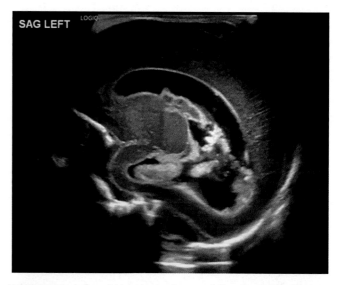

FIGURE 13-2. Left ventricular hemorrhage and dilated ventricle with increased ependymal lining, due to chemical ventriculitis in a 26-week neonate.

ventricular enlargement (Figs. 13-1 and 13-2). With grade IV IVH, a parenchymal bleed is present.

GERMINAL MATRIX HEMORRHAGE, SUBEPENDYMAL

The subependymal germinal matrix of the lateral ventricle is the most common intracranial bleed site in premature infants. Subependymal germinal matrix hemorrhage is rarely seen in term infants and is typically only visualized when term infants are small for gestational age.

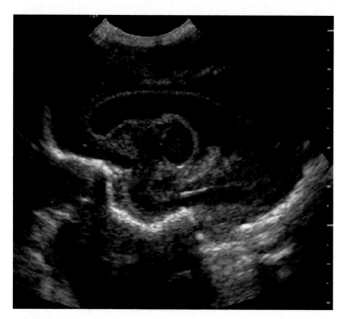

FIGURE 13-1. Left ventricular hemorrhage and dilated ventricle.

CEREBELLAR HEMORRHAGE

Cerebellar hemorrhage occurs more frequently in premature infants less than 32 weeks gestational age due to primary intracerebellar hemorrhage, venous infarction, or extension of intraventricular and subarachnoid hemorrhage into the cerebellum. These bleeds are generally localized, and large hemorrhages may cause brainstem compression and increased intracranial pressure. When occurring in term infants, cerebellar hemorrhage may be due to traumatic delivery, cerebellar laceration, rupture of veins, increased venous pressure from facemask ventilation, and coagulation disorders. During traumatic delivery cerebellar laceration or rupture of cerebellar, posterior fossa, or occipital veins may occur. In term infants, the cerebellar vermis is the predominant bleed site. Sonographic findings include asymmetric echogenicity, echogenic cerebellar mass, loss of interface definition between the cerebellum and fourth ventricle, and lateral and third ventricle dilatation (Fig. 13-3).

PRIMARY SUBARACHNOID HEMORRHAGE

Primary subarachnoid hemorrhage results from traumatic hypoxic events with the rupture of at-risk vessels. Infants with large subarachnoid hemorrhage may present with seizures.

Sonography is insensitive in detecting small subarachnoid bleeds because of similar echogenicity between blood and the brain's surface. Large hemorrhage appears as a fluid collection within the interhemispheric fissure, Sylvian fissure, or subarachnoid cisterns with communicating hydrocephalus.

SECONDARY SUBARACHNOID HEMORRHAGE

Secondary subarachnoid hemorrhage occurs subsequent to extension from subdural, intraventricular, or intracerebellar hemorrhage.

SUBDURAL HEMORRHAGE

Subdural hemorrhage (Fig. 13-4) occurs more frequently in term infants and is commonly a result of birth trauma such as breech birth, forcep use, or vacuum extraction delivery. Subdural hemorrhage can also be seen as an incidental finding in asymptomatic infants. With trauma, veins can rupture in the subdural space and bleeding results within the cerebellum or venous sinus. Subdural hemorrhage is seen at a rate of 12.8 per 100,000 children <2 years of age, annually. Subdural hemorrhage can occur in various locations including over the cerebellar hemispheres, along the tentorium, along the interhemispheric fissure, and over the parietooccipital and occipital lobes. Hydrocephalus can result as bleeds evolve.

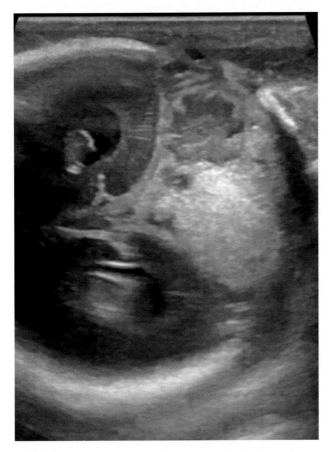

FIGURE 13-3. Transmastoid view of a 24-week neonate with a grade IV intracranial hemorrhage and extensive cerebellar hemorrhage.

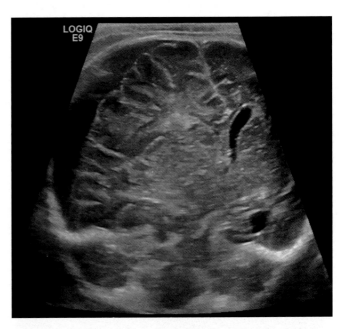

FIGURE 13-4. Full-term infant at day 1 of life. There is large hypoechoic extra-axial fluid collection, consistent with subdural hemorrhage involving the right hemisphere. Significant midline shift and effacement of the lateral ventricular system on the right, and mild enlargement of the ventricular system on the left is present. These findings are consistent with transfalcine herniation.

EPIDURAL HEMORRHAGE

Epidural hemorrhage is rare and usually caused by traumatic delivery. The origin of epidural hemorrhage can be arterial or venous, and supratentorial or infra-tentorial in location. Sonographic findings include an acute hematoma with echogenic fluid collection between the brain and skull with parenchymal displacement. This hemorrhage is best demonstrated with computed tomography (CT) or magnetic resonance imaging (MRI).

PARENCHYMAL HEMORRHAGE

Parenchymal hemorrhage results from ischemia, hypotension, birth trauma, coagulation defects, vein of Galen malformation, hypertension, emboli, polycythemia, and extracorporeal membrane oxygenation (ECMO). Premature infants are particularly at risk for parenchymal hemorrhage. Sonographic findings include a focal echogenic or hypoechoic mass in the cerebral cortex ganglia (Figs. 13-5(a)-(c)).

CHOROID PLEXUS HEMORRHAGE

Choroid plexus hemorrhage occurs more commonly in term than preterm infants. Sonographic findings include an enlarged lobulated choroid plexus with irregular margins, and possible extension of the bleed into the occipital horn. This extension may demonstrate a choroid plexus thrombus. Choroid plexus hemorrhage can resolve completely via central liquefaction, well-defined cyst, or rupture into the ipsilateral ventricle.

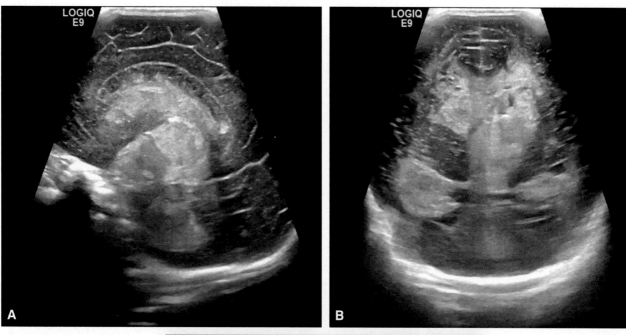

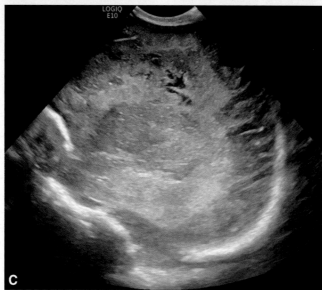

FIGURE 13-5. Full-term infant with grade 4 hemorrhage (parenchymal).

INTRACRANIAL INFECTIONS

Meningitis

Gram-negative bacilli *Escherichia coli (E. coli)* and group B Streptococcus (GBS) bacteria account for a large percentage of all bacterial meningitis infections acquired in newborns. *E. coli* is the most common early-onset cause of meningitis and sepsis in premature neonates measuring less than 1,500 grams at birth. The neonatal population is at high risk for bacteremia which can lead to neonatal bacterial meningitis. This risk is associated with an immature immune system and because infants must be a minimum age of 2 months before receiving their first meningococcal vaccination. Along with E. coli, other bacteria which cause late-onset meningitis infection in premature or very low birth weight (VLBW) infants is *Pseudomonas aeruginosa*, methicillin-resistant *Staphylococcus aureus*, *Klebsiella*, and coagulase-negative staphylococci. Late-onset meningitis may be caused by way of nosocomial spread, therefore proper precautions should be taken when imaging and caring for premature and VLBW infants. Ascending infection can result from penetrating trauma or surgery, spread of adjacent infection such as sinusitis, or by hematogenous spread. Additional contributing factors include mothers who are positive for GBS bacteria or sexually transmitted disease prior to birth or who pass *Listeria* to their infant. Mothers who are positive for GBS are administered antibiotics in the intrapartum period to reduce occurrence of GBS infection in the neonate. Meningeal infection starts as a choroid plexus infection leading to inflammation of the ventricles, meninges, subarachnoid, and subdural spaces. Meningeal inflammation causes vessel occlusion, edema, and cortical infarction. Diagnosis is based on lab results from a sample of cerebrospinal fluid (CSF). Sonographic findings include extra-axial fluid collection, cerebral edema, abscess formation, hydrocephalus, and white matter atrophy.

Ventriculitis

Ventriculitis is an intracranial infection where inflammatory exudate organisms gain ventricular access via route of the choroid plexus. Sonographic findings include ventricular dilatation, thickened ependymal lining, intraventricular septations and debris, and increased echogenicity of the choroid plexus (Figs. 13-6(a) and (b)).

INTRACRANIAL MASSES

Brain tumors are rare in neonates with teratoma, primitive neuroectodermal tumor, astrocytoma, and choroid plexus papilloma being the most frequent of the rare tumors in the first year of life. Clinical findings include increasing head circumference, vomiting, lethargy, and neurologic signs that depend on the location of the tumor.

Arachnoid Cyst

Arachnoid cysts account for 1% of childhood intracranial masses. Arachnoid cysts occur due to abnormal splitting of leptomeninges with CSF collection between two layers of arachnoid membrane. These cysts do not communicate with surrounding subarachnoid CSF or the ventricles. Arachnoid cysts are asymptomatic unless they become large, in which case they can compress adjacent structures causing hydrocephalus and intracranial hypertension. Sonographic appearance includes an

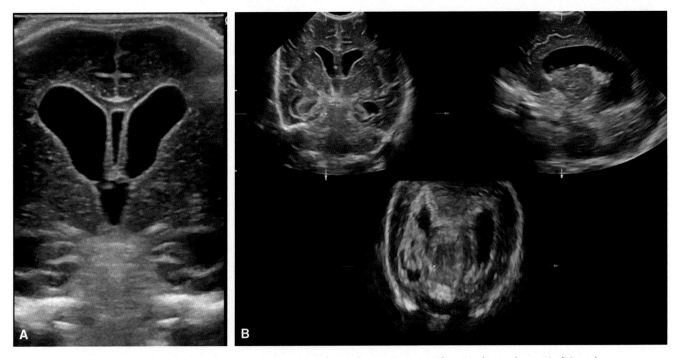

FIGURE 13-6. A 27-week infant. The 3D image depicts post-hemorrhagic supratentorial ventriculomegaly, ventriculitis, and evolving grade III hemorrhage.

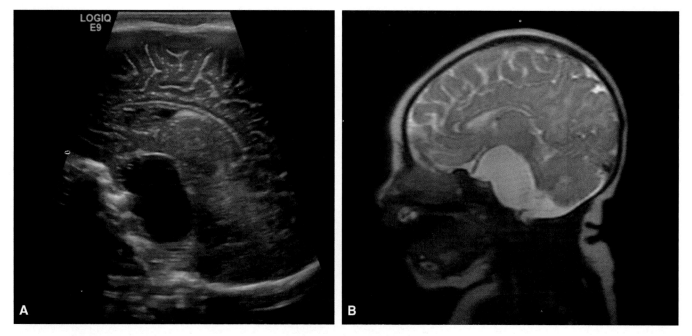

FIGURE 13-7. A 1-month-old male with prenatally diagnosed cystic lesion. Ultrasound and MRI demonstrate a large arachnoid cyst anterior to the brainstem and extending into the suprasellar cistern.

anechoic lesion with indiscernible walls (Fig. 13-7(a) and (b)). Differentiation between arachnoid cyst and Dandy-Walker complex is made by determining if the cyst is separate from the fourth ventricle or if the cyst is the dilated fourth ventricle. If the cyst is separate from the fourth ventricle it is an arachnoid cyst. If the cyst appearance is a dilated fourth ventricle, it is consistent with Dandy-Walker complex.

Subependymal Cyst

Subependymal cysts result from germinal matrix hemorrhage in premature neonates due to ischemia and TORCH infection (acronym for *T*oxoplasmosis, *O*ther agents, *R*ubella, *C*ytomegalovirus, and *H*erpes simplex). These are typically found incidentally and often seen in patients with no previously known infection or hemorrhage. Sonographic appearance includes a discrete anechoic lesion in the subependymal ventricular lining.

Choroid Plexus Cyst

The choroid plexus functions to produce CSF. Choroid plexus cysts (CPC) are small CSF-filled pseudocysts within the trigone of the choroid plexus. Isolated CPC have no clinical significance or association with other CNS abnormalities or developmental delay postnatally. CPC are usually singular and measure less than 1 centimeter. When measuring greater than 1 centimeter or occurring bilaterally, it has been noted in literature CPCs can be a "soft marker" associated with chromosomal disorders such as trisomies 18 and 21, Aicardi syndrome and Klinefelter syndrome. However, in more recent studies, it has been debated whether formation of CPCs exhibit true aneuploidy association. This sonographic finding is now correlated to prenatal maternal serum screening methods to determine whether aneuploidy risk is present in the fetus. Sonographic appearance of a CPC

includes a cystic mass with well-defined walls within the choroid plexus. By 28 weeks gestational age, the vast majority of CPCs regress. Most CPCs which persist postnatally or are identified in the neonate during a neonatal intracranial sonogram were noted to spontaneously resolve.

> **Hint:** An isolated "soft marker" on obstetrical ultrasound can further be defined as a standalone anatomic finding unrelated to intrauterine growth restriction, structural fetal anomalies, or other sonographic "soft markers" associated with aneuploidy risk (i.e., echogenic bowel, echogenic intracardiac focus, thickened nuchal fold, hypoplastic or absent nasal bone, etc.). It should be noted that visualization of multiple soft markers during obstetric evaluation has greater association with increased risk of congenital abnormalities.

Porencephaly

Porencephaly is an uncommon congenital disorder resulting in porencephalic cysts, cystic degeneration, and encephalomalacia. Porencephalic cysts are areas of focal brain destruction in early and late gestation. Antenatal sonographic appearance includes single or multiple intracranial cysts communicating with the subarachnoid space and/or ventricular system with potential ventricular asymmetry.

Encephalomalacia

Encephalomalacia is an area of focal brain destruction in all age groups following a brain insult. This etiology typically has a cystic sonographic appearance.

Intracranial Teratoma

Intracranial teratoma (Figs. 13-8(a)-(c)) is a neoplasm that varies greatly in clinical presentation and sonographic appearance, depending on intra-axial or extra-axial tumor location and whether the teratoma is immature, mature, or mature with malignant transformation. Intra-axial intracranial teratoma occurs antenatally or in the neonate. Intra-axial intracranial teratoma is usually supratentorial in location and presents as a large mass that may increase head circumference, hindering normal childbirth. Extra-axial intracranial teratoma occurs in childhood through early adulthood, originating in the pineal or suprasellar areas of the brain. This etiology includes a smaller mass and can be associated with hydrocephalus due to obstruction. Serum alpha fetoprotein and carcinoembryonic antigen may be elevated with this tumor.

Astrocytoma

Astrocytoma is a CNS tumor derived from star-shaped glial cells. Of all intracranial tumors, astrocytoma occurs most often, with glioblastoma being the most common form of astrocytoma.

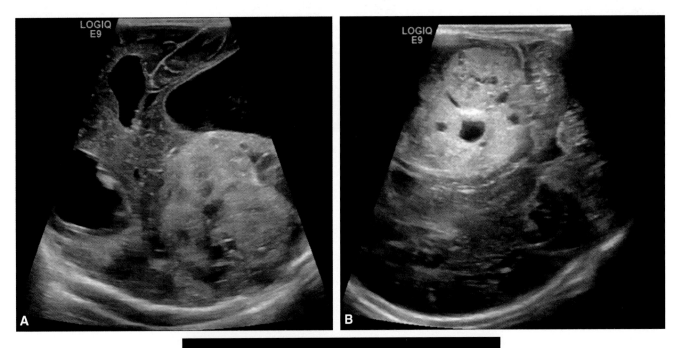

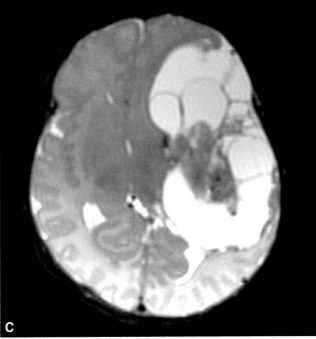

FIGURE 13-8. There is a large mixed solid and cystic consistency multiseptated mass in the left cranial cavity as seen on ultrasound and MRI. Significant mass effect is present with total effacement of left lateral ventricle which is identified only by its choroid plexus. There is a 6 millimeters rightward midline shift with asymmetric mild dilatation of the right lateral ventricle.

There are multiple types of intracranial astrocytoma, ranging from Grades I to IV on the St. Anne-Mayo grading system (also referred to as the *Daumas-Duport grading system*). According to the World Health Organization, Grade I is benign, and Grade IV is the most malignant. Grade I tumors have a 96%, 5-year survival rate. Alternatively, Grade IV tumors indicate a lifespan of approximately 15 months following diagnosis. Forms of Grade I astrocytoma include pilocytic, pleomorphic xantoastrocytoma, and subependymal giant cell. Pilocytic astrocytoma is most often located in the cerebellum. Subependymal giant cell astrocytoma most commonly occurs in pediatric patients and is associated with tuberous sclerosis. Grade II refers to diffuse astrocytoma. Anaplastic astrocytoma is categorized as Grade III. Glioblastoma makes up 60% of all astrocytomas and is categorized as Grade IV. This astrocytoma is aggressive, malignant, and in pediatric patients, progresses quickly in malignancy from a lower-grade astrocytoma. Clinical symptoms include headaches, blurred vision, seizures, impacted speech, weakness of the limbs or clenching of hands, and brain fog. Treatment includes surgical resection, with radiotherapy, chemotherapy with temozolomide, steroids, tumor treating electrical fields, antiseizure medication, and Bevacizumab as adjuvant therapies. Although etiologies may be visualized on ultrasound, astrocytoma is best evaluated by CT and MRI.

CHOROID PLEXUS PAPILLOMA

Choroid plexus papilloma begins in the trigone of the lateral ventricles and is a rare, neuroepithelial intraventricular tumor. These benign tumors are more common in pediatric patients but are also seen in the adult population. Choroid plexus papilloma makes up 2 to 6% of all brain tumors in pediatric patients. Nearly 85% of choroid plexus papillomas occur in children less than 5 years of age. The majority of choroid plexus papilloma cases present with hydrocephalus (80%). Antenatal sonographic appearance includes a bilateral increase in size of the echogenic choroid plexus, ventriculomegaly, and enlargement of the fluid-filled extra-axial spaces.

HYDROCEPHALUS

Hydrocephalus is a dilatation of the ventricular system, associated with increased intraventricular pressure. This dilatation and pressure results from obstruction of ventricular CSF outflow and impaired absorption by the arachnoid villi. The choroid plexus of the lateral, third, and fourth ventricles produces 80 to 90% of CSF. The remaining CSF is produced within the ventricular ependyma and arachnoid lining of the brain and spinal cord.

Hydrocephalus can be communicating (nonobstructive) or noncommunicating (obstructive).

Hydrocephalus from extraventricular obstruction of CSF is referred to as *communicating hydrocephalus*. With communicating hydrocephalus, there is overproduction of CSF, or lack of CSF absorption, and fluid leaves the ventricles. Communicating extraventricular hydrocephalus is usually caused by hemorrhage and infection. If the fourth ventricle or aqueducts are compressed, such as by hematoma, hydrocephalus can result. Up to 80% of Dandy-Walker patients have resulting hydrocephalus.

Hydrocephalus due to intraventricular obstruction of CSF is referred to as *noncommunicating hydrocephalus*. With noncommunicating hydrocephalus, there is an internal obstruction in the flow of CSF, or a ventricular system outflow obstruction. Noncommunicating intra-ventricular hydrocephalus is usually acquired or congenital, such as with Dandy-Walker syndrome. The most common cause of congenital hydrocephalus is aqueductal stenosis.

Ventriculomegaly

Ventriculomegaly is a less specific term for ventricular enlargement or dilatation, secondary to hydrocephalus or brain atrophy.

Callosal Agenesis

Callosal agenesis, also referred to as *dysgenesis of the corpus callosum*, is a partial or complete anomaly that occurs in utero, where the corpus callosum never develops or there is development interference. Callosal agenesis is a congenital anomaly associated with many anomalies, including inborn errors of metabolism, anomalies of the CNS (i.e., hydrocephalus, intracranial lipoma, Dandy-Walker, Chiari II, etc.), aneuploidy (i.e., trisomies), and non-aneuploidy syndromes (i.e., fetal alcohol syndrome, etc.).

Preterm and Term Infant Hypoxic-Ischemic Insults

Decreased oxygenation of blood due to respiratory depression causes a decrease in cerebral blood flow and is a significant cause of neonatal morbidity and mortality. The main cause of neonatal hypoxic-ischemic brain injury is intrapartum, peripartum, or postpartum asphyxia due to congenital heart disease, trauma, meningitis, ECMO, chorioamnionitis, intrauterine infection, or placental inflammation.

Ischemic Lesions in the Premature Neonate

Ischemic lesions in the premature neonate include periventricular leukomalacia and cerebellar ischemia. Periventricular leukomalacia is a bilateral increased echogenicity (Fig. 13-9) of the periventricular white matter. Cerebellar ischemia is increased parenchymal echogenicity with lack of Doppler flow.

Ischemic Lesions in the Term Neonate

Ischemic lesions in the term neonate are commonly located in frontal and parieto-occipital regions. These lesions can include mild ischemic encephalopathy due to edema, poorly defined gyral-sulcal interface, slit-like or enlarged ventricles depending

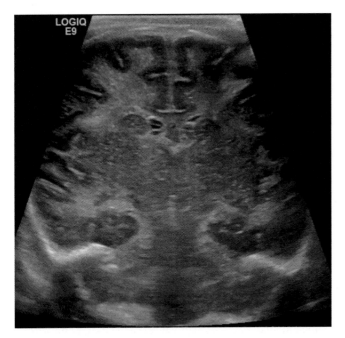

FIGURE 13-9. Increased echogenicity in the white matter of the bilateral cerebral cortex. Pattern of injury is most consistent with moderate to severe hypoxic ischemic injury.

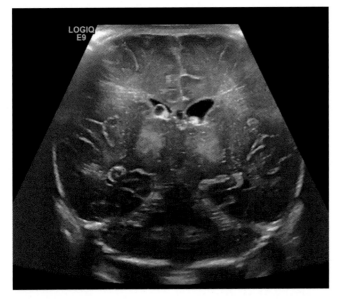

FIGURE 13-10. Increased echogenicity in bilateral thalami consistent with ischemia.

on time of ischemic injury, and cystic changes to the white and gray matter (Fig. 13-10).

PEDIATRIC TRANSCRANIAL DOPPLER

Sickle-Cell Disease

Sickle cell disease is a common cause of acute cerebral ischemic infarction in older infants and children. Sickle cell anemia can cause large vessel occlusion at the base of the brain leading to

cerebral infarction and stroke. This occurs due to vessel damage and abnormal adhesive, clot-forming properties of the sickle-shaped red blood cells. The largest risk factor for cerebral infarct and stroke in sickle cell patients is previous stroke history. Transcranial Doppler (TCD) studies can detect or monitor middle cerebral artery (MCA) vasospasm, aneurysm, basilar artery obstruction, evaluate for internal carotid artery (ICA) stenosis, monitor real-time blood flow to the brain during surgical procedures, and so forth. TCD studies may also be used as an adjunct with other exams (i.e., nuclear medicine perfusion test, computed tomographic angiography) to confirm brain death due to high repeatability and specificity rates, although this is not the most common reason TCD is performed. Cerebral blood flow velocity is an effective stroke predictor. TCD is based on time-averaged mean of maximum velocity (TAMMX) where velocities less than 170 cm/s are considered normal, 170 to 199 cm/s are conditional, and greater than 200 cm/s are read as abnormal. TCD sensitivity for diagnosing stenosis and occlusion is 86 to 94% accurate. When performing a TCD study on a sickle-cell patient, the patient should be asymptomatic and not in crisis during time of exam. A patient experiencing symptoms may skew results.

Imaging Techniques and Patient Positioning for a TCD Study

For the exam, the patient is placed supine on the exam table looking straight up at the ceiling. The position of the head should be adjusted as needed to optimize the spectral Doppler signal. The patient should remain alert throughout the duration of the exam, as sleeping has potential to cause abnormal waveforms, skewing the results of the exam. A transcranial 2 MHz transducer is used through the temporal window (Fig. 13-11), with sample volume at approximately 6 millimeters.

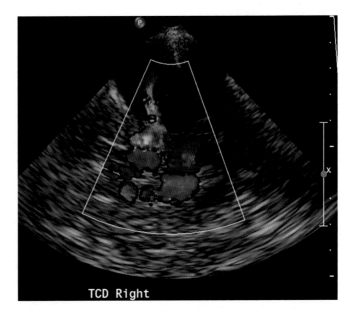

FIGURE 13-11. Transtemporal right acoustic window.

TABLE 13-1 • Transtemporal Depths and Flow Direction

Artery	Direction of Flow	Depth of SV (cm)	Mean Velocity (cm/s)
MCA	Toward Transducer	3.0–6.0 Average 3.0–5.4 (HD 12 cm) 3.0–5.8 (HD 13 cm) 3.4–6.2 (HD 14 cm)	55 +/− 12
MCA/ACA	Bidirectional	5.5–6.5 Average	–
ACA (A1)	Away from Transducer	6.0–8.0 Average 5.0–5.8 (HD 12 cm) 5.2–6.2 (HD 13 cm) 5.6–5.8 (HD 14 cm)	50 +/− 11
PCA (P1)	Toward Transducer	6.0–7.0 Average 4.0–6.0 (HD 12 cm) 4.2–6.6 (HD 13 cm) 4.6–7.0 (HD 14 cm)	39 +/− 10
TICA	Toward Transducer	5.5–6.5 Average 5.0–5.4 (HD 12 cm) 5.2–5.8 (HD 13 cm) 5.6–6.4 (HD 14 cm)	39 +/− 9

HD = Head Diameter. It is important to note that sample volume depth can vary based on age and head diameter of pediatric patient. In example, the PCA in a head diameter of 12 centimeters can be obtained at a SV depth of 4.0 to 6.0 centimeters, versus 4.6 to 7.0 centimeters in a patient with head diameter of 14 centimeters. It is more critical to understand appropriate direction of flow.

Sources: Alexandrov AV, Sloan MA, Wong LK, et al. Practice standards for transcranial Doppler ultrasound: part I—test performance. *J Neuroimaging.* 2007;17(1):11–18; and Reuter-Rice K. Transcranial Doppler ultrasound use in pediatric traumatic brain injury. *J Radiol Nurs.* 2017;36(1):3–9.

Doppler trace images are obtained, scanning through the bilateral temporal windows. Images include the MCA from M1 segment (proximal) to the bifurcation, bifurcation of the MCA (including MCA and/or anterior cerebral artery [ACA]), ACA, distal (terminal) ICA (DICA), posterior cerebral artery (PCA), and top of the basilar artery (TOB) (Table 13-1). A Doppler trace should be obtained scanning through the transforaminal (suboccipital) window of the basilar artery at 7 to 10 centimeters depth (Table 13-2).

A transorbital approach shows the carotid siphon and branches of the ICA which are not routinely imaged on a standard TCD examination, such as the supraclinoid and parasellar arteries (Table 13-3).

The transtemporal window is usually found on the temporal bone, cephalad to the zygomatic arch and anterior to the ear. The sonographer should identify the heart-shaped cerebral peduncles, then apply color Doppler. The PCA course around either side of the peduncles. Just anterior to the peduncles is the star-shaped echogenic interpeduncular suprasellar cistern. Anteriorly and laterally from the basilar artery is the MCA's echogenic fissure. MCA flow will be toward the transducer, or above baseline, creating a positive Doppler shift. The MCA should be followed at 4 millimeters intervals from the shallowest segment (36-40 mm) to area of bifurcation (48-53 mm).

TABLE 13-2 • Suboccipital Depths and Flow Direction

Artery	Direction of Flow	Depth of SV (cm)	Mean Velocity (cm/s)
Vertebral	Away from Transducer	6.0-9.0	38 +/− 10
Basilar	Away from Transducer	8.0-12.0	41 +/− 10

TABLE 13-3 • Transorbital Depths and Flow Direction

Artery	Direction of Flow	Depth of SV (cm)	Mean Velocity (cm/s)
Carotid Siphon	–	6.0–8.0	–
OA	Toward Transducer	4.0–6.0	21 +/− 5
Supraclinoid	Away from Transducer	6.0–8.0	41 +/1 11
Parasellar	Toward Transducer	6.0–8.0	47 +/− 14
Genu	Bidirectional	6.0–8.0	–

The sample volume should always be placed in the center of the vessel. The highest velocity should be documented at each segment. Listening to the waveform, the sonographer should adjust the transducer at each segment to obtain the highest velocity (particularly if velocity is in the mean 170-200 cm/s range). Two measurements should be recorded at each level for RI, peak systolic velocity, and average. The sonographer may average 2 to 3 waveforms in a run. After the bifurcation, record two measurements in the ACA with flow going away for RI, peak systolic velocity, and average measurements. The ICA should be at a greater depth and just posterior to the bifurcation (frequently seen as a "curve" extending 4 millimeters deep from the area of bifurcation). The MCA should be imaged at the bifurcation. At this level the sonographer angles down slightly to visualize a small vessel out of plane of the MCA (4 mm deeper). The PCA is imaged toward the transducer around the cerebral peduncles, obtaining two or more measurements for the RI, peak systolic velocity, and average.

Still Images

1. MCA (M1) begin at 36 mm and obtain an image at every 2 mm to the bifurcation (Figs 13-12 and 13-13)
2. MCA bifurcation (Fig. 13-14)
3. ACA, 2 mm past the bifurcation, taking images at 2 mm increments (Fig. 13-15)
4. DICA, 2 mm past the bifurcation, taking images at 2 mm increments (Fig. 13-16)
5. PCA, 2-4 mm past the bifurcation, taking images at 2 mm increments to the TOB
6. TOB (Fig. 13-17).
7. Basilar artery, taking images at 2 mm increments

Note: Repeat protocol through both the right and left transtemporal windows (Figs. 13-18 and 13-19). If an abnormality such as increased velocity or bruit is present, the sonographer should take additional images as needed. In cases of suboptimal visualization of the intracranial vessels, the sonographer should remove color Doppler, returning to B-mode, and reidentify anatomical landmarks before resuming color Doppler. Color gain should be increased until color confetti appears on the image, then slightly decreased to maximize color sensitivity.

Please refer to Chapter 10, "Sonographic Intracranial Vasculature in Pediatrics" for additional TCD information.

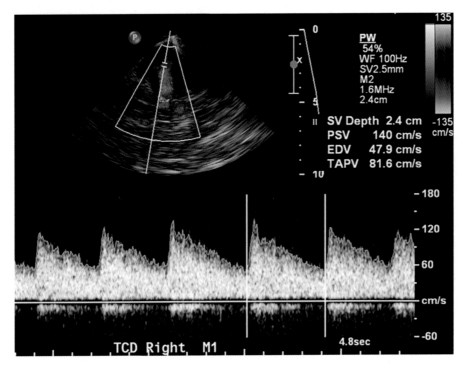

FIGURE 13-12. M1.

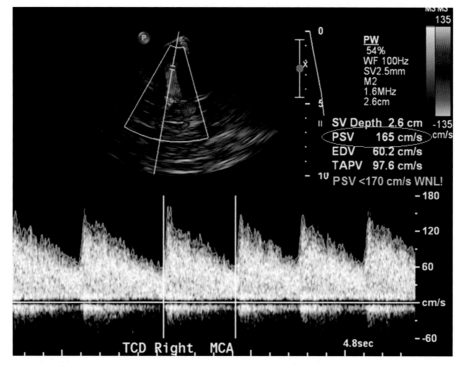

FIGURE 13-13. MCA flow direction toward transducer and above baseline.

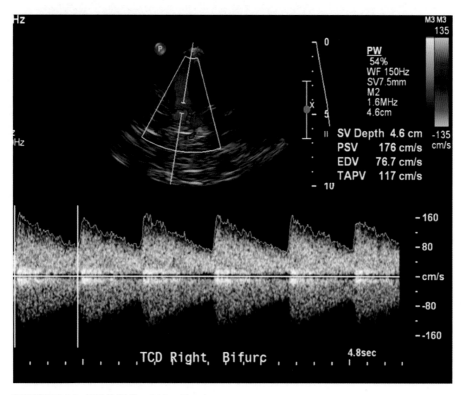

FIGURE 13-14. MCA/ACA flow bidirectional.

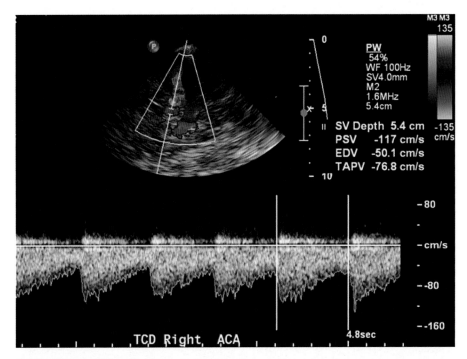

FIGURE 13-15. ACA flow direction away from transducer and below baseline.

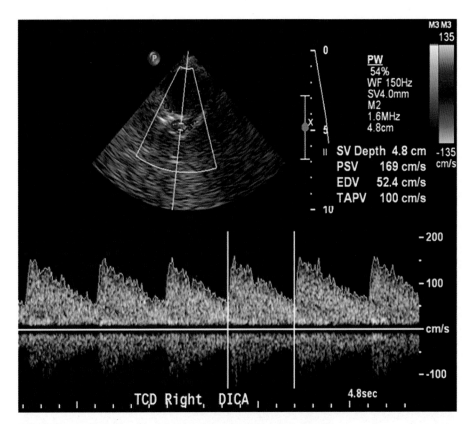

FIGURE 13-16. DICA flow direction toward transducer and above baseline.

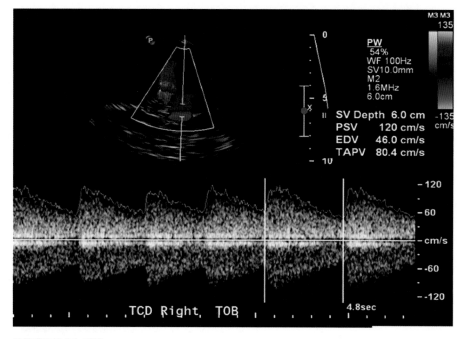

FIGURE 13-17. TOB.

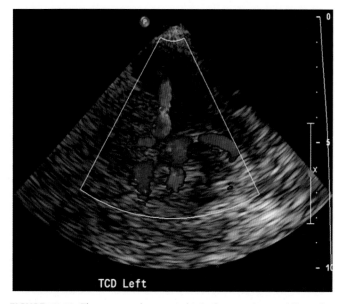

FIGURE 13-18. The sonographer must obtain the same images bilaterally, taking multiple samples at each location for a mean PSV.

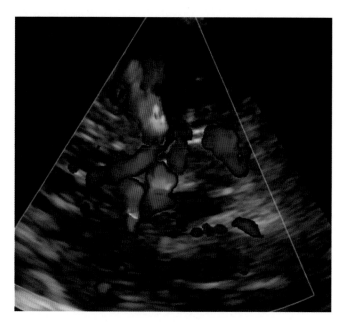

FIGURE 13-19. Circle of Willis in an 8-year-old patient with sickle cell disease.

14

Spinal Malformations

NEURULATION

Neurulation is closure of the neural tube which occurs when the neural plate or neural ectoderm thickens at 17 days gestational age to form the neural folds. These neural folds then come together at midline and fuse to separate the ectoderm from the neural tissue. This then forms the neural crest, dorsal to the neural tube. The neural crest cells migrate to form dorsal root ganglia. Errors in disjunction during neurulation can lead to the development of spinal malformations.

VARIANTS OF THE LUMBAR SPINE

When performing an evaluation of the infant spine for presence of spinal malformation, it is not uncommon to encounter anatomical spinal variants. These include filar cyst (Figs. 14-1 to

14-6), prominent filum terminale, ventriculus terminalis, pseudosinus tract, cauda equina pseudomass, and dysmorphic coccyx. The sonographer should be aware of these normal variants as to not confuse them with true spinal abnormalities.

A filar cyst is a common observation during sonogram of the neonatal lumbar spine. The filum terminale is a thin, threadlike fiber of connective tissue continuous with the spinal pia mater. It continues inferiorly toward the sacrum from the apex of the conus medullaris. A filar cyst is a normal developmental variant of the filum terminale. Sonographically, a filar cyst appears as an anechoic elongation caudal to the conus medullaris. It is located within the midline filum terminale. The true presence of a filar cyst has been pondered by various authors, as this sonographic finding is not reproducible on spinal magnetic resonance imaging (MRI) and is not identifiable on autopsy. Although often

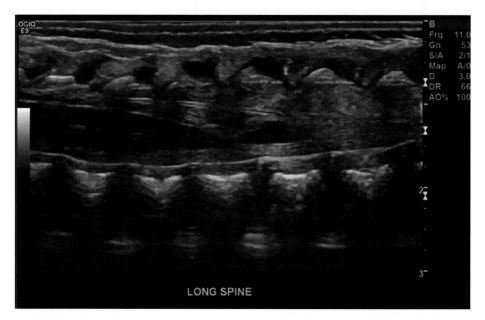

FIGURE 14-1. Filar cyst.

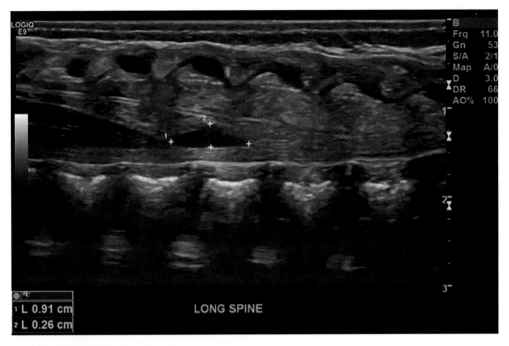

FIGURE 14-2. Filar cyst with sagittal measurement.

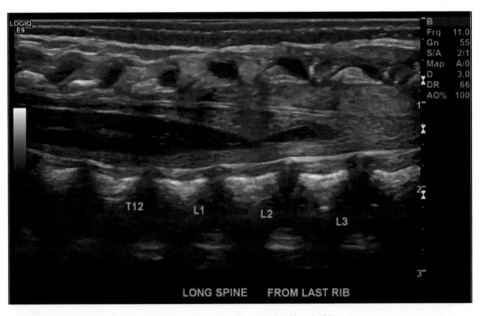

FIGURE 14-3. Vertebrae labeling demonstrating lumbar vertebral level of filar cyst.

identified via sonogram, it is questionable whether this finding is artifactual versus a true anatomic structure.

A prominent filum terminale is an uncommon anatomic variant in which the filum terminale appears increased in echogenicity compared to surrounding nerve roots. A prominent filum terminale in symptomatic patients can be caused by a tethered cord or spinal dysraphism and is termed *fatty filum terminate, filar lipoma,* or *lipoma of the filar terminale.* The anatomic variant counterpart, which is identified as an incidental

finding in the asymptomatic patient, is solely referred to as a *prominent filum terminale.* Sonographic confidence in distinguishing prominent filum terminale from filar lipoma is achieved when the filum terminale sustains its usual midline course and appropriate thickness.

Ventriculus terminalis is also called *terminal ventricle of Krause, persistent terminal ventricle,* or fifth ventricle. It is related to incomplete regression of the embryonic terminal ventricle of Krause in the conus medullaris during the fetal period.

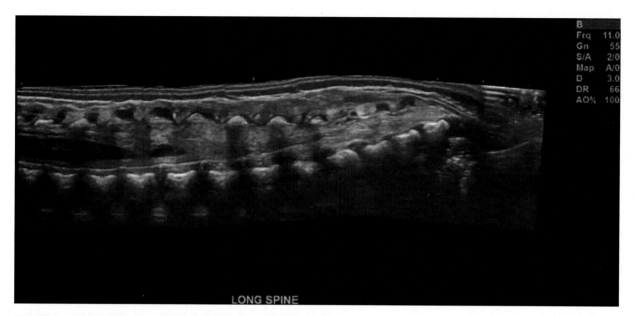

FIGURE 14-4. Panoramic view of sagittal spine demonstrating filar cyst.

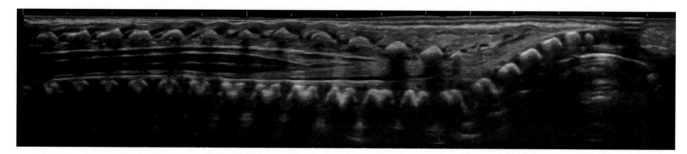

FIGURE 14-5. Normal variant, filar cyst noted in newborn at L2-L3.

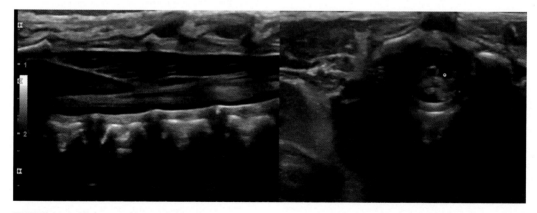

FIGURE 14-6. Filar cyst in long and transverse.

Ventriculus terminalis appears as a fusiform dilation of the spinal cord's terminal central canal. While a filar cyst is based within the filum terminale, ventriculus terminalis is not. Ventriculus terminalis is identified as extending from the region of the conus medullaris tip to the filum terminale origin. This can be seen sonographically in the neonatal period or on MRI in children less than 5 years of age. However, persistent terminal ventricle often regresses during the first few weeks of life.

Pseudosinus tract is a threadlike fibrous tissue remnant that courses from a visible skin dimple toward the coccyx. A pseudosinus tract does not communicate with the thecal sac and is not associated with seepage of cerebrospinal fluid (CSF). This finding is considered a normal variant and is most commonly located between a dimple overlying the sacral spine region and the coccyx. The sonographer should meticulously evaluate for presence of CSF or a mass within a visualized tract, which indicates a true dermal sinus tract is present. If a true dermal sinus tract is identified, MRI is the gold standard for imaging evaluation. It is important to note, true dermal sinus tracts occur less often at the coccygeal tip region and are more often identified cranially.

Cauda equina pseudomass is a positional artifactual "mass" of the nerve roots. This occurs when an infant is sonographically evaluated in decubitus position and nerve roots appear bundled together, falsifying the appearance of a mass. This pseudomass resolves when the infant is rescanned in prone position, and nerve roots lie in their proper position.

The coccyx is the most inferior segment of the vertebral column. Position and shape of the coccyx is variable, although in most of the population it exhibits a slight ventral curve following the sacral curvature. Dysmorphic coccyx is a variance in the shape of the coccygeal tip, mimicking a spinal mass upon physical palpation of the spine.

SPINAL MALFORMATIONS

Spinal Dysraphism

Spinal dysraphism includes a group of disorders from embryologic origin in which there is incomplete or absent fusion of posterior midline structures. Some diseases in this group of spinal malformations include spina bifida and occult spinal dysraphism. Spina bifida aperta is a non-skin covered open neural tube defect, whereas occult spinal dysraphism is a skin-covered defect. If left untreated, these processes can lead to progressive cord traction as the cord elongates, leading to tethering of the spinal cord (Fig. 14-7). Symptoms of tethered cord syndrome may include incontinence, lower extremity symptoms such as weakness and limp, back pain, and back problems such as scoliosis. Signs of occult dysraphism include hair growth over

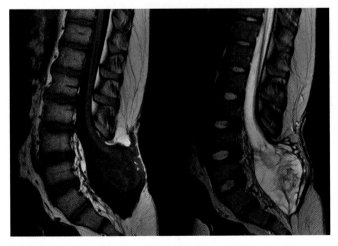

FIGURE 14-7. MRI of the pediatric lumbar spine without contrast in a 10-year-old spina bifida patient. Images demonstrate a large area of spinal dysraphism at L4-L5, with a low-lying conus. The spinal cord appears to extend to and into the defect, correlating with tethered cord clinical symptoms.

the lumbosacral spine, skin tags, hemangiomas, and dimples. A dimple may be considered low risk for occult dysraphism, whereas multiple stigmata are of higher risk.

Occult Spinal Dysraphism

Occult spinal dysraphism is a skin-covered (closed) spinal malformation that can occur with or without an accompanying mass.

Occult malformations with a subcutaneous mass may include lipomyelocele, lipomyelomeningocele, intradural lipoma, terminal myelocystocele, limited dorsal myeloscisis, meningocele, and fibrolipoma of the filum terminale.

Lipomyelocele is typically seen near the thoracolumbar region as a fatty mass underneath the skin. Lipomyelocele is one of the most common occult spinal malformations and is twice as common as a lipomyelomeningocele.

Unlike lipomyeloceles, lipomyelomeningoceles are typically located above the intergluteal cleft or along the spinal canal. Lipomyeloceles and lipomyelomeningoceles occur from premature disjunction of the neural tube allowing mesenchymal cells to reach ependymal lining of the neural tube. This induces differentiation of mesenchyme into fat, causing tethering of the neural tissue. Both lipomyeloceles and lipomyelomeningoceles contain a component of fat, hence the Greek prefix "lipo-."

Occult malformations without a subcutaneous mass may include intradural lipoma, tight filum terminale, filar lipoma, posterior spina bifida, persistent terminal ventricle, disorders of midline notochordal integration, and disorders of notochordal formation. Disorders of midline notochordal integration include neurenteric cyst, dorsal dermal sinus or enteric fistula, split cord malformations such as diastematomyelia and diplomyelia. Disorders of notochordal formation include segmental spinal dysgenesis, and caudal regression syndrome, types I and II.

Diastematomyelia is a split cord malformation characterized by a sagittal cleft in the spinal cord which divides the spinal cord into two hemi-cords. Each hemicord is surrounded by its own pia mater and central canal. This malformation is known to be more common in females.

Simple Meningocele

Simple meningoceles are posterior herniations through a bony vertebral defect. These herniations are simple, thus only CSF filled. This causes the appearance of a cyst-like mass within the posterior subcutaneous tissues.

Myelocystocele

Myelocystoceles are rare skin-covered lesions characterized by a meningocele and hydromyelic cord which terminates as a large cyst. A hydromyelic cord is dilated, and these lesions are most common in females. Should this lesion contain a fat component, it would be termed a *lipo*myelocystocele.

Overt-Aperta Spinal Dysraphism

Overt or aperta spinal dysraphism is a non-skin covered (open) malformation including myeloceles, myelomeningoceles (98%), hemimyelomeningoceles, and hemimyeloceles. These are among the most common congenital malformations of the spine, although with use of prenatal maternal folic acid, the incidence is decreasing. These disease processes result from failure of primary disjunction where the neural plate fails to fold, leaving it exposed and in continuity with the ectoderm on the skins surface.

Some helpful prefixes and suffixes are listed in Table 14-1.

For imaging protocol of the infant spine, please refer to Chapter 2, "Sonographic Anatomy of the Pediatric Spine."

TABLE 14-1 • Prefixes and Suffixes
Lipo-Fat
Myelo-Spinal cord or bone marrow
Meningo-Meninges including dura, arachnoid, and pia mater
Cyst-Cyst, sac
Hemi-Half
-cele Hernation, pouching

15

Pancreatic Pathology

CYSTIC FIBROSIS

Cystic fibrosis is caused by an autosomal recessive gene on the long arm of chromosome 7. This chromosome codes for a polypeptide of 1,480 amino acids called *cystic fibrosis transmembrane conductance regulators* (CFTR). In vertebrates, CFTR is a chloride channel and membrane protein encoded by the CFTR gene. The role of CFTR in the biliary epithelium is to help water and solute movement and promote bile flow. With cystic fibrosis, there is abnormally thick luminal secretions which lead to pancreatic duct obstruction, glandular atrophy, fibrosis, fatty replacement, and exocrine dysfunction. This can lead to symptoms of abdominal pain, fat intolerance, steatorrhea, and failure to thrive in 90% of cystic fibrosis or affected patients. The sonographic appearance of cystic fibrosis within the pancreas can include a hyperechoic fatty pancreas, possible cyst formation, calcifications, and atrophy.

ACUTE PANCREATITIS

Acute pancreatitis is an acute inflammatory process of the pancreas with local tissue and remote organ system involvement. Causes of acute pancreatitis include abdominal trauma, medications, and infections such as HIV, viral infection, or ascariasis. Structural pancreatic abnormalities that alter pancreas secretion drainage such as choledochal cyst, pancreas divisum, annular pancreas, and duodenal duplication may also cause acute pancreatitis. Lastly, hereditary disease processes such as cystic fibrosis, hereditary pancreatitis, and multisystem diseases including Kawasaki disease and inflammatory bowel disease can lead to development of acute pancreatitis. Acute pancreatitis can be caused by unknown reasons in up to 30% of children. After the first acute episode of acute pancreatitis, recurrent acute pancreatitis can be seen in up to 10% of children.

Mild acute pancreatitis is characterized by interstitial edema, small echogenic foci, acinar cell necrosis, and minimal to no pancreatic inflammation. Clinical symptoms of mild pancreatitis include abdominal pain, elevated pancreatic enzymes, vomiting, and fever. Mild acute pancreatitis is seen to improve in clinical findings 48 to 72 hours after initial onset.

Severe acute pancreatitis includes macroscopic necrosis, hemorrhage, ductal disruption, extensive inflammation, major organ failure such as gastrointestinal bleed, renal insufficiency, pulmonary insufficiency, low serum calcium, pseudocyst formation, pancreatic abscess, and elevated amylase and lipase values. Approximately 50% of children with severe acute pancreatitis have extra-pancreatic fluid collections that lack a well-defined capsule. Other extra-pancreatic abnormalities associated with severe acute pancreatitis are bowel wall thickening, gallbladder wall thickening, pericholecystic fluid, and splenic involvement including infarct, hemorrhage, or abscess. Pseudocyst formation is the most common complication of acute pancreatitis. Pseudocyst of the pancreas requires 4 to 6 weeks to form.

Multiple treatment options are available in the event that the pancreatic pseudocyst (Figs. 15-1 to 15-3) does not regress without treatment. Less commonly used is percutaneous catheter drainage. This method is controversial due to concern of fistula formation or reaccumulation in patients with severe pancreatitis, although multiple institutions report high level of efficacy and safety. Pancreatic cysts that are noncommunicating with the pancreatic duct are not likely to create a fistula and typically are non-recurring. More commonly performed treatments options include endoscopic drainage and open surgical debridement. A Roux-en-Y jejunal loop is used for open surgical debridement or cystenterotomy. Endoscopic drainage through the duodenum or stomach is referred to as a *cyst-gastrostomy*.

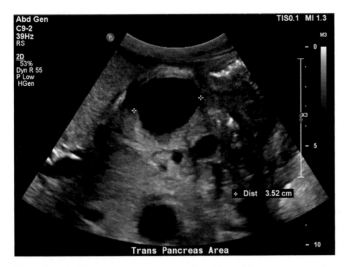

FIGURE 15-1. Transverse pancreas pseudocyst formation.

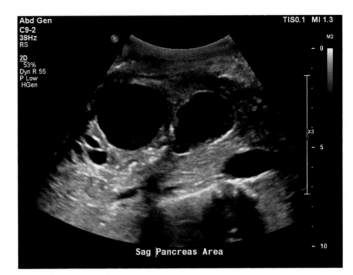

FIGURE 15-3. Anechoic and complex peripancreatic cystic masses, representing pseudocyst formation.

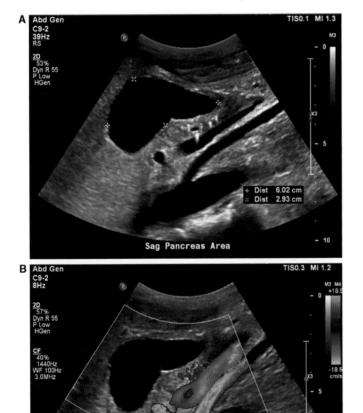

FIGURE 15-2. Sagittal pancreas pseudocyst formation.

Additionally, an infusion of octreotide can also aid in decreasing the amount of pancreatic secretions. Pseudoaneurysm and venous thrombosis formation are rare complications of acute pancreatitis in children.

CHRONIC PANCREATITIS

Chronic pancreatitis is an inflammatory process characterized by progressive destruction of the pancreatic parenchyma. Chronic pancreatitis may result from recurrent acute pancreatic episodes. Clinical symptoms include recurrent abdominal pain and obstructive jaundice from fibrosing pancreatitis. Sonographic evidence of chronic pancreatitis includes pancreatic calcification with or without acoustic shadowing, irregular pancreatic duct, glandular atrophy, and biliary duct dilatation.

HEREDITARY PANCREATITIS

Hereditary pancreatitis is an autosomal dominant disorder characterized by recurrent episodes of acute pancreatitis beginning in childhood and continuing over many years. Late complications may include exocrine or endocrine insufficiency, pseudocyst formation, and adenocarcinoma.

IDIOPATHIC FIBROSING PANCREATITIS

Idiopathic fibrosing pancreatitis is characterized as chronic pancreatitis of unknown cause, where pancreatic parenchyma begins to replace with fibrous tissue. This replacement can cause obstructive jaundice as fibrotic tissue narrows the common bile duct. Idiopathic fibrosing pancreatitis is associated with inflammatory bowel disease and is not associated with pseudocyst formation.

CONGENITAL PANCREATIC CYSTS

True pancreatic cysts are lined with epithelium and are not associated with the pancreatic ducts, compared to other ductal-communicating cysts of the pancreas. Congenital pancreatic cysts may result from abnormal segmentation of the primitive ductal system during development. Most congenital pancreatic cysts are found within the tail of the pancreas, with the most common congenital cystic mass of the pancreas being a pseudocyst. Clinical findings include abdominal distension, palpable mass, vomiting, or jaundice related to compression of adjacent structures. Congenital pancreatic cysts are associated with polycystic kidneys and renal tubular ectasia.

PANCREATOBLASTOMA

Pancreatoblastoma is a slow-growing exocrine infantile pancreatic carcinoma. Although these masses are rare, they are the most common childhood pancreatic neoplasm and generally present prior to 10 years of age (i.e., average occurrence ~4.5 years of age). These masses are low-grade malignant and typically have a good outcome if identified, with a brighter prognosis compared to adult pancreatic adenocarcinoma. In 35% of cases, pancreatoblastoma metastasizes to the liver and lymph nodes.

Pancreatoblastoma is a large, solitary, well-defined vascular lesion. Pancreatoblastoma may have a hyperechoic or hypoechoic heterogeneous sonographic appearance. These masses can range anywhere from 1.5 to 20 centimeters in size and rarely invade the liver or adjacent vessels. Computed tomography (CT) and magnetic resonance imaging (MRI) are alternative modalities that aid in evaluation. Clinical findings may include abdominal pain, nausea, vomiting, pancreatic and biliary ductal dilatation, and jaundice. Pancreatoblastoma has a slight male prevalence and is associated with increased levels of alpha-fetoprotein. Treatment includes complete surgical resection. When this is not possible (i.e., due to lesion size, location, involvement, etc.), patients may require neoadjuvant chemotherapy.

PANCREATIC LYMPHANGIOMA

Pancreatic lymphangioma is a non-epithelial neoplasm and congenital mass that occurs due to obstruction of the fetal lymphatic system. This mass generally has a hypoechoic sonographic appearance. A pancreatic lymphangioma may be septated, multi-cystic, and filled with a serous or chylous fluid. This mass is typically surrounded by a thin capsule and may be hemorrhagic if debris or internal echoes are visualized.

PANCREATIC CYSTIC TERATOMA

Pancreatic cystic teratoma is a non-epithelial neoplasm. These masses are large and may measure up to 8 to 12 centimeters. Clinical findings may include a palpable abdominal mass. Pancreatic cystic teratomas are cystic tumors with a consistency of fat, bone, soft tissue, and calcification. On sonogram, tip-of-the-iceberg or dermal mesh sign may be visualized.

Pancreatic cystic teratomas develop from pluripotential cells of embryonic remnants of the ectoderm. Teratomas in general originate from germ cells and have the capability of creating tissues from all three germinal layers, including the endoderm, mesoderm, and ectoderm. Furthermore, teratomas can be categorized as immature or mature, depending on tumor makeup and whether the tumor contains immature neuroectodermal components.

PANCREATIC LYMPHOMA

Pancreatic lymphoma is a non-epithelial neoplasm that is rare in children but can occur more commonly as a non-Hodgkin lymphoma. This pathology has a sonographic appearance of a diffusely enlarged homogeneous, hypoechoic pancreas with possible anechoic masses that can mimic pancreatic cysts. Pancreatic lymphoma may be seen along with splenomegaly and widespread lymph node enlargement.

PANCREATIC ADENOCARCINOMA

Pancreatic carcinomas very rarely occur in the pediatric population. However, this etiology may be encountered as a distractor on the registry exam. Pancreatic adenocarcinoma is an exocrine pancreatic carcinoma. This exocrine tumor is most commonly ductal or acinar in origin. The ductal variation of this etiology is the most common pancreatic neoplasm in adults; however, when occurring in the pediatric population the acinar variation may be seen in adolescents. These masses are large ranging between 2 and 30 centimeters. They typically have a heterogeneous, hypoechoic poorly defined sonographic appearance (Fig. 15-4). Local extension into surrounding areas and metastasis is common with adenocarcinoma of the pancreas, and surgical excision is currently the only possibility of cure. Vascular invasion, ascites, and pancreatic or biliary ductal dilation is not uncommon.

PANCREATIC SOLID PSEUDOPAPILLARY TUMOR

Solid pseudopapillary tumor, formerly known as the *Frantz tumor*, is an exocrine pancreatic tumor. Solid pseudopapillary tumors are low-grade malignant and arise from the pancreatic tail. These exocrine lesions are large, generally measuring around 9 centimeters. They have a well-defined, complex sonographic appearance with areas of hemorrhage and cystic degeneration (Figs. 15-5 and 15-6). Clinical symptoms may include abdominal pain or jaundice. Solid pseudopapillary tumors may contains sheets of epithelial cells and pseudopapillae within. The average age of presentation is around 22 years. This tumor is more common in adolescent girls and young women than in their male counterparts.

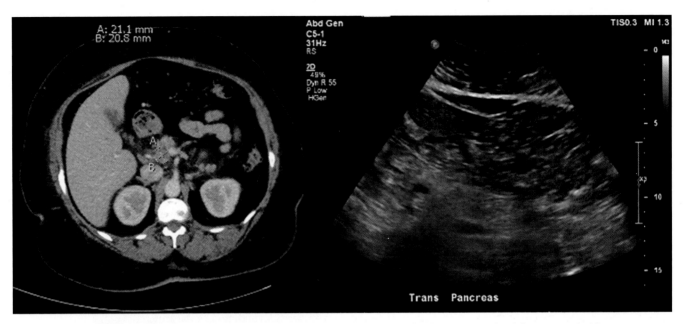

FIGURE 15-4. Biopsy-proven adenocarcinoma of the pancreatic head, ill-defined on ultrasound and demonstrated with measurement on computed tomography of the abdomen.

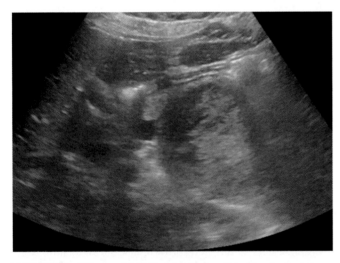

FIGURE 15-5. Ultrasound depicting a solid pseudopapillary tumor in a 12-year-old girl with left upper quadrant pain.

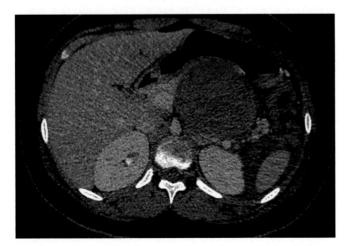

FIGURE 15-6. CT depicting a solid pseudopapillary tumor in a 12-year-old girl with left upper quadrant pain.

ENDOCRINE FUNCTIONING ISLET-CELL TUMOR

Endocrine tumors arise from the neural crest tissue that give rise to islet of Langerhans cells. These tumors are hormonally active and produce polypeptide hormones. Polypeptide hormones produced include insulin, gastrin, glucagon, vasoactive intestinal peptide, and somatostatin. Endocrine tumors can sometimes be seen with Von-Hippel Lindau syndrome, MEN type 1, and phakomatoses patients.

ENDOCRINE NONFUNCTIONING ISLET-CELL TUMOR

Nonfunctioning endocrine tumors are hormonally inactive, nonfunctioning, non-insulin-producing tumors. These lesions may involve calcification, cystic changes, or malignant behavior that can cause pain leading to diagnosis.

INSULINOMA

Insulinoma is a pancreatic endocrine and functioning islet-cell tumor. This tumor is small, typically measuring around 2 centimeters. Insulinomas have a homogeneous, hypoechoic sonographic echotexture and may present with a hyperechoic capsule. These tumors can be hypervascular and are generally solitary and benign. Clinical findings may include hypoglycemia and elevated serum insulin. Insulinoma is the most common islet cell tumor seen in approximately 47% of pancreatic endocrine tumor patients.

GASTRINOMA

Gastrinoma is a pancreatic endocrine and functioning islet-cell tumor. This tumor is generally larger than an insulinoma measuring around 4 centimeters. Gastrinomas have a heterogeneous sonographic appearance with areas of necrosis and calcification. Clinical findings may include associated peptic ulcer disease, gastric acid hypersecretion, and diarrhea. Gastrinoma is the second most common islet-cell tumor, seen in approximately 30% of pancreatic endocrine tumor patients. Gastrinomas have a higher likelihood of malignancy as opposed to insulinomas.

GLUCAGONOMA, SOMATOSATINOMA, AND VIPOMAS

This class of pancreatic endocrine and functioning islet-cell tumors secrete vasoactive intestinal peptide. These tumors are very rare and are more likely to be malignant due to high incidence of vascular invasion. Although uncommon, these etiologies may be encountered as distractors on the registry exam. Glucagonoma, somatostatinoma, and vasoactive intestinal peptide tumors (VIPomas) are large, measuring up to 5 centimeters and have a heterogeneous sonographic appearance with areas of calcification and cystic change.

MISCELLANEOUS PANCREATIC TUMORS

Additional pancreatic tumors that may appear large, heterogeneous, or contain areas of necrosis and cystic change include pseudotumor, schwannoma, neurofibroma, lipoma, leiomyoma, or hemangioendotheliomas. These listed pancreatic tumors may vary in sonographic echogenicity.

MISCELLANEOUS PANCREATIC CYSTIC LESIONS

Miscellaneous cystic lesions of the pancreas that can cause dilation of the main pancreatic duct include microcystic and serous cystadenoma, macrocystic and mucinous cystadenoma, and intraductal papillary mucinous neoplasm. These lesions are all very rare in children, however, may be encountered as distractors on the registry exam.

METASTATIC LESIONS

Metastatic lesions of the pancreas may be secondary to a retroperitoneal tumor, most commonly sarcomas.

16

Hepatic Pathology

The purpose of this section is to review the many pathologies associated with the liver throughout childhood. Abnormalities of the liver can be categorized as genetic conditions, congenital abnormalities, benign or malignant pathologies, or infectious processes.

There are numerous genetic conditions of the liver. Some of these conditions include Niemann-Pick disease, cystic fibrosis, primary (hereditary) hemochromatosis, lipid storage disorders, glycogen storage disorders, galactosemia, Wilson disease, and Gaucher disease. Niemann-Pick disease is an inherited lipid storage disease. Cystic fibrosis is an autosomal recessive disorder which affects the lungs and digestive system. Gaucher disease is a genetic lysosomal storage disorder.

Congenital liver defects often involve the bile duct(s) and are disorders of the liver which are present at the time of birth. Some congenital abnormalities of the liver include congenital hepatic fibrosis, Caroli's disease, Alagille syndrome, and heterotaxy syndrome. Caroli's disease is an abnormal widening (i.e., multifocal cystic dilation) of the intrahepatic bile ducts paired with renal cysts. The cause of Caroli's disease is unknown, with result being congenital hepatic fibrosis. Heterotaxy syndrome is an abnormality of abdominal and thoracic organ location. These patients may demonstrate a midline liver, intrahepatic vessel variants, and cardiac abnormalities. Many of the hereditary abnormalities associated with the liver and their sonographic appearances are discussed throughout this section.

The sonographic appearance of liver disease and clinical significance of ultrasound as it relates to liver function are outlined in this section. This section also reviews liver transplantation and covers the various obstructive processes of the liver. Occlusion of the portal vein, hepatic vein(s), and inferior vena cava may require surgical intervention and/or stent placement. The normal and abnormal peak flow velocities associated with placement of a transjugular intrahepatic portosystemic shunt are reviewed and the normal mean diameter of the portal vein, which varies with age, height, weight, and gender, are discussed.

FATTY INFILTRATION

Non-alcoholic fatty liver disease (NAFLD) is a chronic condition related to steatosis of the liver. Non-alcoholic steatohepatitis (NASH) is steatosis which occurs alongside fibrosis, inflammation, and necrosis of the liver. Fatty infiltration is also seen with Reye's (Reye) syndrome.

FOCAL FATTY SPARING

Focal fatty sparing is a form of diffuse parenchymal disease. With focal fatty sparing (Fig. 16-1), normal areas of liver parenchyma appear as hypoechoic masses in a diffusely infiltrated echogenic fatty liver.

MICROVESICULAR STEATOSIS

Microvesicular steatosis is a fatty degenerative diffuse parenchymal disease involving excessive accumulation of triglycerides within liver hepatocytes. Hepatocytes contain small fat droplets that do not displace the nucleus from the center of the cell. Microvesicular steatosis is associated with acute fatty liver during pregnancy, Reye's (Reye) syndrome, cystic fibrosis, and massive tetracycline therapy. Clinical findings include acutely ill patients with a painful liver, vomiting, jaundice, and/or coma. This disease is rarely reversible. Sonographic findings include hepatomegaly, diffuse or focal fatty infiltration, increased parenchymal echogenicity and sound beam attenuation, nonvisualization of the diaphragm and vessels, and possible areas of focal fatty sparing that may mimic a mass.

MACROVESICULAR STEATOSIS

Macrovesicular steatosis is a fatty degenerative diffuse parenchymal disease involving excessive accumulation of triglycerides within the liver hepatocytes. Hepatocytes contain large fat

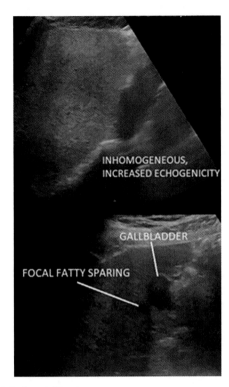

INHOMOGENEOUS,
INCREASED ECHOGENICITY

GALLBLADDER

FOCAL FATTY SPARING

FIGURE 16-1. Fatty infiltration.

vacuoles that fill the cell, pushing the nucleus against the cell wall. Macrovesicular steatosis is associated with nutritional abnormalities, metabolic disorders, drug therapy, cystic fibrosis, and viral infections. Nutritional abnormalities may include starvation, obesity, or intestinal bypass, while metabolic disorders include diabetes and hyperlipidemia. Clinical findings are asymptomatic, and this disease is reversible. Sonographic findings include hepatomegaly, diffuse or focal fatty infiltration, increased parenchymal echogenicity and sound beam attenuation, non-visualization of the diaphragm and vessels, and possible areas of focal fatty sparing that may mimic a mass.

CONGENITAL HEPATIC FIBROSIS

Hepatic fibrosis is a diffuse parenchymal disease involving fibrosing of the liver tissue. Clinical findings include hepatomegaly and portal hypertension. Sonographic findings include increased parenchymal echogenicity in the periportal region or diffusely throughout the liver. Images obtained with a high-frequency linear transducer may demonstrate irregularity of the liver surface and capsule. Bile duct dilation and signs of cirrhosis and portal hypertension may be seen. Hepatic fibrosis is associated with congenital conditions including autosomal recessive polycystic kidney disease, Caroli disease, Meckel-Gruber, and Ivemark syndromes.

PRIMARY HEMOCHROMATOSIS

Primary hemochromatosis is a diffuse parenchymal disease involving presence of increased iron storage in the liver. Primary hemochromatosis is a human leukocyte antigen–linked

inherited disorder where a mucosal defect in the intestinal wall leads to increased absorption of ingested iron. This iron is then deposited within the hepatocytes. Sonographic appearance is nonspecific. Primary hemochromatosis is best diagnosed and quantified with magnetic resonance imaging (MRI).

SECONDARY HEMOCHROMATOSIS

Secondary hemochromatosis is an acquired diffuse parenchymal disease involving presence of increased iron storage in the liver. Secondary hemochromatosis is associated with red blood cell breakdown related to hemolytic anemia. The sonographic appearance includes decreased echogenicity of the liver parenchyma or a normal liver appearance. Secondary hemochromatosis is best diagnosed and quantified with MRI.

TRANSFUSIONAL IRON OVERLOAD HEMOCHROMATOSIS

Transfusional iron overload hemochromatosis is a type of secondary hemochromatosis and diffuse parenchyma disease involving presence of increased iron storage in the liver due to multiple blood transfusions. With transfusional iron overload hemochromatosis, iron begins to deposit in the liver, spleen, and bone marrow. The sonographic appearance includes decreased echogenicity of the liver parenchyma or a normal liver appearance. MRI is the test of choice for diagnosis.

CIRRHOSIS

Cirrhosis is a chronic diffuse parenchymal disease that involves destruction of liver parenchyma, liver scarring, fibrosis, and nodular degeneration with lobular and vascular architecture disorganization (Fig. 16-2(a) and (b)). Cirrhosis is caused by chronic hepatitis, cystic fibrosis, metabolic disease, prolonged total parenteral nutrition, Budd-Chiari syndrome, and biliary atresia. Clinical findings include hepatomegaly, jaundice, and ascites. The sonographic appearance includes a small right hepatic lobe with a hypertrophied left and caudate lobe, coarse heterogeneous parenchyma, increased echogenicity, decreased penetration of the sound beam, and ascites. The liver appears nodular with an irregular capsule; it is helpful to use a high-frequency linear transducer to demonstrate the liver's surface. A newer method of assessing liver fibrosis uses shear-wave elastography. Elastography is a noninvasive quantitative tool which measures the speed of shear waves across tissue to determine liver stiffness and elasticity. Elastography (Fig. 16-2(c)) can measure increased stiffness influenced by fibrosis, hepatic congestion, portal hypertension, and inflammation. Increased values correlate with increased stiffness. With cirrhosis, aspartate transferase, alanine transaminase, and lactic dehydrogenase lab values are elevated.

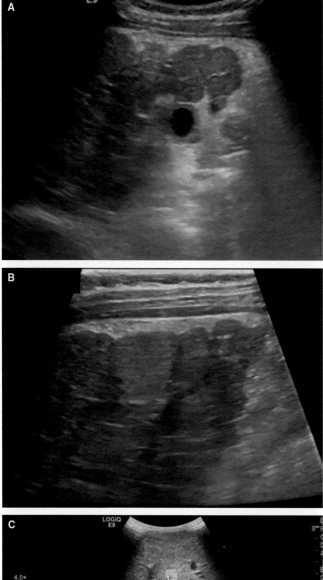

FIGURE 16-2. A 12-year-old male with histoy of autoimmune hepatitis and chronic liver failure, now with cirrhosis. Elastography values greater than 2.04 m/s (12.5 kPa) are suggestive of cirrhosis.

CYSTIC FIBROSIS

Cystic fibrosis is a metabolic liver disease. With this genetic abnormality, an abnormal cystic fibrosis transmembrane conductance regulator inadequately facilitates water and solute movement via chloride secretion to promote bile flow, resulting in biliary cirrhosis, portal hypertension, and abnormal sodium and chloride transport. This causes thick, viscous secretions affecting many organ systems, particularly the lungs and exocrine glands of the gastrointestinal tract. Clinical and sonographic findings in pediatric patients may include increased liver parenchymal echogenicity due to steatosis, fibrosis, cirrhosis, and portal hypertension.

GLYCOGEN STORAGE DISEASE

Glycogen storage disease is a family of metabolic storage diseases. This autosomal recessive disorder is the most common carbohydrate metabolism inborn error characterized by excessive glycogen deposition in hepatocytes and proximal renal tubules. Type I glycogen storage disease is known as Von Gierke disease and is the most common form of glycogen storage disease in pediatrics. Von Gierke disease manifests in the neonatal period with marked hepatomegaly and hypoglycemia. Sonographic findings include hepatomegaly, increased parenchymal echogenicity secondary to fatty infiltrate, hepatic adenoma, and hepatocellular carcinoma in long-term disease. Clinical treatment involves hypoglycemia dietary management.

GALACTOSEMIA

Galactosemia is a metabolic liver disease and autosomal recessive disorder caused by deficiency of galactose-1-phosphate uridyltransferase. Clinical findings include liver failure, jaundice, and hypoglycemia in the neonatal period. Sonographic appearance includes cirrhosis, portal hypertension, hepatomegaly, and increased parenchymal echogenicity secondary to fatty infiltrate.

GAUCHER DISEASE

Gaucher disease is a metabolic liver disease and the most common lysosomal storage disorder which is caused by deficiency of B-glucosidase and accumulation of glucosylceramide. Clinical findings include hepatosplenomegaly, abdominal pain, hepatic or splenic infarction, and growth retardation. Sonographic findings include liver fibrosis, hepatomegaly, and increased parenchymal echogenicity.

WILSON DISEASE

Wilson disease is a metabolic liver disease. This autosomal recessive abnormality is characterized by excessive copper deposition in the liver, brain, and cornea. Sonographic findings include a diffusely enlarged heterogeneous echogenic liver.

HEPATIC INFARCTION

Hepatic infarction is very rare due to the liver's dual blood supply. Sonographic findings of hepatic infarction are similar to the spleen in which a round, oval, or wedge-shaped hypoechoic area with nondistinctive margins and no blood flow is present.

PELIOSIS HEPATIS

Peliosis hepatis is a sinusoidal dilatation associated with human immunodeficiency virus (HIV), certain medications, and underlying conditions including Marfan syndrome, malnutrition, cystic fibrosis, adrenal gland tumors, congenital cardiopathy, Fanconi anemia, and myotubular myopathy. Clinical findings include hepatomegaly, ascites, portal hypertension, acute hepatic failure, and intraperitoneal hemorrhage. Sonographic findings include diffuse heterogeneous liver with multiple hyperechoic and hypoechoic areas throughout.

OBSTRUCTION

Acute Portal Vein Thrombosis

The main portal vein (MPV) forms at the junction of the superior mesenteric and splenic veins, entering the liver at the porta hepatis. Occlusion of the MPV is described as acute or chronic, with progression leading to variance in sonographic and clinical findings. Clinical findings of acute portal vein thrombosis (PVT) include acute abdominal pain and splenomegaly. Patients with acute PVT more often present with fever and abdominal pain compared to those with chronic PVT. Sonographic findings include enlargement of the portal vein, hypoechoic or anechoic intraluminal thrombosis, and absence of color Doppler flow. Normal portal vein diameter varies with patient's age, weight, height, and gender (see Tables 16-1 to 16-3). Portal vein enlargement should be assessed based on normal patient parameters.

Tables 16-1, 16-2 and 16-3 display the normal diameter of portal vein based on parameters including patient's age, weight, height, and gender for assessment of enlargement associated with portal vein thrombosis.

Chronic Portal Vein Thrombosis

Clinical findings of chronic PVT include acute abdominal pain and splenomegaly. Sonographic findings include periportal collateral vein formation to increase hepatopetal flow, referred to as cavernous transformation. Cavernous transformation entails multiple tortuous vessels filling the portal vein bed. Nonvisualization of the MPV, antegrade, or bidirectional portal venous waveforms in the cavernoma, and increased hepatic arterial diameter and flow may be seen.

Major Hepatic Vein Occlusion

Major hepatic vein occlusion can be idiopathic or secondary to hepatocellular carcinoma, Wilms tumor, or hepatoblastoma. Sonographic findings include hepatomegaly, hypoechoic or echogenic thrombus within the hepatic veins or inferior vena cava (IVC), absence of hepatic vein flow on Doppler exam, caudate lobe enlargement, and possible right lobe atrophy with collateral pathway development.

TABLE 16-1 • Mean Diameter of Portal Vein Relating to Age and Gender				
Age	Mean Diameter (mm)	Male (mm)	Female (mm)
1–4 Weeks	3.4	3.3	3.5
1–3 Months	3.9	3.9	3.8
3–6 Months	4.0	4.1	4.1
6–11.9 Months	4.3	4.4	4.2
12–23 Months	4.8	4.8	4.7
2–4 Years	5.2	5.2	5.2
4–6 Years	6.0	5.9	6.0
6–9 Years	6.0	6.1	6.0
9–10 Years	7.2	7.2	7.2
10–12 Years	7.7	7.7	7.6

Source: Ghosh T, Banerjee M, Basu S, Das R, Kumar P, De S, Ghosh MK, Ganguly S. Assessment of normal portal vein diameter in children. *Trop Gastroenterol*. 2014 Apr-Jun;35(2):79–84. PMID: 25470869.

TABLE 16-2 • Mean Diameter of Portal Vein Relating to Height and Gender				
Height (cm)	Mean Diameter (mm)	Male (mm)	Female (mm)
<80	3.9	3.9	4.0
80–100	4.9	4.9	4.9
100–120	6.2	6.2	6.3
120–140	7.3	7.3	7.2
>140	8.1	8.2	8.0

Source: Ghosh T, Banerjee M, Basu S, Das R, Kumar P, De S, Ghosh MK, Ganguly S. Assessment of normal portal vein diameter in children. *Trop Gastroenterol*. 2014 Apr-Jun;35(2):79–84. PMID: 25470869.

Inferior Vena Cava Occlusion

Doppler findings of IVC occlusion include absent flow in an obstructed vena cava and decreased or reversed hepatic vein flow upon spectral Doppler evaluation. The segment of IVC distal to the level of obstruction is generally dilated.

Hepatic Veno-Occlusive Disease

Hepatic veno-occlusive disease occurs secondary to toxins, radiation, chemotherapy, and bone marrow transplant. With hepatic veno-occlusive disease, sublobular veins become obstructed.

TABLE 16-3 • Mean Diameter of Portal Vein Relating to Weight and Gender			
Weight (kg)	Mean Diameter (mm)	Male (mm)	Female (mm)
<10	3.9	3.9	3.9
10–20	5.4	5.4	5.5
20–30	6.9	6.8	7.0
30–40	7.7	7.7	7.6
>40	8.6	9.0	8.5

Source: Ghosh T, Banerjee M, Basu S, Das R, Kumar P, De S, Ghosh MK, Ganguly S. Assessment of normal portal vein diameter in children. *Trop Gastroenterol.* 2014 Apr-Jun;35(2):79–84. PMID: 25470869.

Portosystemic Hypertension, Collaterals, and Shunts

Portal hypertension results from increased intrahepatic resistance to hepatopetal portal venous flow or from an arteriovenous fistula causing increased portal blood flow. Clinical findings include ascites, splenomegaly, hematemesis, esophageal varices, and prominent abdominal veins. When there is increased intrahepatic resistance to portal venous flow, portosystemic collateral pathways will open to drain the portal venous system. Some collaterals may include the left gastric, short gastric, superior, and inferior mesenteric veins. Developed collaterals are a last response and include recanalization of the preexisting vessels. Recanalization may occur within the paraumbilical, splenorenal, and splenoretroperitoneal veins that lack functional communication with the portal venous system. The left gastric vein, also called the coronary vein, is the most important portosystemic shunt because it is responsible for forming esophageal varices, which can lead to gastrointestinal bleeds and hematemesis. The left gastric vein connects the systemic and portal venous systems as it communicates via anastomotic channels with the lower esophageal veins, drains the anterior and posterior gastric walls, and traverses the lesser omentum emptying into the portal vein.

Transjugular Intrahepatic Portosystemic Shunt

Transjugular intrahepatic portosystemic shunt (TIPS) procedure is performed to prevent or reduce the risk of recurrent gastrointestinal bleed in cirrhotic patients with portal hypertension and multiple collaterals, particularly esophageal varices. During this procedure, a catheter is inserted into the internal jugular vein and advanced into the hepatic veins, where a stent is then inserted to create a tract between the hepatic and intrahepatic portal veins (Fig. 16-3(a)). Ultrasound imaging should demonstrate a patent shunt filling entirely with color (Fig. 16-3(b)). The portal vein branches should demonstrate reversed flow

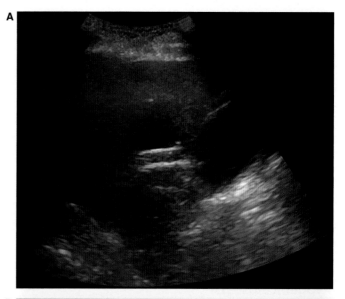

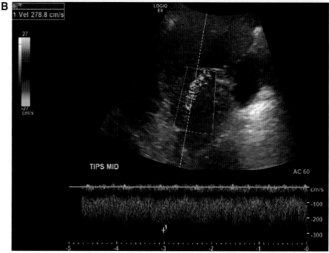

FIGURE 16-3. TIPS.

moving into the shunt, toward the systemic veins. Normal peak flow velocity should be documented between 90 and 130 cm/s within the stent. A complication of TIPS procedure is stent thrombosis, which is an absence of flow and velocity of <90 or >220 cm/s is seen.

Budd-Chiari Syndrome

Budd-Chiari syndrome includes an acute hepatic vein occlusion at the level of the major hepatic veins or the IVC near the hepatic vein ostia, causing postsinusoidal hypertension. Clinical findings include ascites, right upper quadrant pain, jaundice, and hepatomegaly.

INFECTION

Viral Hepatitis (A, B, C, D, and E)

Usually of viral origin, clinical findings of viral hepatitis include jaundice, liver failure, and abdominal pain. Sonography cannot diagnose hepatitis but can determine whether the cause of jaundice is cholestatic or obstructive in nature. Normal liver parenchyma is seen in cases of mild hepatitis. In more severe cases of hepatitis, sonographic findings include hepatomegaly, increased portal venule wall echogenicity known as a "starry sky" liver, enlarged porta hepatic nodes, gallbladder wall thickening with intraluminal sludge, and hypoechoic liver parenchyma may be prevalent. With chronic hepatitis a coarse hyperechoic liver is generally seen. Hepatitis A and E are transmitted via fecal-oral route. Hepatitis B, C, and D are transmitted via bloodborne route. Hepatitis A is the most common viral hepatitis in the United States. Hepatitis D is uncommon in the United States and is primarily a problem when infected with Hepatitis B. Hepatitis E is also uncommon in the United States, and frequently resolves without permanent effects. Vaccines are available to prevent both Hepatitis A and B.

Pyogenic Abscess

Pyogenic abscess results from penetrating injuries then spreads from adjacent organs including the lung, bowel, and remote sites via the portal venous system. The most common organism to cause pyogenic abscess is Escherichia coli in neonates and staphylococcus infection in infants and children. Clinical findings include fever, abdominal pain, hepatomegaly, and elevated liver function tests. Approximately 80% of pyogenic abscess cases are found within the posterior right lobe of the liver. The sonographic appearance includes round hypoechoic masses with thick irregular walls, varying presence of through-transmission, internal debris and septation, hyperechoic gas pockets with acoustic shadowing and reverberation artifact. Pyogenic abscess is treated via percutaneous aspiration or catheter drainage and antibiotic therapy.

Fungal Abscess

Fungal abscess is found in immunocompromised children due to Candida albicans or Aspergillus fungi. The sonographic appearance of fungal abscess includes multiple small, homogeneous, hypoechoic lesions with a hyperechoic "wheel within a wheel" or bullseye pattern throughout the liver, spleen, and kidneys. Fungal infection can mimic metastases, lymphoma, and other diseases.

Hydatid Disease (Echinococcosis)

Hydatid disease, or echinococcosis, is a parasitic infection usually occurring in the Middle East and southern United States. Hydatid disease is obtained through ingestion of food contaminated with feces of a host, such as dog or sheep, containing echinococcosis eggs from an adult tapeworm. Clinical findings include enlarged liver, abdominal pain, and jaundice if the bile duct is obstructed. The sonographic appearance includes a complex cyst with multiple internal daughter cysts, called the "water lily" sign. These complex cysts contain septations and debris, as well as calcifications and possible biliary duct dilatation. Hydatid disease is diagnosed via serologic testing and treated with surgical or percutaneous drainage.

Amebic Abscess

Amebiasis is caused by Entamoeba histolytica parasite, endemic to tropical and subtropical climates. The intestines are the most common site of involvement, with the liver being the most common extraintestinal amebic abscess site. Clinical findings include hepatomegaly and right upper quadrant pain. The sonographic appearance includes round, unilocular masses with smooth or irregular margins and fine low-level echoes in the right lobe near the liver dome. Treatment involves surgical or percutaneous drainage along with medical therapy.

Ascariasis

Ascariasis lumbricoides colonizes to form an abscess in the liver parenchyma. Ascariasis appears as a hypoechoic lesion with central echogenicity and poorly defined margins.

Schistosomiasis

Schistosoma reach the liver via the portal vein and start a granulomatous reaction that occludes the portal vein branches, causing portal hypertension. The sonographic appearance includes hepatomegaly and echogenic portal tracts. Schistosomiasis, amebiasis, and hydatid disease are quite uncommon in the United States and other developed countries.

Chronic Granulomatous Disease

Chronic granulomatous disease is an X-linked recessive disorder characterized by the inability of leukocytes to lyse phagocytized bacteria. The sonographic appearance of chronic granulomatous disease includes hypoechoic lesions that can become echogenic and calcify over time, with possible acoustic enhancement.

Cat-Scratch Disease

Cat-scratch disease is characterized by granulomatous or suppurative reaction to gram-negative bacillus. Hepatic involvement occurs in less than 10% of patients scratched by a domestic cat. Clinical findings include fever and lymph node enlargement. The sonographic appearance includes of multiple small hypoechoic lesions within the liver measuring between 3 millimeters and 2 centimeters.

Acquired Immunodeficiency Syndrome (AIDS)

Sonographic abnormalities in liver parenchyma which are associated with acquired immunodeficiency syndrome include hepatomegaly, punctuate hyperechoic foci, diffuse patchy echogenicity resulting from steatosis and fatty degeneration, and focal mass lesions. Biliary tract abnormalities including gallbladder dilatation, wall thickening, sludge, and biliary duct dilatation.

BENIGN LESIONS

Infantile Hepatic Hemangioma

Infantile hepatic hemangioma, earlier known as hepatic infantile hemangioendothelioma, is the most common benign hepatic tumor in infants less than 6 months of age. Infantile hepatic hemangioma is derived from endothelial cells with initial rapid growth followed by slow spontaneous growth over many years. Clinical findings include normal or slightly elevated serum alpha-fetoprotein, cardiac failure, vascular malformation, and hemoperitoneum resulting from tumor rupture. Sonographic appearance is variable; however, color Doppler readily demonstrates increased flow due to prominent vascular channels throughout the mass.

Cavernous Hemangioma

Cavernous hemangioma is a benign small asymptomatic lesion in adolescents, usually discovered as an incidental finding. Cavernous hemangioma has no malignant potential but can cause hepatomegaly in the case of large lesions. These lesions are comprised of a large network of endothelium-lined vascular spaces filled with red blood cells, separated by fibrous septa. The sonographic appearance includes a hyperechoic, homogeneous mass with well-defined margins and slow blood flow (Figs. 16-4 and 16-5 (a) and (b)). Cavernous hemangioma is most commonly found in the right lobe of the liver.

Mesenchymal Hamartoma

Mesenchymal hamartoma is also called "lymphangioma" and "bile cell fibroadenoma." This benign lesion is a congenital abnormality originating in portal tract connective tissue. Mesenchymal hamartoma is more common in males, affecting patients between 2 and 3 years of age. Clinical findings include a palpable mass, abdominal enlargement, and possible congestive heart failure due to tumor arteriovenous shunting. Sonographic findings include multilocular encapsulated mass greater than 8 centimeters containing mucoid gelatin and solid material with echogenic septa. If arteriovenous shunting is present, the proximal aorta and hepatic veins will be dilated.

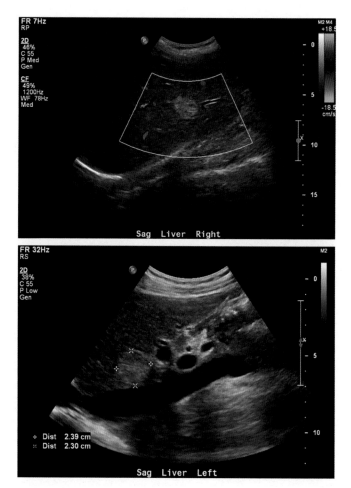

FIGURE 16-5. Cavernous hemangioma.

Focal Nodular Hyperplasia (FNH)

Resulting from a preexisting vascular malformation, FNH is a developmental hyperplastic response of normal hepatocytes. This mass is comprised of Kupffer cells, fibrous connective tissues, abnormally arranged hepatocytes, and bile duct elements. FNH most commonly occurs in young adolescent to middle-aged patients, with a strong female predominance. Clinical findings include hepatomegaly, abdominal pain, and normal serum alpha-fetoprotein levels. The sonographic appearance includes a well-defined isoechoic, non-encapsulated mass with central stellate scar formed by bile ducts, Kupffer cells, and normal hepatocytes (Figs. 16-6 and 16-7).

Hepatic Adenoma

Hepatic adenoma is associated with oral contraceptive use, obesity, type I and type III glycogen storage disease, metabolic syndrome, diabetes mellitus, and use of anabolic steroids—particularly in young males. Patients are usually asymptomatic or may have abdominal pain with hepatomegaly. This mass is also made up of abnormal hepatocytes but does not contain Kupffer cells. The sonographic appearance includes a solitary, heterogeneous, well-defined, hypoechoic, or hyperechoic encapsulated tumor made up of hepatocytes.

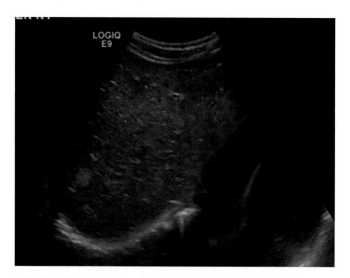

FIGURE 16-4. A 1.1-centimeter hyperechoic lesion in the right hepatic lobe incidenally detected in a 12-year-old female.

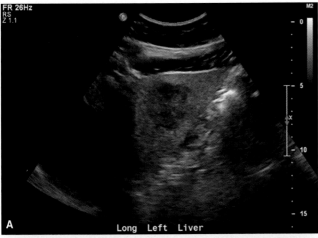

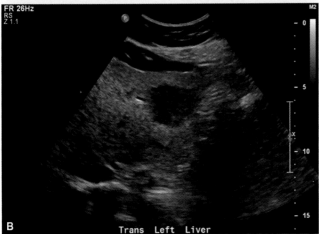

FIGURE 16-6. Hypoechoic mass visualized on ultrasound confirmed with MRI as focal nodular hyperplasia in segment 2 of the liver. In this example, the mass appears hypoechoic, however these lesions are more often isoechoic in appearance.

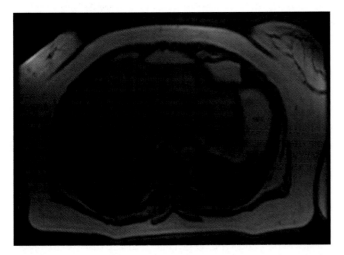

FIGURE 16-7. Hypoechoic mass visualized on ultrasound confirmed with MRI as focal nodular hyperplasia in segment 2 of the liver.

Nodular Regenerative Hyperplasia

Nodular regenerative hyperplasia is a benign regenerative nodular lesion that forms within a non-cirrhotic liver due to myeloproliferative and lymphoproliferative syndromes, immune

related disorders, and long-term steroid or antineoplastic agent use. Sporadic occurrence of nodular regenerative hyperplasia in children occurs around 8 years of age. Clinical findings include hepatomegaly. The sonographic appearance includes multiple, well-defined, hypervascular nodules of varying echogenicity within the liver parenchyma.

Fatty Tumor

Benign fatty tumors include angiomyolipoma, lipoma, and adenoma. Angiomyolipoma is associated with tuberous sclerosis and exhibits a target-like appearance in the liver. Lipoma and adenoma appear as isolated lesions.

Simple Hepatic Cyst

Simple hepatic cysts are uncommon in pediatrics. Sonographic appearance includes solitary, epithelial-lined anechoic structures filled with serous fluid. Clinical findings include hepatomegaly and abdominal pain secondary to mass effect in large cysts. Multiple cysts can be associated with autosomal dominant polycystic kidney disease, Von Hippel-Lindau disease, Byler syndrome, Turner syndrome, and tuberous sclerosis.

MALIGNANT LESIONS

Hepatoblastoma

Hepatoblastoma is the most common malignant liver tumor in children. Up to 90% of cases are seen in patients less than 5 years of age, with peak occurrence between infancy and 2 years of age. This malignancy contains small primitive epithelial cells and mesenchymal elements. Hepatoblastoma occurs unifocally in the right lobe of the liver and commonly invades vasculature such as the portal vein. Elevated serum alpha-fetoprotein is seen 80 to 90% of cases. The sonographic appearance includes a well-marginated echogenic mass. A large hepatoblastoma can have variable echogenicity, but remain well-defined (Fig. 16-8(a) to (c)). Hepatoblastoma is associated with Beckwith-Wiedemann syndrome, hemihypertrophy, fetal alcohol syndrome, prematurity, and low birth weight, familial adenomatosis polyposis, and Gardner syndrome.

Hepatocellular Carcinoma

Hepatocellular carcinoma (HCC), or hepatoma, is the second most common malignant pediatric liver tumor. This malignancy most commonly occurs between 5 and 15 years of age. Clinical findings include elevated serum alpha-fetoprotein, right upper quadrant mass, and abdominal distention. The sonographic appearance includes a hyperechoic multifocal or diffuse infiltrating mass with hypoechoic rim, commonly in the right lobe with vascular invasion, areas of calcification or necrosis, and metastases (Fig. 16-9(a) to (e)). Hepatocellular carcinoma contains large pleomorphic multinucleated cells and is associated with preexisting liver disease including hepatitis B, cirrhosis, hemochromatosis, type I glycogen storage disease, and Wilson disease.

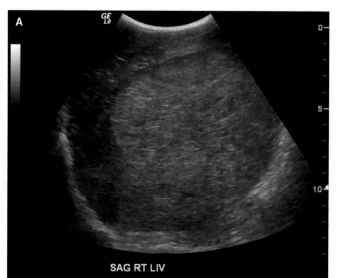

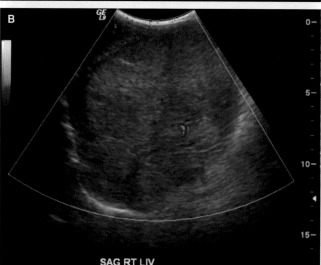

FIGURE 16-8. Hepatoblastoma demonstrated in the right liver lobe of a 3-year-old pediatric patient. Patient presented with abdominal distension and elevated liver enzymes.

Fibrolamellar Hepatocellular Carcinoma

Fibrolamellar hepatocellular carcinoma (FL-HCC) is a sub-type of HCC characterized by eosinophilic-laden hepatocytes surrounded by parallel fibrous bands. Although FL-HCC can occur in pediatric patients, it is more commonly seen in adults between 20 and 40 years of age. This malignant form of hepatocellular carcinoma is not associated with preexisting liver disease. Clinical findings include normal serum alpha-fetoprotein levels, hepatomegaly, and abdominal pain. The sonographic appearance is variable but may include a solitary, well-margin-ated tumor of varying echogenicity with focal calcifications and possible central scar. In contrast-enhanced ultrasound there can be inhomogeneous enhancement during the arterial phase and decreased echogenicity in the portal-venous phase of imaging.

Undifferentiated Embryonal Sarcoma

Undifferentiated embryonal sarcoma is also known as "hepatic mesenchymal sarcoma" and "malignant mesenchymoma." This mesenchymal myxoid matric spindle cell tumor contains cystic and cellular areas. Measuring between 7 and 20 centimeters, undifferentiated embryonal sarcoma affects children between 6 and 10 years of age and has a poor prognosis with survival rate less than 1 year. Clinical findings include normal serum alpha-fetoprotein levels, abdominal mass, and abdominal pain. The sonographic appearance includes a solitary solid or complex mass with septations, cystic spaces, and echogenic components.

Angiosarcoma

Angiosarcoma is a rare malignant endothelial cell tumor. Sonographic appearance includes a large heterogeneous cystic and solid mass with multiple satellite nodules.

Hepatic Leiomyosarcoma

Hepatic leiomyosarcoma is a rare malignant mesenchymal tumor associated with AIDS. The sonographic appearance includes a solid mass with cystic components, representing hemorrhage and necrosis.

Rhabdomyosarcoma

Rhabdomyosarcoma is a rare malignant tumor with nonspecific clinical imaging findings. Rhabdomyosarcoma may appear as a large solid tumor sonographically.

Metastases

Malignant tumors that most frequently metastasize to the liver include Wilms tumor, neuroblastoma, rhabdomyosarcoma, and lymphoma. The sonographic appearance includes a round hypoechoic mass with smooth, well-defined margins, and possible internal echoes related to hemorrhage.

Post-transplantation Lymphoproliferative Disorder

Post-transplantation lymphoproliferative disorder is a solid organ transplant complication that can be seen in many organs.

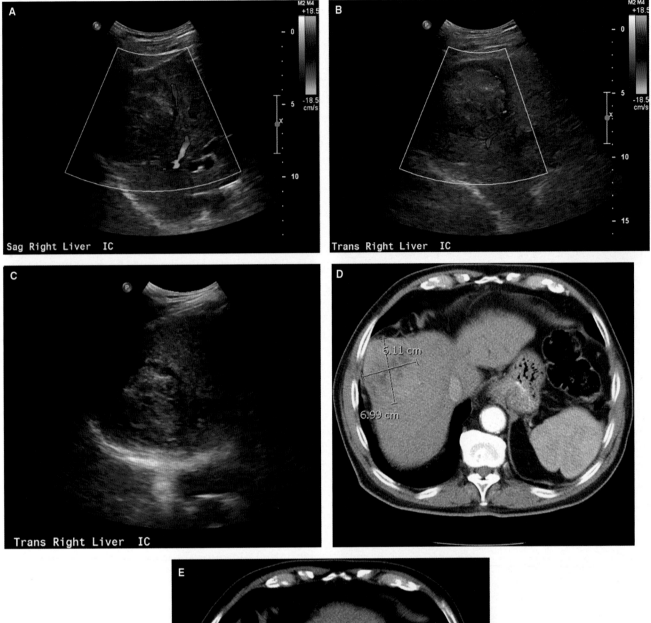

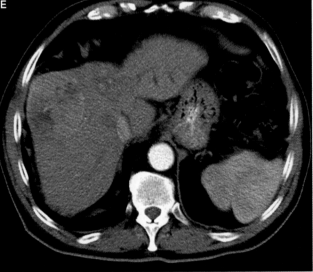

FIGURE 16-9. A sonographic heterogeneous mass determined to be hepatocellular carcinoma (HCC) in the right lobe of the liver. This mass correlates on CT as a solid hyperenhancing mass.

In the abdomen, the liver is most affected. This can also be visualized in the small bowel, colon, and stomach, although post-transplantation lymphoproliferative disorder is less common in the colon and stomach. This disorder can also affect the lungs, head, neck, primary central nervous system, cutaneous, and less commonly osseous structures. Post-transplantation lymphoproliferative disorder appears as a single or diffuse hypoechoic nodules with homogeneous or heterogeneous echotexture and well-defined margins within the transplanted liver. Periportal infiltration and biliary destruction may be present.

Lymphoma

Secondary to non-Hodgkin lymphoma, this malignancy appears as well-defined, homogeneous nodules of hypoechoic to anechoic echogenicity within an enlarged liver. Possible nodule septations may be present.

Leukemia

Leukemia appears as hepatosplenomegaly with para-aortic lymph node enlargement, ascites, and hypoechoic or hyperechoic lesions throughout the liver.

LIVER TRANSPLANT

Liver transplant is the only treatment for end-stage liver disease and is performed via whole cadaveric allograft, split cadaveric allograft, or living related donor allograft. With living related donor allograft, the right or left lobe is taken from the living donor and transplanted to the child recipient. Sonography is used to determine post-transplant anatomy, size, and patency of the liver and portal vein to evaluate for proper direction of flow. Hepatic artery thrombosis occurs in 40% of allografts in the first two post-operative months. PVT occurs in 3 to 10% of pediatric liver transplants. IVC thrombosis occurs in less than 1% of cases. Parenchymal complications of transplant include infarct, abscess, hematoma, biloma, seroma, and rejection.

Sonogram of a liver transplant involves evaluation of the transplant in its entirety including patency of vasculature. The native liver prior to transplant, the intraoperative, and postoperative transplanted liver should be carefully evaluated for optimal patient outcome.

Preoperative Transplant Imaging Technique

Still images:

1. Preoperatively, the sonographer should document diameter and patency of the extrahepatic portal vein in long-axis.
2. Using color and spectral Doppler, document direction of flow within the portal vein in long-axis.
3. Measurement should be obtained at the widest location (typically halfway between the splenic and SMV confluence and the portal bifurcation).
4. If portal venous diameter measures less than 4 millimeters, the diameter should also be measured at the confluence.
5. Evaluate patency of the IVC. IVC patency can be affected in patients with biliary atresia, involving interruption of a short segment below the confluence of the hepatic veins.
6. The sonographer should evaluate the preoperative liver in 2 imaging planes for hepatic masses, portal hypertension, and collateral routes.

Note: Pre-transplantation evaluation of the native hepatic artery and hepatic veins are of less importance. Hepatic veins in the native liver are generally only evaluated pre-transplantation if observing specifically for Budd Chiari syndrome, which is uncommon in pediatric patients. Arterial issues more commonly arise in the donor liver and are cared for at the time of transplant by way of conduit grafts or arterial reconstruction. If a hepatic mass is found in the pre-transplant liver, it should be documented. If there are any pancreatic abnormalities, such as history of pancreatitis, the sonographer should also image the pancreas. If present, the gallbladder, and any presence of biliary ductal dilatation should be imaged. If hydronephrosis is present, this may need to be resolved prior to liver transplantation and therefore the kidneys should also be surveyed.

INTRAOPERATIVE TRANSPLANT IMAGING TECHNIQUE

Intraoperatively, ultrasound may be requested by the surgeon to identify the portal vein, hepatic vein, and hepatic artery patency, demonstrating adequate liver graft function. If ultrasound is needed, the sonographer should inquire with the operating room (OR) staff where to connect the ultrasound unit to power supply. The ultrasound unit should not be connected to power supply with existing OR equipment already in use.

A sterile sleeve should cover the transducer. A 5-MHz curved array or sector transducer should be used for adolescents and larger habitus patients. A 7-MHz sector or linear transducer should be used for young or smaller habitus patients.

Often the surgeon or radiologist handles the transducer. If a radiologist is present and scrubs into the case, the radiologist will guide the surgeon's transducer placement and orientation. The sonographer should assist the radiologist or surgeon in capturing optimal images and obtaining cine clips as necessary in handling of the ultrasound unit.

Still Images:

1. Sagittal evaluation of the extrahepatic portal vein and hepatic artery, with and without color and spectral Doppler
2. Imaging of the right and left portal vein and hepatic artery branches, with and without color and spectral Doppler
3. The IVC and hepatic veins are evaluated only if requested by the surgeon

Early Postoperative Imaging Technique

Before performing the initial post-operative study, the sonographer should contact the surgeon or review the operative record for anastomoses-type to reduce probability of diagnostic errors. This initial examination is limited to the liver and surrounding areas.

Still images:

1. Liver parenchyma, evaluating for appropriate echogenicity, focal abnormalities, presence of biliary ductal dilation, and positioning of the biliary stent.
2. Patency of vasculature, evaluating in grayscale, color, and spectral Doppler waveforms the MPV, hepatic artery, hepatic veins, and IVC.

The long axis of the MPV including anastomosis-site, portal venous bifurcation demonstrating the "Y" of the right and left branches, IVC-hepatic vein confluence in transverse plane, and sagittal view of the IVC should be demonstrated. RI should be obtained in the main, right, and left hepatic arteries. If anastomosis is visualized, image pre- and post-anastomosis in the main hepatic artery. The sonographer should also document any presence of intraluminal thrombus, anastomotic narrowing, portal venous jets or eddy currents, and flow in the IVC.

3. Ascites and fluid collections within the liver or in close proximity to vessels, ruling out pseudoaneurysm versus collections.
4. Any presence of right adrenal hemorrhage.
5. Coronal and transverse images of the spleen, observing for splenic infarcts.

Late Postoperative Imaging Technique

Late postoperative exams should address any specific clinical problems and tailored to the patient's unique case. If exam indication is unclear, it is the sonographer's responsibility to consult with the radiologist or ordering physician prior to examination.

1. The liver parenchyma should be re-evaluated, carefully observing vasculature and the biliary ductal system.
2. Reobserve for ascites and fluid collections.
   a. Check the right and left lower quadrants, pelvis, and cul-de-sac for presence of ascites.

If child has an unexplained fever, the entire abdomen should be surveyed for presence of collections, ruling out possibility of abscess.

Gallbladder and Biliary Pathology

CHOLELITHIASIS

Cholelithiasis is the presence of stones, or calculi, within the gallbladder. Gallstones are formed because of elevated liver cholesterol secretion or decrease in bile salts from irregular enterohepatic circulation. When bile cholesterol secretion exceeds its ability to hold a soluble form, small crystals result and solidify, becoming gallstones. In the pediatric population, gallstones are more commonly seen in adolescents. Clinical symptoms include right upper quadrant abdominal pain, jaundice, and vomiting. These symptoms may be more pronounced following a meal. Sonographic findings include highly attenuating, hyperechoic, nonvascular, spheric structures with posterior acoustic shadowing (Figs. 17-1 and 17-2). A phenomenon known as a "wall-echo-shadow" (WES) sign (Fig. 17-3) occurs in the presence of numerous, small gallstones or a single, large gallstone which fills the lumen of a partially visualized or contracted gallbladder. An anterior curved, hyperechoic line is visualized at the gallstone's surface, just beneath the gallbladder lumen. Posterior to the highly attenuating gallstone's surface, a large acoustic posterior shadow is produced. When imaging the gallbladder, the sonographer should demonstrate whether gallstones are mobile or non-mobile by imaging in two patient positions, such as supine and left lateral decubitus.

BILIARY SLUDGE

Biliary sludge is made of calcium salts, cholesterol crystals, calcium bilirubinate, and other bile precipitates layered along the dependent portion of the gallbladder. Sonographic findings include non-shadowing, nonvascular, low-medium echoes in the dependent gallbladder, or a fluid-fluid level that changes with patient position (Fig. 17-4).

HYDROPS

Hydrops is a distension of the gallbladder without inflammation. Hydrops of the gallbladder measures greater than 3 centimeters in length in infants less than 1 year of age, and greater than 7 centimeters in length in adolescents (Fig. 17-5).

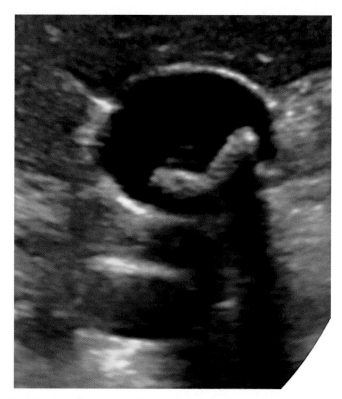

FIGURE 17-1. Transverse gallbladder with dependant cholelithiasis (gallstones) creating posterior shadowing artifact.

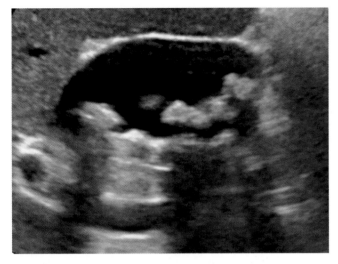

FIGURE 17-2. Sagittal gallbladder with dependant cholelithiasis (gallstones) creating posterior shadowing artifact.

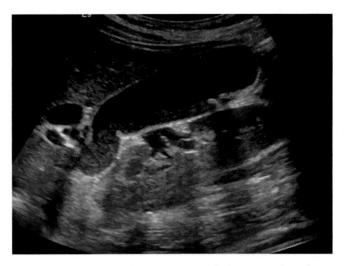

FIGURE 17-4. Low-level echoes representing sludge present throughout gallbladder neck and body in a 13-year-old.

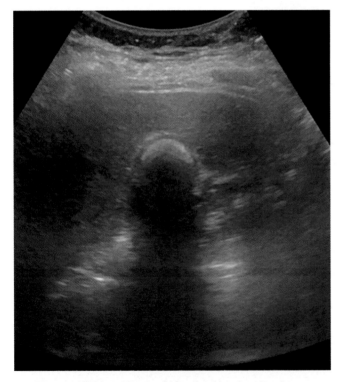

FIGURE 17-3. WES in an 18-year-old female with epigastric pain.

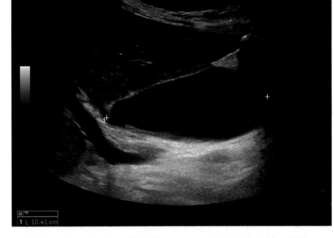

FIGURE 17-5. Hydropic gallbladder in a 9-year-old with sickle cell disease and acute myeloid leukemia measuring up to 10.4 cm.

NEONATAL CHOLESTASIS

Cholestasis in the neonate results from bile flow impairment due to intra- or extrahepatic disorders. Cholestasis is conjugated hyperbilirubinemia caused by unconjugated and indirect reacting bilirubin deposit in the reticuloendothelial system. Clinical symptoms include jaundice, hepatomegaly, elevated bilirubin, dark yellow urine, and acholic stools. Sonographic findings include biliary duct dilation, sludge, and/or hyperechoic gallstones.

CHOLECYSTITIS

Cholecystitis is inflammation or infection of the gallbladder.

CHRONIC CHOLECYSTITIS

Chronic cholecystitis is a long-term inflammation of the gallbladder resulting from intermittent cystic duct blockage.

ACALCULUS CHOLECYSTITIS

Acalculus cholecystitis is inflammation of the gallbladder without the presence of gallstones (Figs 17-6 and 17-7).

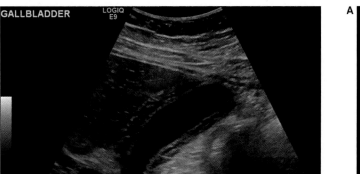

FIGURE 17-6.   Sagittal gallbladder with marked wall thickening in an immunocompromised 13-year-old male with acute onset right upper quadrant pain and positive Murphy's sign.

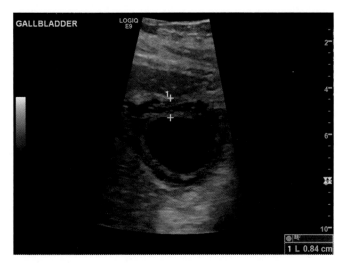

FIGURE 17-7.   Transverse gallbladder with marked wall thickening in an immunocompromised 13-year-old male with acute onset right upper quadrant pain and positive Murphy's sign.

ACUTE CALCULUS CHOLECYSTITIS

Acute calculus cholecystitis is an acute inflammation of the gallbladder due to gallstone obstruction of the gallbladder neck or cystic duct. Acute calculus cholecystitis is the most common cause of pain in the right upper quadrant of the abdomen.

CHOLEDOCHOLITHIASIS

Choledocholithiasis is a complete or partial obstruction of the bile ducts due to the presence of calculi, with the common bile duct (CBD) most often affected (Fig. 17-8(a) and (b)). Stones within the bile ducts commonly originate from the gallbladder.

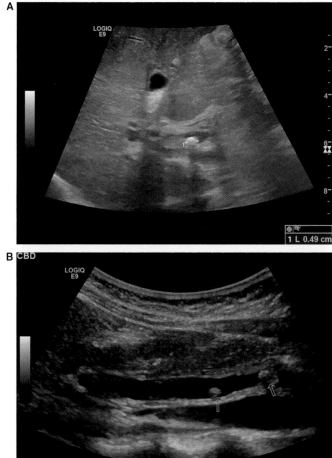

FIGURE 17-8.   Multiple stones present in the common bile duct in a 3-year-old female status post cholecystectomy with hereditary spherocytosis.

MIRIZZI SYNDROME

Mirizzi syndrome is an obstruction of the extrahepatic biliary tree resulting from a blocked cystic duct. Mirizzi syndrome is associated with cystic duct inflammatory processes or as a result of extrinsic compression.

BILE PLUG SYNDROME

Also known as "inspissated bile syndrome," bile plug syndrome is an extrahepatic syndrome of the bile duct resulting from sludge.

SCLEROSING CHOLANGITIS

Sclerosing cholangitis is a chronic inflammation resulting in fibrosis of the extrahepatic and intrahepatic biliary ducts.

CHOLEDOCHAL CYST

Choledochal cyst is a rare congenital disorder of unknown etiology involving cystic dilation of the biliary tree. A classification system created by Todani et al categorizes choledochal cysts into five types with additional subtypes. It is suspected some subtypes of choledochal cyst are associated with anomalous formation at the junction of the pancreas and biliary ducts, creating an enlarged shared channel that drains the pancreatic and biliary ducts. This disorder has a slight predominance in female patients of East Asian descent, with a 1:4 male to female ratio. Approximately 60% of choledochal cysts are discovered in patients less than 10 years of age. Sonographic findings include a saccular dilation of the common hepatic duct or CBD. Clinical symptoms include jaundice, abdominal pain, and least commonly a palpable abdominal mass.

BILIARY ATRESIA

Biliary atresia is a congenital disorder involving biliary system obstruction with absence of extrahepatic bile ducts and intrahepatic bile duct proliferation. The patient may present with jaundice, a distended abdomen, and darkened urine. Sonographic findings include an abnormal-appearing or absent gallbladder, hepatomegaly, increased diameter of the hepatic artery, difficulty visualizing the biliary system, and echogenic triangular cord sign (triangular fibrous tissue at the porta hepatis).

18

Splenic Pathology

SPLENOMEGALY

Splenomegaly (Fig. 18-1(a) and (b)) refers to enlargement of the spleen. Common disorders associated with splenomegaly are infectious processes such as Epstein-Barr virus, cat-scratch disease, leukemia, and lymphoma. Other causes of splenic enlargement may include portal hypertension, portal vein thrombosis, and storage disorders such as Gaucher disease and Neimann-Pick disease. Hematologic elements secondary to extracorporeal oxygenation (ECMO) related to splenic pooling of red blood cells that are damaged during ECMO may also cause splenomegaly.

POLYSPLENIA

Polysplenia is the presence of multiple splenic nodules in the right or left upper quadrant (Fig. 18-2). Polysplenia may be associated with other abdominal and thoracic anomalies such as short pancreas, bowel rotation, and cardiac abnormalities. The sonographic appearance of polysplenia may include multiple small isoechoic nodules of splenic tissue within the right upper quadrant or two large spleens with multiple smaller splenic nodules in the left upper quadrant.

ACCESSORY SPLEEN

An accessory spleen is a normal anatomic variant, which occurs more commonly than polysplenia. This variant occurs secondary to failure of embryonic splenic tissue bud fusion in the dorsal mesogastrium. The accessory spleen is usually located near the splenic hilum or along the vessels, but can also be found in the scrotum or attached to the left ovary due to close relationship during development in utero. An accessory spleen has no clinical significance and has the same sonographic appearance as normal splenic tissue.

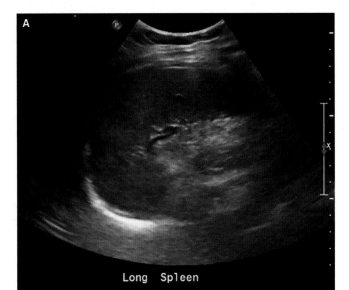

FIGURE 18-1. Splenomegaly in a 12-year-old patient measuring 13.9 cm. The normal range for splenic dimensions in patients 11 to 12.9 years of age is between 7.5 and 11.5 cm.

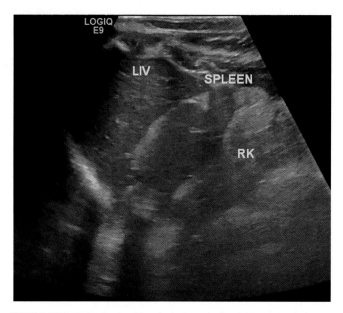

FIGURE 18-2. Polysplenia with splenic tissue in the right upper quadrant in a patient with heterotaxy.

WANDERING SPLEEN

A wandering spleen has no fixed ligamentous attachments, resulting in a highly mobile spleen that may change position in the abdomen. The ligaments that normally hold the spleen in place consist of the gastrosplenic and splenorenal ligaments. A wandering spleen can also rotate centrally or inferiorly, causing intermittent torsion and abdominal pain or infarct. Intermittent splenic torsion may present as a palpable mass on clinical examination. Sonographic findings of a wandering spleen include absence of the spleen in its normal location or a mass elsewhere in the abdomen with splenic tissue echotexture.

SPLENIC INFARCTION

Splenic infarction (Fig. 18-3(a) to (c)) is an occlusion of the splenic artery or its branches. Splenic infarction results most commonly from hematologic disorders, hypercoagulable states (i.e., factor V Leiden), and embolic events. Splenic infarction from hematologic disorders (i.e., sickle cell disease) is more common in young patients, while infarct from embolic events (i.e., marantic endocarditis, infective endocarditis) is more common in older patients. Additional etiologic factors that contribute to splenic infarction include splenic arterial aneurysms, collagen vascular disease, granulomatosis with polyangiitis, compression of the splenic artery (i.e., by tumor of the pancreas), and leukemia. Splenic infarction appears as an avascular wedge-shaped hypoechoic lesion.

SPLENIC TORSION

Splenic torsion occurs when the spleen rotates, reducing or terminating normal blood flow. Complications of splenic torsion and infarct include abscess formation, bowel obstruction,

pancreatitis, or necrosis of the pancreatic tail, and if venous congestion is present, gastric varices may develop. Surgical treatment is required for splenic salvage and splenectomy is reserved as a final resort.

SPLENOSIS

Splenosis is an acquired condition resulting from splenic rupture secondary to trauma or auto transplantation of splenic tissue surgery. Splenic tissue can be found most commonly in the peritoneum, as well as the abdomen or chest. The sonographic appearance of splenosis includes round masses indistinguishable from an accessory spleen.

ASPLENIA

Asplenia is simply the absence of splenic tissue. Asplenia is associated with total or partial situs inversus, microgastria, and intestinal malrotation.

SPLENIC CYSTS

Clinical findings of splenic cysts may include a palpable mass within the patient's left upper quadrant, epigastric fullness, low grade pain from organ compression, or acute pain from cyst rupture or infection. Congenital splenic cysts, otherwise known as true epidermoid cysts, are lined with epithelium. These cysts are solitary, unilocular, contain a smooth fibrous wall, and appear as a well-defined hypoechoic or anechoic lesion with through-transmission and absent blood flow (Fig. 18-4). Whether the cyst is filled with protein, blood, fat, or cholesterol will determine if it has a turbid hypoechoic or clear anechoic sonographic appearance.

SITUS INVERSUS OF THE SPLEEN

Situs inversus is a mirror-image anomaly of single or multiple organs. Situs inversus of the spleen will have a sonographic appearance of solid and vascular splenic tissues within the right upper quadrant, rather than the typical left upper quadrant (Figs. 18-5 and 18-6).

INFECTIONS

Pyogenic Abscess

Pyogenic abscess can result from penetrating injuries and hematogenous seeding of infection, however, hepatic abscess can occur from other routes. The most common organism to cause pyogenic abscess is Escherichia coli in neonates and staphylococcus infection in infants and children, but streptococcus and salmonella can also result in splenic abscess formation. Clinical findings include fever and abdominal pain. Sonographic appearance includes a hypoechoic complex mass with internal

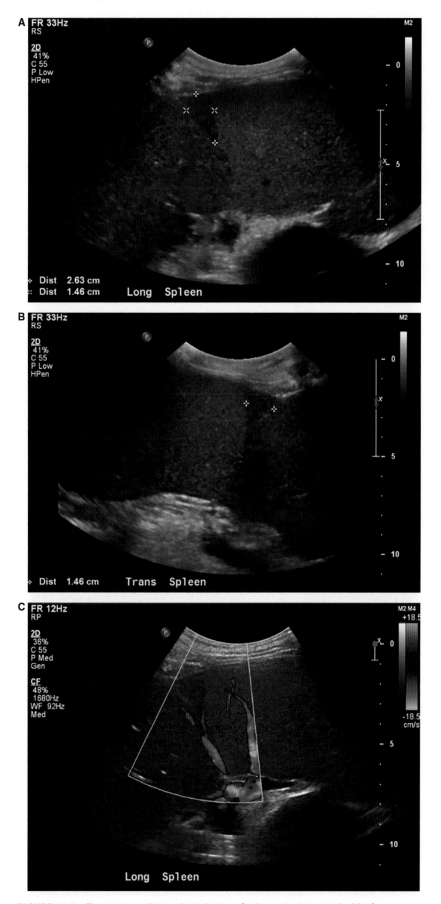

FIGURE 18-3. Chronic vague hypoechoic density of spleen, consistent with old infarct.

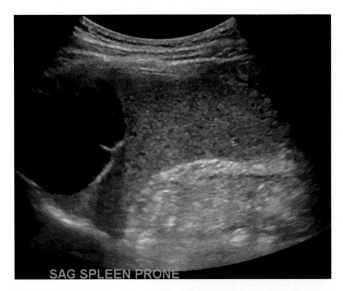

FIGURE 18-4. Splenic cyst in a 16-year-old patient with thin, single partial septation.

echoes, fluid-fluid level, septations, and echogenic foci with shadow and ring-down artifact resulting from gas within the abscess cavity. Surrounding lymphadenopathy may also be visualized. Pyogenic abscess is treated via percutaneous aspiration or catheter drainage and antibiotic therapy.

Fungal Abscess

Fungal abscess can occur in immunocompromised children due to Candida albicans or Aspergillus fungi. Sonographic appearance includes multiple small, homogeneous, hypoechoic lesions with a hyperechoic "wheel within a wheel" or bullseye patterns throughout the liver, spleen, and kidneys. Echogenic foci with acoustic shadowing may also be present. Fungal infection may mimic metastases, lymphoma, and other diseases.

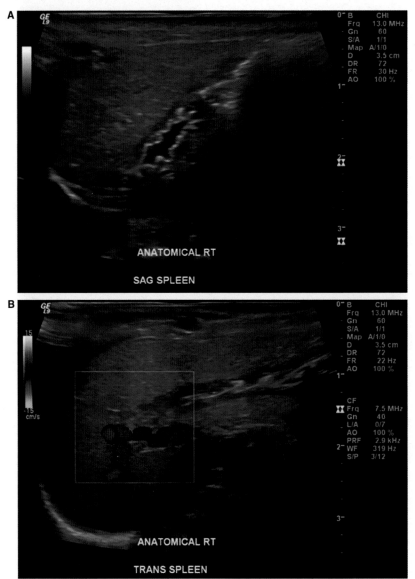

FIGURE 18-5. Situs inversus with demonstration of the spleen in the patient's anatomical right abdomen.

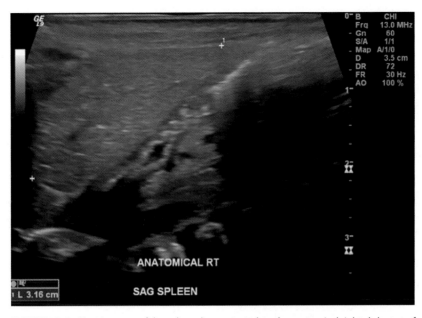

FIGURE 18-6. Situs inversus of the spleen demonstrated on the anatomical right abdomen of a 1-day old premature infant, born at 29-weeks, 6-days gestational age.

Acquired Immunodeficiency Syndrome (AIDS)

Patients with acquired immunodeficiency syndrome (AIDS) have increased risk of developing splenic abscess due to their immunocompromised state. Patients with AIDS may develop abscess secondary to Candida albicans, tuberculosis, and cytomegalovirus. Sonographic appearance is similar to fungal abscess, and may include multiple small homogeneous, hypoechoic, lesions with hyperechoic wheel within a "wheel or bullseye" patterns throughout the liver, spleen, and kidneys.

BENIGN LESIONS

Hemangioma

Hemangioma is the most common primary splenic neoplasm. This benign mass is comprised of red blood cells, a single endothelial layer, and multiple vascular channels. Sonographic appearance includes a well-defined homogeneous, hyperechoic, hypervascular lesion (Fig. 18-7(a) and (b)). Splenic hemangioma can be associated with Beckwith-Wiedemann and Klippel-Trenaunay-Weber syndromes. With these syndromes, hemangioma is seen along with port-wine stain, venous varicosities, and overgrowth of extremity soft tissue and bone.

Littoral Cell Angioma

Littoral cell angioma is a rare benign vascular neoplasm. Littoral cell angioma arises from splenic red pulp sinus lining and littoral cells with branching vascular channels. Sonographic appearance includes lesions of varying size and echogenicity with vascular flow. Although rare, this etiology may be encountered as a distractor on the registry exam.

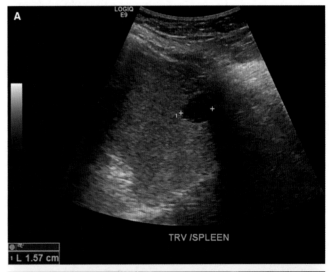

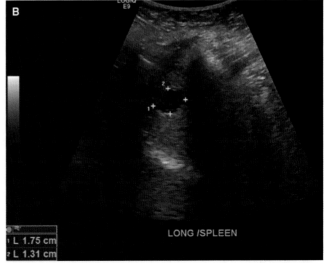

FIGURE 18-7. Atypical hypoechoic hemangioma in a 16-year-old pediatric patient with history of spina-bifida.

Peliosis

Peliosis is a rare benign neoplasm consisting of multiple blood-filled spaces without endothelial lining throughout the spleen. Peliosis is associated with HIV, tuberculosis, hematologic malignancy, and use of anabolic steroids. Sonographic appearance includes small hypoechoic lesions that have potential to form into a large multiloculated, septated mass. Although rare, this etiology may be encountered as a distractor on the registry exam.

Lymphangioma

Lymphangioma is a benign congenital malformation of the lymphatic system composed of endothelial lined lymph-filled spaces separated by fibrous bands. Sonographic appearance includes a multilocular cyst containing hypoechoic and anechoic locules, echogenic septations with calcified components, and avascularity noted on Doppler examination. When the multilocular cyst is hypoechoic, hemorrhagic components are involved.

Hamartoma

Hamartoma is a benign solid lymphoid tissue lesion with disorganized congested splenic sinuses, or red pulp. Sonographically, hamartoma appears as well-defined, vascular, hypoechoic masses with complex or cystic change. This neoplasm is associated with Beckwith-Wiedemann syndrome and tuberous sclerosis.

Inflammatory Pseudotumor

Inflammatory pseudotumor is a rare benign fibroblastic inflammatory pseudotumor composed of stroma, polymorphous inflammatory cells, plasma cells, lymphocytes, neutrophils, and eosinophils. Sonographic appearance includes a well-defined hypervascular, hypoechoic mass with possible calcification in the matrix or wall of the lesion. Although rare, this etiology may be encountered as a distractor on the registry exam.

MALIGNANT LESIONS

Lymphoma

Lymphoma is the most common malignant splenic neoplasm occurring in Hodgkin and non-Hodgkin patients. Sonographic findings include an enlarged spleen with solitary or multiple avascular hypoechoic to anechoic masses without acoustic enhancement. Surrounding lymphadenopathy may be present in the splenic hilum and retroperitoneum.

Leukemia

During active stages or remission leukemia can involve the spleen's red pulp. This malignant neoplasm causes discrete nodules and splenomegaly.

Langerhans Cell Histiocytosis

Langerhans cell histiocytosis is a malignant neoplasm that may cause splenomegaly or multiple hypoechoic nodules within the spleen.

Angiosarcoma

Angiosarcoma is a rare malignant splenic tumor composed of disorganized anastomosing vascular channels lined by endothelial cells with large irregular nuclei and high mitotic rate. Angiosarcoma frequently leads to early widespread metastases to lymph nodes, bone, liver, and lung tissues. Sonographic appearance includes solid or complex mass with Doppler flow in the solid echogenic portions of the tumor. Although rare, this etiology may be encountered as a distractor on the registry exam.

19

Intestinal Pathology

PYLORIC STENOSIS

Hypertrophic pyloric stenosis (HPS) is considered an acquired gastric outlet obstruction of the pylorus' circular muscle, resulting in narrowing of the pyloric channel. Pyloric stenosis appears as a hypervascular target or bullseye sign in the transverse imaging plane (Fig. 19-1). This bullseye represents the thick hypoechoic muscle surrounding the echogenic mucosa. In the sagittal imaging plane, pyloric stenosis resembles a hypervascular thickened pyloric muscle (Fig. 19-2) which surrounds an elongated, narrow pyloric channel (Fig. 19-3). The *antral nipple sign* presents when the pyloric channel mucosa prolapses into the gastric antrum. Positive findings of HPS include inability to view gastric emptying (Fig. 19-4(a) and (b)), a pyloric wall thickness equal to or greater than 3 millimeters, and an elongated pyloric channel measuring greater

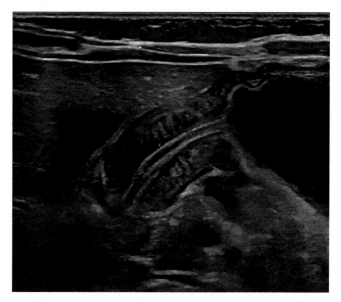

FIGURE 19-2. Long axis view of hypertrophic pyloric stenosis, markedly thick wall.

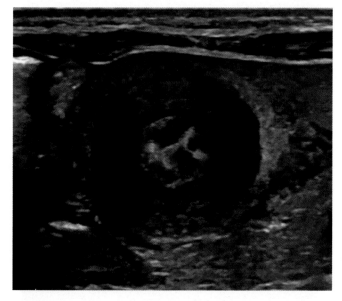

FIGURE 19-1. Short axis view of hypertrophic pyloric stenosis, markedly thick wall.

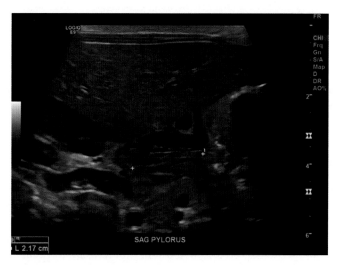

FIGURE 19-3. Lengthened pyloric channel.

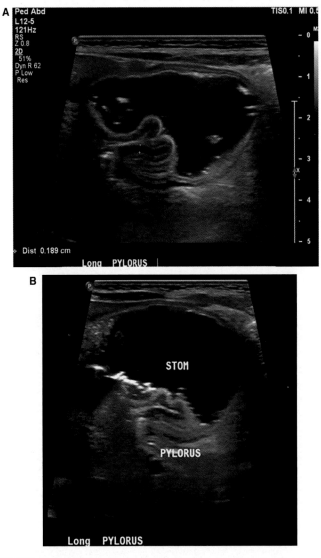

FIGURE 19-4. Gastric contents not visualized passing through pyloric channel.

TABLE 19-1 • Criteria for Pyloric Stenosis
Abnormal pylorus measurements:
Pyloric channel >17 mm
Anterior muscle wall thickness >3 mm
In previous years, a pyloric channel measuring > 14 millimeters was considered abnormal. Current sources note that a pyloric channel is lengthened when > 17 millimeters. However, a pyloric channel measuring between 15 and 17 millimeters may be abnormal and should be closely evaluated.

than 17 millimeters (Table 19-1). Symptoms typically present between 2 and 6 weeks of age and may continue up to 5 months. Clinical findings include projectile nonbilious vomiting, a palpable olive-shaped mass in the epigastrium region, and gastric hyperperistalsis. HPS is 4 to 5 times more likely to occur in males. Pyloric stenosis also has a familial predisposition and occurs in approximately three out of every 1,000 children. The

current treatment for HPS is pyloromyotomy, also called the "Ramstedt procedure." This procedure splits the hypertrophic muscle longitudinally without affecting the pyloric mucosa. While scanning for pyloric stenosis, it is pertinent to not mistake pyloric stenosis with pylorospasm or antral dyskinesia, in which the antrum and pyloric channel spasm. This spasm may cause delayed gastric emptying and nonbilious vomiting in infants, as well as possible thickening of the muscle during the spasm. This muscle thickening should resolve upon spasm completion, thus ruling out pyloric stenosis.

Ultrasound of the pylorus is a common exam ordered for evaluation of HPS. It is preferred that the patient be fasting for 2 hours prior to exam. This exam should be performed between 0 and 4 months of age. The protocol for pyloric ultrasound involves imaging of the pylorus in supine or right posterior oblique position. The pylorus is first evaluated prior to the patient being fed sterile water or Pedialyte. The sonographer should document images of the pylorus in sagittal and transverse imaging planes to include length of the pyloric channel and thickness of the pyloric muscle wall. If the pyloric channel appears lengthened and measures greater than 17 millimeters or the anterior muscle wall appears thickened and measures greater than 3 millimeters, the sonographer should call a pediatric radiologist prior to giving the patient fluids. If pyloric measurements are within normal limits, the baby should be fed 1 oz of fluids and rescanned (Figs. 19-5 and 19-6). The sonographer

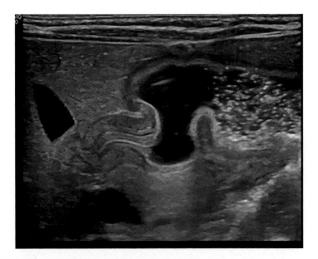

FIGURE 19-5. Pylorus post-Pedialyte, long-axis.

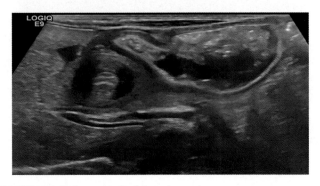

FIGURE 19-6. Pylorus post-Pedialyte, short axis.

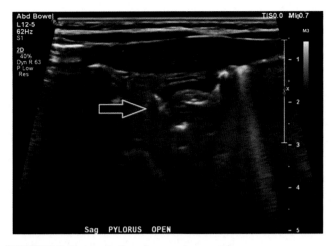

FIGURE 19-7. Demonstration of a normal, open pylorus. If the exam is negative, images of the transverse pancreas should be obtained to show the relationship of the SMA and SMV. Pyloric stenosis is also a gradual thickening of the pylorus. If measurements are borderline, a follow up scan may be recommended at a minimum of 48 hours (preferably 72 hours) following the initial scan.

should document images of the gastric antrum as it fills with fluid, surveying if the pyloric muscle opens or if it appears thickened. Static images and cine loops of fluid flowing through the antrum and pylorus should be obtained (Fig. 19-7).

Still images:

1. Sagittal pylorus
2. Sagittal pylorus with pyloric channel measurement
3. Tranverse pylorus
4. Transverse pylorus with pyloric wall measurement

> **Note:** If measurements are above normal limits, the sonographer should include a color Doppler image of the pylorus and call a pediatric radiologist prior to giving the patient fluids. If measurements are within normal limits, the sonographer should proceed with administering 1 oz of fluids orally to the patient prior to rescanning.

5. Sagittal antrum as it fills with fluid, adjacent to the pylorus (Fig. 19-5)
6. Sagittal image of an open pylorus, with fluid passing through the pyloric channel (Fig. 19-7)
7. Transverse relationship of the superior mesenteric artery (SMA) and superior mesenteric vein (SMV)(Fig. 19-8)

> **Note:** To determine the cause of gastrointestinal obstruction and infantile vomiting, the SMA/SMV relationship is evaluated to rule out malrotation in the scenario of a negative pylorus examination. Ultrasound may demonstrate inversion of the SMA/SMV if the SMV is on the patient's anatomic left and the SMA is on the patient's anatomic right. A *whirlpool* sign may be visualized when malrotation is present (Fig. 19-9(a) and (b)).

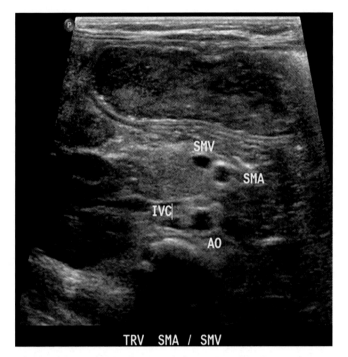

FIGURE 19-8. Normal SMA/SMV relationship. The SMA/SMV is evaluated to rule out malrotation anomaly during a negative pylorus examination. Ultrasound may demonstrate inversion of the SMA/SMV in transverse imaging plane if the SMV is demonstrated on the patient's left (right of screen) and the SMA is on the patient's right (left of screen).

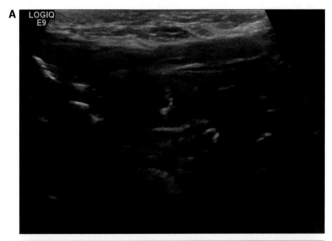

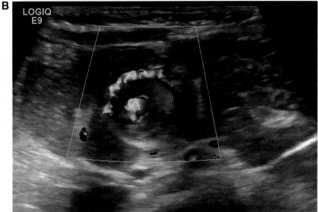

FIGURE 19-9. Images of an abnormal SMA/SMV relationship with a classic whirlpool sign, in a 3-month-old male: (a) Gray scale image; (b) Color Doppler Image.

Cine clips:

1. Fluid flowing through the antrum and open pyloric channel.

MALROTATION AND MIDGUT VOLVULUS

Malrotation is a congenital, anatomical anomaly resulting from abnormal intestinal rotation during embryogenesis. Normally, the SMA is located to the left of the SMV (Fig. 19-8). Inversion of the SMA and SMV is a sign for malrotation. Volvulus is a twisting of the bowel that impedes blood flow. As a result of blood flow impedance, there is cessation of normal peristalsis of bowel contents. Bowel obstruction and ischemia may result as the bowel twists. As the SMA and SMV become compressed and engorged, edematous tissue results from the lack of perfusion. Sonographic findings for volvulus include the whirlpool sign, free fluid, fluid-filled small bowel loops due to obstruction proximally and thickened abnormal bowel wall distal to the site of obstruction. The treatment option for malrotation involves prompt, planned (urgent, but not emergent) surgical intervention using a Ladd's (Ladd) procedure to prevent volvulus. If volvulus occurs, left untreated, it can lead to an entire midgut infarction. Surgical intervention for volvulus is critical to prevent gut infarction and is considered an emergency.

If malrotation is present, it may be associated with additional abdominal anomalies including defects of the digestive system, congenital diaphragmatic herniation, heterotaxy, gastroschisis, omphalocele, duodenal atresia, duodenal web, duodenal stenosis, choanal atresia, abnormalities of other organs including the liver or spleen, and heart defects.

INTUSSUSCEPTION

Intussusception is telescoping of a proximal segment of intestine, the intussusceptum, into a caudal segment of bowel, the intussuscipiens (Fig. 19-10). Intussusception is the most common acute abdominal disorder of early childhood. This disorder is most common between 3 months and 3 years of age, with peak occurrence between 5 and 9 months. Approximately 90% of intussusceptions are ileocolic in location, with no pathologic lead points for the intussusception to occur.

Although many cases of intussusception are idiopathic, a notable correlation has been made following episodes of gastroenteritis and other viral or bacterial gastrointestinal tract infections. With infection, lymph-tissue swells, creating a pressure that can pull the intussusceptum into the intussuscipiens. Additionally, lead points such as a tumor, enlarged lymph nodes, and blood-vessel abnormalities may cause bowel to catch during peristalsis, increasing the likelihood of intussusception occurrence (Figs. 19-11 and 19-12).

Sonographic findings include a transverse donut or target sign. This target sign represents a complex mass with concentric hypoechoic and hyperechoic rings. The echogenic portion of these rings consists of mucosa and submucosa, with the hypoechoic portion being the muscularis. Some other sonographic findings associated with intussusception include inversion of mesenteric vessels, peritoneal fluid, and dilation of small bowel proximal to the site of intussusception. In an elongated sagittal view intussusception exhibits a pseudokidney sign (Figs. 19-13 and 19-14).

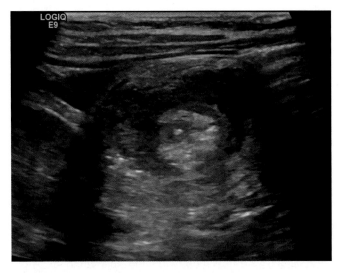

FIGURE 19-11. Intussusception containing appendix.

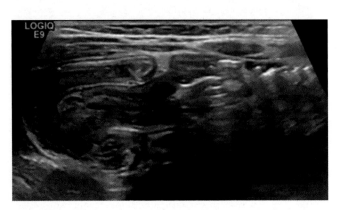

FIGURE 19-10. Intussusceptum and intussuscipiens.

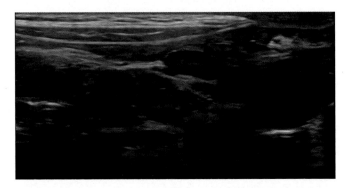

FIGURE 19-12. Surrounding lymph nodes visualized with SBI.

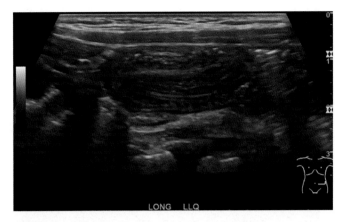

FIGURE 19-13. SBI, pseudokidney sign in sagittal plane.

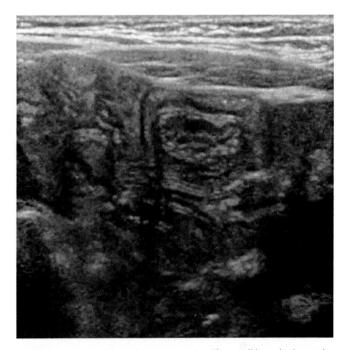

FIGURE 19-15. Small bowel intussusception. The small bowel is located centrally, versus the peripheral large bowel. Small bowel intussusception typically measures less than 2.5 centimeters. Intussusceptum of a transient small bowel intussusception intermittently slides in and out of the intussuscipiens. SBI generally reduce themselves and may be considered an incidental finding, particularly with cases of enteritis or Henoch-Schoenlein purpura.

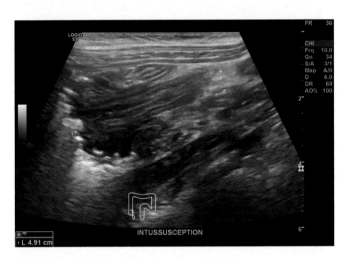

FIGURE 19-14. LBI pseudokidney sign in sagittal plane.

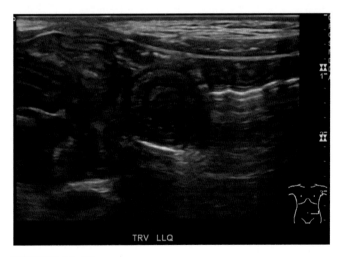

FIGURE 19-16. SBI.

Clinical signs and symptoms of intussusception may include stool changes such as diarrhea or a "currant jelly" stool appearance, resulting from a combination of blood and mucous in the stool. Additionally, clinical presentation of intussusception can have variation based on age. Infants tend to be lethargic, have stool changes, and swelling of the abdomen. Young children more often experience vomiting and will draw the knees upward and cry during intermittent spells of abdominal pain.

The most noticeable difference between benign and complicated intussusception is the dimension of the intussusception. The measurement of a transient small bowel intussusception is smaller in diameter (Figs. 19-15, 19-16, and 19-17) compared to the diameter of a large bowel intussusception (Figs. 19-18, 19-19, and 19-20(a)-(b)). Mean lesion diameter of an ileocolic large bowel intussusception is 2.63 centimeters in diameter, ranging between 1.3 and 4.0 centimeters. Comparatively, mean lesion diameter for a small-bowel intussusception is 1.42 centimeters, ranging between 0.8 and 3.0 centimeters. The presence of blood flow in a large bowel intussusception is suggestive of reducibility (Fig. 19-21). Current treatment options consist of air reduction, called "pneumatic reduction," hydrostatic reduction which involves the use

of a water-soluble contrast, or reduction using a barium contrast agent using fluoroscopic guidance. In 90% of cases, air or barium enema is successful in reduction of intussusception. For an intussusception reduction procedure, the patient is placed in a supine position, a catheter is inserted rectally, and a form of contrast agent (i.e., barium, Cysto-Conray II) is introduced into the colon via gravity until the intussusception is encountered. Sonographic guidance, although less commonly used, is now an accepted method of performing hydrostatic reduction of intussusception using Ringer's lactate solution,

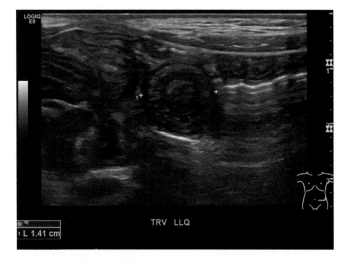

FIGURE 19-17. Transient SBI.

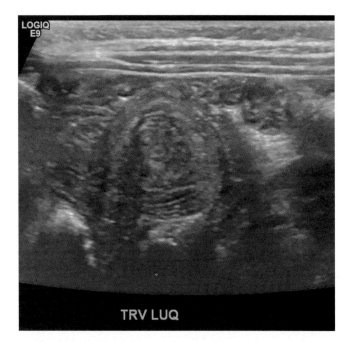

FIGURE 19-18. Large bowel intussusception.

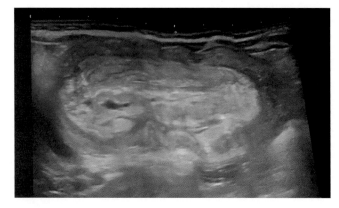

FIGURE 19-19. Panoramic view of large bowel intussusception.

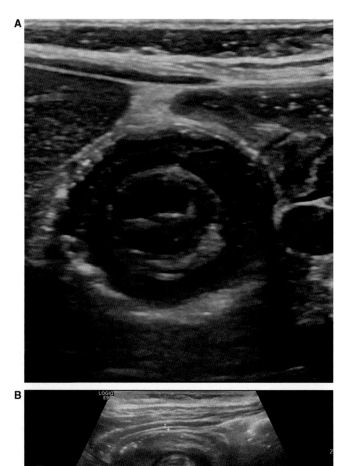

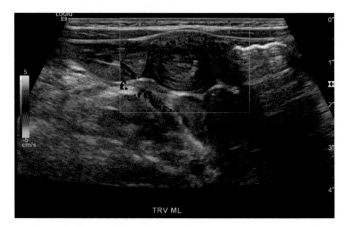

FIGURE 19-20. LBI.

FIGURE 19-21. Color Doppler present with LBI.

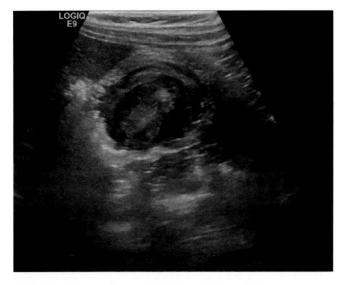

FIGURE 19-22. Pre-reduction under sonographic guidance.

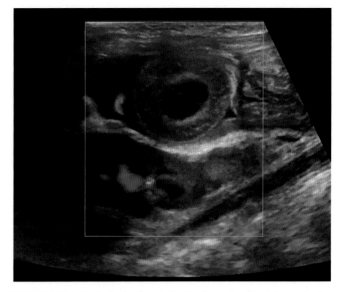

FIGURE 19-24. Lack of color flow, indicating long standing intussusception (and ischemia) which failed fluoroscopic reduction and required surgical guidance. Right kidney is seen below.

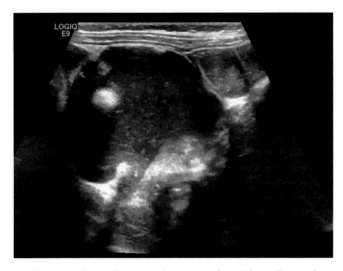

FIGURE 19-23. Post-reduction under sonographic guidance. Factors that predict non-reducibility include trapped intraperitoneal fluid, a lead point and lack or absence of blood flow raising likelihood of ischemia. Note that a lead point is rare but may cause intussusception in older children.

saline, or plain tap water (Figs. 19-22 and 19-23). Surgical intervention is reserved as a last resort when prior methods are unsuccessful or when there is any suspicion for ischemia or perforation (Fig. 19-24).

An ultrasound for evaluation of intussusception is a common exam ordered in the acute care setting and should be ordered STAT (from the Latin term *statim*, which translates to immediately). A 10 MHz linear transducer should be selected for infants and young children and a 5-7 MHz curvilinear or sector transducer should be selected for larger habitus children.

The protocol for intussusception involves a sonographic evaluation of the small and large intestine using graded compression with the imaging transducer. The purpose of graded compression is to disperse bowel gas, optimizing intestinal visualization. The sonographer should begin midline in the central abdomen, surveying the area of the small intestine. The terminal ileum should then be located in the right lower quadrant of the abdomen. Following the large intestine from the ileocecal junction, the sonographer should evaluate the ascending, transverse, and descending colon to the rectum. The sonographer can survey the abdomen in a grid pattern to ensure all bowel is evaluated. The sonographer should provide static images in each quadrant in two orthogonal imaging planes (i.e., sagittal and transverse). It is beneficial for the sonographer to provide cine loops for radiologist evaluation. If intussusception is visualized, the sonographer should use color Doppler to document if blood flow is present. The presence of intestinal blood flow suggests reducibility. A lack of perfusion can indicate ischemic bowel which leads to necrosis and may require surgical intervention. If a positive intussusception is visualized, the sonographer should notate the location and measure the outer-to-outer diameter to determine whether it is a potential large versus small bowel intussusception. If a large bowel intussusception is suspected, the sonographer should promptly call a radiologist to review the examination for expedited patient care. If a positive small bowel intussusception is visualized, the sonographer should evaluate for transient (self-reducing) intussusception and provide image documentation of reduction prior to calling the radiologist (Fig. 19-25). This may require delayed imaging and 20 minutes is a reasonable interval for re-evaluation of the suspected small bowel intussusception.

Still images:

1. Sagittal right lower quadrant
2. Transverse right lower quadrant
3. Sagittal right upper quadrant

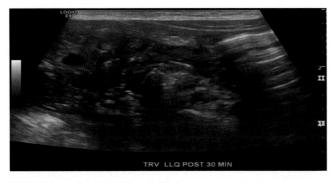

FIGURE 19-25. Transient SBI—resolved.

4. Transverse right upper quadrant
5. Sagittal left upper quadrant
6. Transverse left upper quadrant
7. Sagittal left lower quadrant
8. Transverse left lower quadrant

Note: These images are obtained following the route of the large intestine from ascending, transverse, to descending colon using graded compression and surveying for intussusception. If intussusception is visualized, measure the outer-to-outer diameter to differentiate between a potential large versus small bowel intussusception, and provide color Doppler images.

Cine clips:

1. Tansverse right upper quadrant to right lower quadrant
2. Transverse midline superior to inferior
3. Transverse left upper quadrant to left lower quadrant
4. Sagittal right upper quadrant to left upper quadrant

Note: The transverse midline superior to inferior cine clip provides documentation of the central abdomen and primary location of the small intestine. It is important this area is thoroughly assessed with graded compression before cine clip documentation.

NECROTIZING ENTEROCOLITIS

Necrotizing enterocolitis (NEC) is an ischemic disease of the bowel resulting from hypoxia and superimposed infection, primarily visualized in premature neonates less than 36 weeks gestational age with a very low birth weight (VLBW) of less than 1000 grams (Fig. 19-26(a) to (d)). NEC is the most frequently occurring gastrointestinal condition among premature neonates and is a notable cause of neonatal morbidity and mortality. The neonatal bowel wall is permeable and vulnerable to bacterial infection, which can lead to inflammation and ischemia.

Left untreated, NEC can escalate to bowel perforation and subsequent peritonitis, sepsis, and disseminated intravascular coagulation (DIC). When occurring in full-term infants, NEC is usually associated with heart disease, sepsis, or bowel obstruction that predisposes the infant to bowel ischemia. Compared to the ~90% of NEC cases presenting in premature neonates, a smaller percentage of ~10% of cases occur in full-term infants.

NEC begins in the mucosa and submucosa and can extend through all bowel layers, with the distal ileum and right colon most often involved. The first stage of bowel ischemia is reversible ischemic enteritis. With NEC progression, fibrotic stricture can develop as necrosis of the mucosal and submucosal layers ensues. A higher rate of mortality is associated with the final stage of bowel ischemia, where all layers of the bowel wall are affected. Symptoms of NEC include abdominal distention, vomiting, bloody stool, and irritability.

For evaluation of NEC, the sonographer should survey the central abdomen and all four abdominal quadrants, assessing the echogenicity and thickness of the bowel wall, the presence or absence of peristalsis, air in the abdominal (peritoneal) cavity called "pneumoperitoneum," and abdominal fluid collections. Normal thickness of the bowel wall ranges between 1.1 and 2 mm. The small bowel should produce peristaltic contractions at a minimum rate of 11 movements per minute. Sonographic findings include initial hyperemic, thick-walled, fluid-filled bowel loops, pneumatosis intestinalis (PI), portal vein gas, and pneumoperitoneum. A bowel wall thickness of greater than 2.7 mm which coincides with hyperechoic bowel echogenicity is considered abnormal. As NEC progresses, a lack of color Doppler can be noted, indicating that the bowel is nonviable due to the onset of transmural necrosis. With lack of sufficient blood flow, the bowel wall begins to thin. The measurement of an ischemic bowel wall is abnormally thin, measuring less than 1 mm. Hepatic portal venous gas (HPVG) closely coincides with bowel ischemia and pneumatosis intestinalis. To assess for the presence of gas in the portal vein, the sonographer examines the portal vein, surveying for spherical ~1 mm echogenic particles flowing through the portal circulation.

Still images utilizing a high frequency linear transducer:

Note: Observe for presence of free fluid and any bowel or omental abnormalities, such as increased echogenicity, PI, and lack of peristalsis.

1. Sagittal right lower quadrant
2. Transverse right lower quadrant
3. Sagittal right upper quadrant
4. Transverse right upper quadrant
5. Sagittal left upper quadrant
6. Transverse left upper quadrant
7. Sagittal left lower quadrant

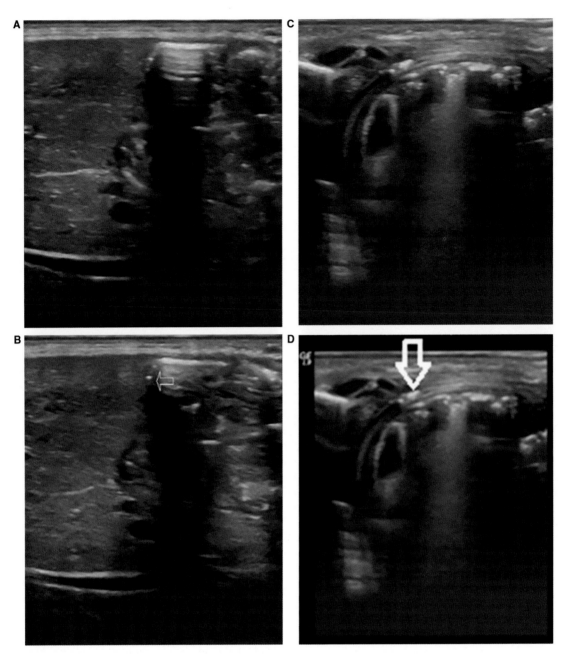

FIGURE 19-26. (a, b, and c): Eight-day old pediatric patient positive for NEC. Tiny echogenic flecks representing air seen within the fluid adjacent to the abdominal wall, with pneumatosis present in bowel loops below the liver. (d) Arrow depicting pneumatosis.

8. Transverse left lower quadrant

9. Measurement of bowel wall thickness

10. Color Doppler of bowel wall perfusion

    a. Normal color Doppler of the bowel wall produces 1 to 9 color Doppler signal dots/cm^2

    b. Hyperemia of the bowel wall produces a 'zebra', 'ring, or 'Y pattern

    c. Lack of perfusion suggests transmural necrosis

11. Sagittal hepatic portal vein

12. Transverse hepatic portal vein

13. Transverse hepatic-diaphragmatic junction, assess for echogenic free abdominal gas

14. Spectral Doppler of the superior mesenteric artery (SMA)

    a. In sagittal plane obtain a minimum of two spectral Doppler samples of the SMA, increased peak systolic velocity of ~100-120 cm/s or greater and elevated end diastolic velocity is suggestive toward NEC

Cine clips:

1. Demonstrate peristaltic contractions of the bowel

APPENDICITIS

Appendicitis is an acute inflammation of the appendix and the most common cause of emergent abdominal surgery in childhood. Ultrasound of the appendix is an exam which is frequently encountered in the acute care setting when patients present with pain in the right lower abdominal quadrant. No patient preparation is required; however, a full bladder can be a useful sonographic window for optimal visualization of the pelvic and lower abdominal cavity. The sonographer should review patient lab values prior to performing the exam if they are available. An elevated white blood cell count indicates infection or inflammation, which may be present with acute appendicitis or abscess associated with a ruptured appendix.

The protocol for appendiceal ultrasound involves evaluation of the right lower abdominal quadrant and caudal extension of the peritoneal cavity, called the "pouch of Douglas (cul-de-sac)." Using a sector transducer, the sonographer should survey the right lower abdominal quadrant and pelvic region in two imaging planes for the presence of abscess, free fluid, and any bowel or omental abnormalities (see Table 19-2). Appendiceal perforation is more prevalent in pediatrics than in the adult population due to the challenge associated with identifying abdominal pain and its cause in early childhood. Additionally, because the omentum continues developing throughout childhood, appendiceal rupture is not as likely to remain as a localized collection and generalized peritonitis can develop, which can be fatal if left untreated.

Following a generalized abdominal survey, the sonographer should switch to a high frequency linear transducer for greater imaging resolution. The sonographer should locate the appendix to assess compressibility and obtain an anteroposterior (AP) diameter measurement. The region of the right iliopsoas muscle and iliac vessels is a good starting point for locating the appendix, as the appendix is frequently "draped" over this area. Graded compression can be used to disperse bowel gas and more easily identify the appendix. Using this technique, particularly in the region of McBurney's point, it is not uncommon for patients with true acute appendicitis to experience rebound tenderness, which is caused by the release of pressure from the imaging transducer.

When the appendix is identified, the sonographer should demonstrate the blind-ending appendiceal tip. This provides confidence that the sonographer is truly evaluating the appendix and not a surrounding segment of intestine, like the terminal ileum, which can mimic the appearance of the appendix when compressed. An image of the appendix in relation to the cecum may also be provided and an AP measurement of the appendix in long and short-axis views should be obtained. A normal appendiceal measurement is 6 millimeters or less. A split-screen image with and without compression should be acquired. The normal appendix is compressible. An appendix which is non-compressible, along with other positive findings, is suggestive of appendicitis (Fig. 19-27). Color Doppler images of the appendix should be taken using the low flow setting and evaluating for the presence of increased vascularity. At 20 cm/s, even a hyperemic appendix may not be well demonstrated with color Doppler, therefore it is important to set scale low (Fig. 19-28). Scale is also called "pulse repetition frequency," or "PRF," and the labeling on the ultrasound unit varies by vendor.

If the appendix is not visualized due to overlying bowel gas artifact, or rupture is suspected and presence of abscess and/or free fluid is identified, representative static images should be taken. The sonographer should also provide cine clips when allowable that will benefit radiologist evaluation, including an anterior transverse cine clip of the right hemiabdomen from the colonic hepatic flexure to the right lower abdominal quadrant and a transverse posterior approach cine clip of the right hemiabdomen demonstrating the region of Morison's pouch and scanning inferiorly toward the right lower abdominal quadrant. A sagittal cine clip from the right lower abdominal quadrant at the region of the right iliopsoas muscle toward the midline bladder should also be acquired for review. Documentation of any surrounding lymph nodes should be obtained (Fig. 19-29).

Still images utilizing a sector transducer:

Note: Observe for presence of free fluid and any bowel or omental abnormalities.

15. Sagittal right lower quadrant
16. Transverse right lower quadrant
17. Sagittal right upper quadrant
18. Transverse right upper quadrant
19. Sagittal left upper quadrant
20. Transverse left upper quadrant
21. Sagittal left lower quadrant

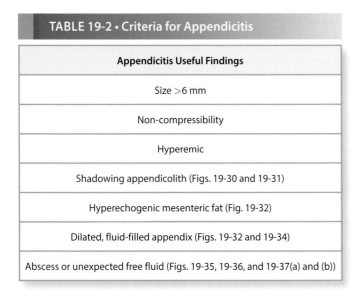

TABLE 19-2 • Criteria for Appendicitis
Appendicitis Useful Findings
Size >6 mm
Non-compressibility
Hyperemic
Shadowing appendicolith (Figs. 19-30 and 19-31)
Hyperechogenic mesenteric fat (Fig. 19-32)
Dilated, fluid-filled appendix (Figs. 19-32 and 19-34)
Abscess or unexpected free fluid (Figs. 19-35, 19-36, and 19-37(a) and (b))

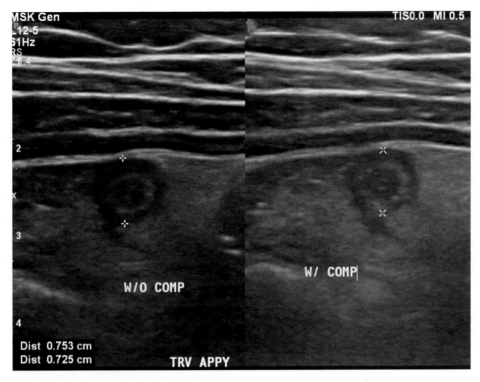

FIGURE 19-27. Noncompressible.

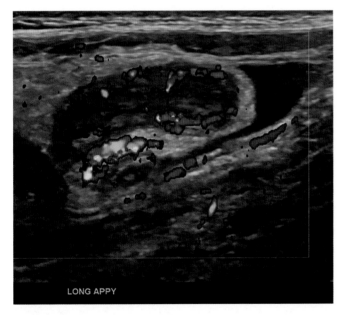

FIGURE 19-28. Hyperemia.

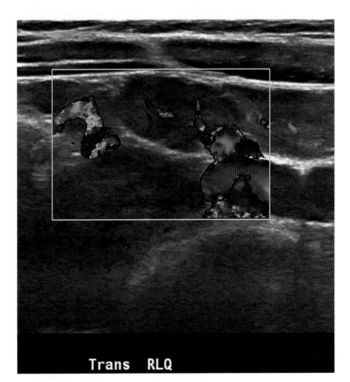

FIGURE 19-29. Surrounding lymph nodes.

22. Transverse left lower quadrant

23. Sagittal cul-de-sac/bladder region

24. Transverse cul-de-sac/bladder region

Cine clips:

1. Transverse superior to inferior anterior approach, colonic hepatic flexure to right lower quadrant

2. Transverse superior to inferior posterior approach, Morison's pouch to right lower quadrant

3. Sagittal right lower abdominal quadrant toward midline bladder and cul-de-sac

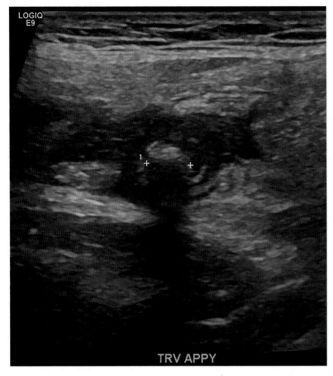

FIGURE 19-30. Appendicolith.

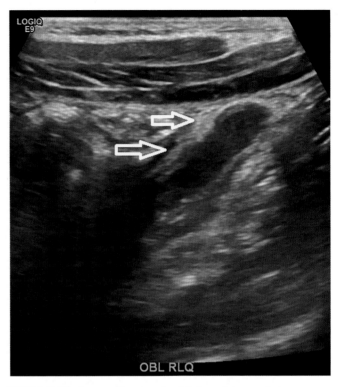

FIGURE 19-32. Surrounding stranding fat, tissue is hyperechoic.

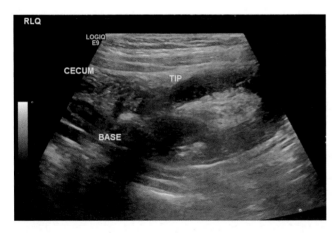

FIGURE 19-31. Dilated appendix with appendicolith at the base.

Still images utilizing a high-frequency linear transducer:

Note: Document images of the appendix and surrounding locations.

4. Long-axis image of the cecal tip
5. Sagittal right lower quadrant, demonstrating region of the ililopsoas muscle and iliac vessels
6. Transverse right lower quadrant, demonstrating region of the ililopsoas muscle and iliac vessels
7. Sagittal appendix
8. Sagittal appendix with AP measurement
9. Sagittal appendix with color Doppler

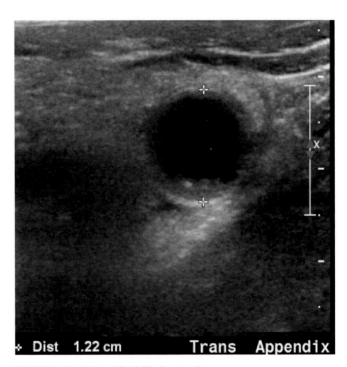

FIGURE 19-33. Dilated, fluid-filled appendix.

10. Transverse appendix
11. Transverse appendix with AP measurement
12. Transverse appendix with color Doppler
13. Transverse appendix utilizing split-screen function, with and without compression (Fig. 19-27)

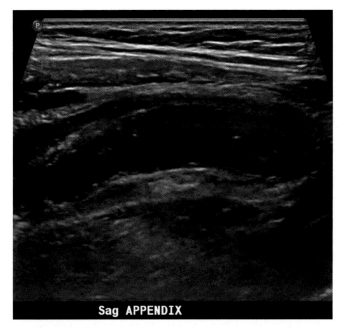

FIGURE 19-34. Loss of gut signature.

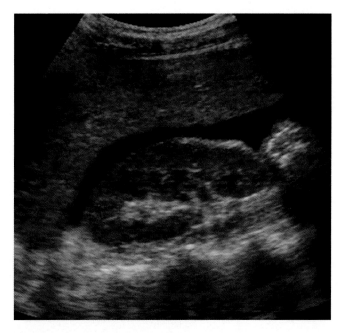

FIGURE 19-36. Fluid in Morison's pouch.

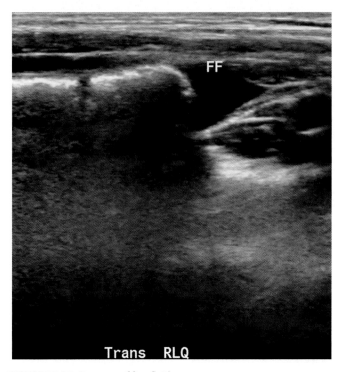

FIGURE 19-35. Presence of free fluid.

Cine clips:

1. Sagittal appendix
2. Transverse appendix, documenting blind end
3. Transverse appendix, with compression

Note: Protocol may vary by institution.

Please refer to Chapter 3, "Sonographic Anatomy of the Abdomen" for additional information pertaining to the appendix.

MECKEL'S DIVERTICULUM

Meckel's diverticulum is an insidious cause of right lower quadrant pain. It is the most common congenital anomaly of the gastrointestinal tract; but the majority of patients remain asymptomatic. Complications and clinical symptoms of Meckel's diverticulum occur more commonly in children than adults. About 60% of Meckel diverticula become symptomatic before patients reach 10 years of age. When children present with vague abdominal pain and there is no obvious cause, the sonographer can look for hidden Meckel's diverticulum which may be seen as a fluid-filled structure with a gut signature (Fig. 19-38) in the mid to lower abdomen (Fig. 19-39) which does not communicate with the small bowel. Surrounding bowel loops will be seen peristalsing around this fluid-filled structure.

MECONIUM ILEUS

Meconium ileus is a distal ileum bowel obstruction in newborns resulting from thick, impacted meconium. This may occur from gut immaturity. Meconium ileus is usually diagnosed and treated with a contrast enema. Sonographic findings include lack of peristalsis, increased bowel echogenicity, and dilated bowel loops. Meconium ileus is strongly associated with cystic fibrosis.

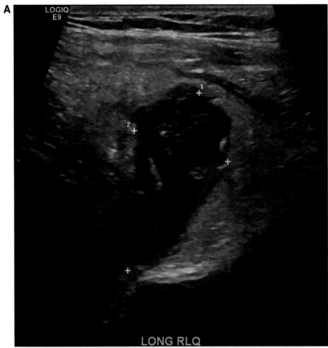

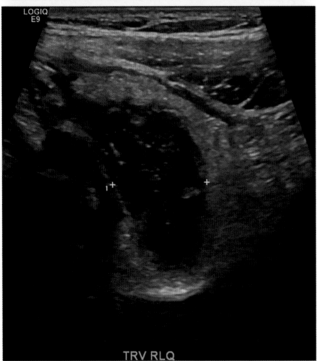

FIGURE 19-37. Abscess, potential for ruptured appendix.

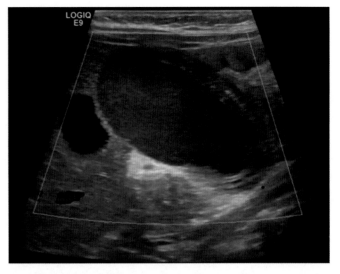

FIGURE 19-38. Meckel's diverticulum in a 10-month-old male with emesis, pain, and bloody stool. Note the gut signature.

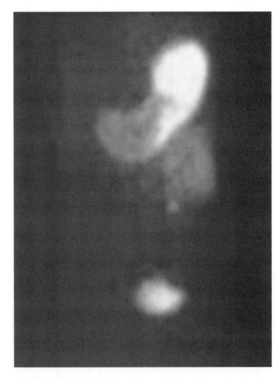

FIGURE 19-39. Nuclear medicine exam shows radiotracer accumulation in the lower abdomen confirming the diagnosis of Meckel's.

MESOTHELIAL CYST

Mesothelial cyst is a rare benign, anechoic mesenteric cyst lined with mesothelial cells (Fig. 19-40(a) and (b)). These cysts may rupture and cause significant bleeding. Immunohistochemical analysis must be done to differentiate a mesothelial cyst from other cysts. Mesothelial cysts may be monitored with imaging and labwork or resected.

DUPLICATION CYSTS

A duplication cyst is a spherical or tubular structure that is lined with gastrointestinal epithelium and contains smooth muscle in its wall. Enteric duplication cysts may occur anywhere along the gastrointestinal tract and are usually attached directly to the bowel, sharing the bowel's blood supply. Clinical symptoms can include a palpable abdominal mass, pain, or gastrointestinal hemorrhage. Enteric duplication cysts may be a lead point for

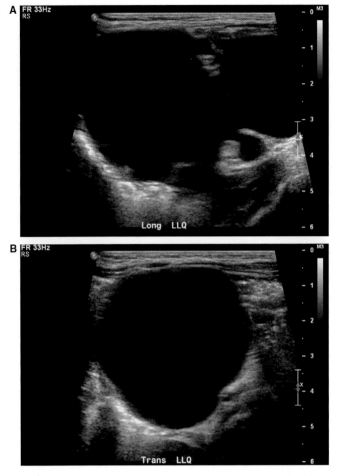

FIGURE 19-40. Mesenteric cyst with lobulated contours in 7-week-old pediatric patient.

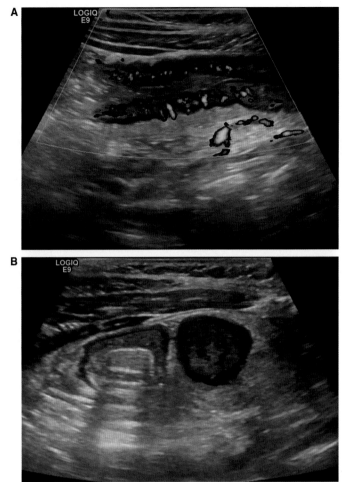

FIGURE 19-41. Thickened, hypervascular bowel loop with infiltrative mesenteric edema in a 12-year-old with Crohn's.

intussusception and can cause pancreatitis if located close to the ampulla of Vater. Esophageal duplication or bronchogenic cysts can be found in the lower neck region which may compress the trachea, causing stridor. Duplication cysts can also occur in the colon, although are more common in the small intestine. When occurring in the colon, these cysts have the same appearance as they do in the small intestine. Sonographically, duplication cysts appear as a sphere or tube-like structure lined with gastrointestinal epithelium. They have an inner layer of mucosa with an echogenic appearance, and a hypoechoic outer rim consisting of the smooth muscle wall.

CROHN'S DISEASE

Crohn's disease is a chronic irritation and swelling of the intestinal lining, most commonly affecting the ileum. Sonographic findings of Crohn's disease includes a hypervascular thickened bowel wall, decrease in peristalsis, bowel target pattern, and loss of bowel compressibility (Fig. 19-41(a) and (b)). Severity of Crohn's disease can be assessed with ultrasound through demonstration and assessment of intramural vascularity, architecture of the bowel wall, presence of intraperitoneal fluid, and

proliferation of mesenteric fatty conjunctive tissue. Much like a survey for other bowel etiologies, a standard abdominal survey should first be performed using a convex 3 to 5 MHz transducer, looking for the presence or absence of free-fluid, abscess, and any bowel or omental abnormalities. The sonographer should then switch to a 5 to 10 MHz linear transducer for a detailed evaluation of the intestine. Higher frequencies provide greater resolution and imaging detail of the bowel wall layers. Extramural complications of Crohn's disease that may be identified with ultrasound include a hypoechoic fistula and/or stenosis of the small intestine or colon. It is beneficial if the patient is fasting for intestinal ultrasound to reduce the presence of bowel gas artifact which can inhibit an optimal evaluation. Additionally, graded compression can be used to disperse bowel gas. Another technique which can further enhance visualization of bowel wall layers is to allow the patient to consume a clear liquid, which fills the internal bowel lumen and acts as a sonolucent contrast. This aids in the discovery of intestinal lesions and assessing the structure of the bowel wall in patients with a history of inflammatory bowel conditions.

MASSES

Gastric Teratoma

Gastrointestinal teratomas contain germ cells made up of an ectoderm, endoderm, and mesoderm. These usually benign masses are very rare, occurring in less than 1% of all childhood teratoma lesions which can occur in various locations throughout the body. Sonographic findings include a complex echogenic cystic mass with internal fluid, fat, and calcification representing bone. Although rare, this etiology may be encountered as a distractor on the registry exam.

Gastric Inflammatory Pseudotumor

Gastric inflammatory pseudotumor is also called a "plasma cell granuloma" or "fibroxanthoma." A gastric inflammatory pseudotumor is not a true neoplasm, but rather an inflammatory mass containing plasma cells and lymphocytes. Sonographic appearance of this pseudotumor includes a poorly defined heterogeneous mass secondary to hemorrhage, necrosis, and wall thickening in the greater curvature of the stomach. This tumor is aggressive and will recur if not totally resected. Enlarged lymph nodes may also be seen surrounding the area.

Gastric Focal Foveolar Hyperplasia

Gastric focal foveolar hyperplasia is a rare echogenic mucosal polypoid mass. This mass is formed by inflamed or obstructed pits in the gastric mucosa where deep gastric glands empty. Although rare, this etiology may be encountered as a distractor on the registry exam.

Miscellaneous Benign Gastric Masses

Miscellaneous benign gastric masses that cannot be differentiated via sonography include myofibromatosis, polyps, hematoma, leiomyoma, neurofibroma, hemangioma, carcinoid, and lipoma lesions. These pathologies may all appear as polypoid mucosal masses (Fig. 19-42) or focal gastric wall thickening.

MALIGNANT

Gastric Lymphoma

Gastric lymphoma is the most common malignant gastrointestinal neoplasm in childhood. Most gastric lymphomas are a non-Hodgkin subtype and include a palpable mass with abdominal pain. Sonographic findings include gastrointestinal wall thickening, hypoechoic polypoid mass with intra- or extra-mural extension, splenomegaly, and surrounding lymph node enlargement (Fig. 19-43(a) to (c)). Colonic involvement is rare, but when it occurs the cecum is the most common tumor site.

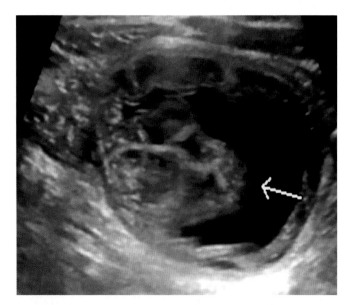

FIGURE 19-42. Jejunal polyp serving as a lead point in a small bowel intussusception.

Gastrointestinal Stromal Tumors (GIST)

GISTs begin in the muscularis propria with intra- and extramural extension. GIST tends to occur in adolescent females and is more common in the antrum and body of the stomach. Clinical symptoms include abdominal pain, hematemesis, melena, and anemia from gastrointestinal bleeding. Sonographic findings include an echogenic heterogeneous mass with nodular cystic areas near the antrum or body of the stomach, with possible areas of hemorrhage and necrosis (Fig. 19-44(a) and (b)).

Gastric Carcinoma

Adenocarcinoma of the colon is rare malignancy in the pediatric population, however, may be encountered as a distractor on the registry exam. Gastric carcinoma is detected directly with colonoscopy evaluation. Lab tests for screening are also available. Fluoroscopic barium enema exam has been used for the evaluation of gastric carcinoma. Sometimes gastric carcinoma can be seen on sonogram as colonic wall thickening, exophytic wall mass, or adjacent mesenteric fat indicating tumor infiltration (Figs. 19-45 and 19-46).

Miscellaneous Malignant Gastric Masses

Leiomyosarcoma and carcinoma rarely occur in the stomach. These malignancies appear as a polypoid mass or focal wall thickening, mimicking benign gastric masses.

ABDOMINAL LYMPHADENOPATHY

In adults, normal retroperitoneal lymph nodes appear hypo- or isoechoic to the muscle and are most often seen adjacent to the abdominal aorta and inferior vena cava as flat oval structures.

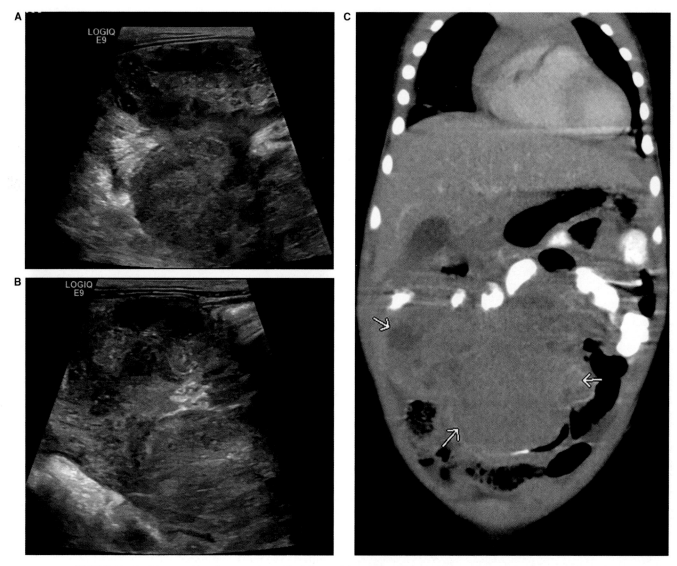

FIGURE 19-43. A 2-year-old male presenting with abdominal distension. CT demonstrates a large heterogeneous mass with areas of central necrosis with encasement of abdominal vessels and extension into adjacent organs. PET scan shows a large tumor burden filling the majority of the abdominal cavity with markedly increased FDG uptake.

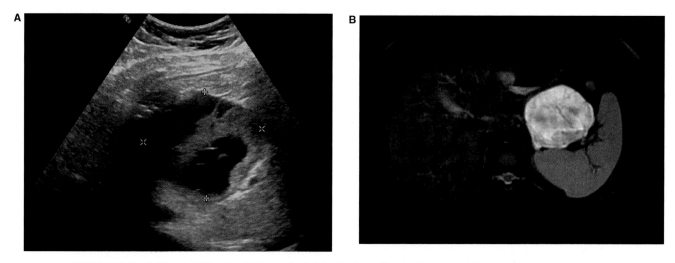

FIGURE 19-44. A 19-year-old female with 1 month of abdominal pain. The dominant mass is located at the greater curvature of the stomach, with a lobulated gastric endoluminal component (not well appreciated on ultrasound).

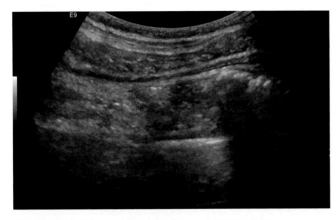

FIGURE 19-45. Ultrasound shows fluid and air-filled bowel loops.

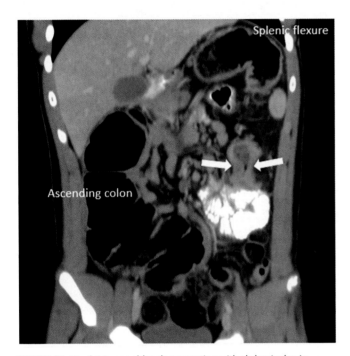

FIGURE 19-46. A 14-year-old male presenting with abdominal pain and vomiting for 5 days. Patient history included difficulty eating and constipation. He was found to have colonic stricture which ultimately became obstructed. Imaging and endoscopic biopsy showed an obstructing lesion in the descending colon. CT demonstrates narrowing of the lumen at the descending colon with upstream dilatation of fecal material at the splenic flexure and ascending colon. Exploratory surgery was performed, and the lesion was resected. Biopsy results were consistent with stage III adenocarcinoma.

In the retroperitoneum, lymph nodes are not generally seen in infants or young children, making the detection of lymphadenopathy important. If detected, pediatric retroperitoneal lymphadenopathy may direct a surgeon to the area of abnormal lymph nodes for surgical sampling to rule out tumor metastasis. In approximately 20% of cases, a local tumor which spreads to the surrounding lymph nodes can occur. Adenopathy refers to the swelling of lymph nodes because of a primary tumor, metastasis, or inflammatory process. Lymph nodes less than 10 millimeters in diameter may be a normal finding in adolescent patients, but multiple nodes greater than 1 centimeter in diameter, or retrocrural lymph nodes, raise suspicion and ultrasound findings should be correlated with clinical symptoms and lab values. Abnormal retroperitoneal lymph nodes have perivascular distribution. Appearance of malignant lymphadenopathy ranges from more than 1 enlarged lymph node to a large confluent mass where individual nodes are no longer detected. Lymph node enlargement has been correlated with decreasing CD4 lymphocyte counts. Pathologic enlargement of nodes can be due to entities such as acquired immunodeficiency syndrome, mononucleosis, cat-scratch disease, Kawasaki disease, Langerhans histiocytosis, general infection, and sarcoidosis.

PERITONEAL FLUID AND ABSCESS

The natural flow of peritoneal fluid is along mesentery and peritoneal pathways. Abscess or metastatic disease tends to form in areas where fluid pools. These areas may include the peritoneal cavity of the pelvis, cul-de-sac, pouch of Douglas, or lateral paravesical recesses. There can be free flow of fluid from the pelvis to the upper abdomen via the right or left paracolic gutters. The most common route is through the right paracolic gutter into the right subhepatic space, near Morison's pouch. Scanning the patient in different positions will determine if fluid is free flowing or loculated. Intraperitoneal abscesses in children are usually caused by appendicitis, Crohn's disease, following abdominal surgery or trauma, or with pelvic inflammatory disease. Patients will have symptoms such as fever, leukocytosis, and abdominal pain. Sonographic findings of abscess include a hypoechoic collection with low-level echoes, septations, fluid-debris level, or gas-bubble areas with an echogenic rim (Figs. 19-47(a) to (c)). Peritonitis is an inflammation of the peritoneal lining and usually occurs in patients with immunologic defenses or due to pancreatitis.

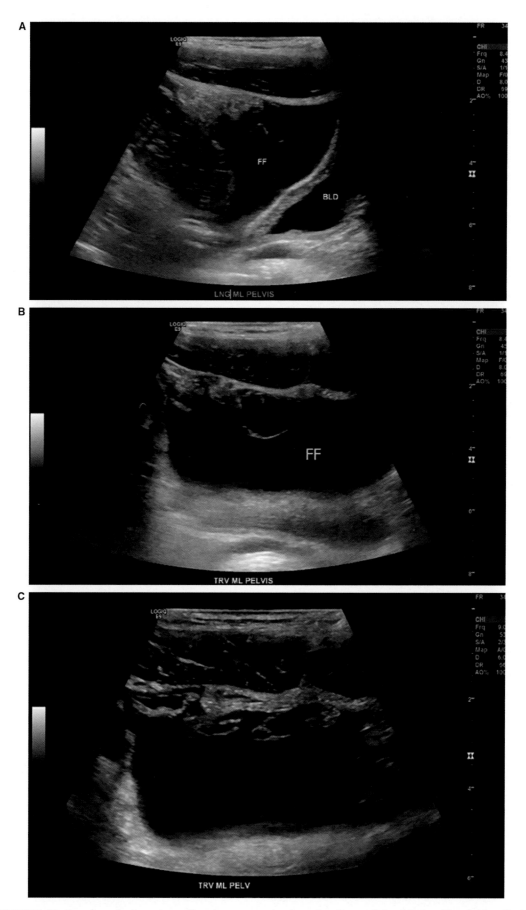

FIGURE 19-47. Complex collection representing abscess secondary to ruptured appendix in a 14-year-old pediatric patient. Clinical symptoms include right lower quadrant pain, fever, and leukocytosis.

20

Hernias

ABDOMINAL HERNIA

Hernia refers to the bulging of contents, generally bowel, fat, and/or other peritoneal structures through a weakened abdominal wall defect. The type of hernia depends on the location. Sonographically, a break will be visualized in the striated muscle wall, accentuated with Valsalva maneuver (Fig. 20-1). During the Valsalva maneuver, bowel or other peritoneal structures further protrude superior through the muscular defect. Depending on hernial contents, appearance may vary; however, commonly bowel will portray a "fluffy cloud" appearance extending superior through the break in striated muscle. When a positive hernia finding is visualized, it is important that the sonographer apply color Doppler to ensure blood flow is present within the bowel. Bowel without flow on color Doppler may be incarcerated, mechanically obstructed, or strangulated. These findings require intervention and reduction may not be possible.

For hernia evaluation, a high frequency linear transducer should be selected.

Still images in supine position include:

1. Sagittal and transverse region of interest in grayscale
2. Sagittal and transverse region of interest with color Doppler
3. Sagittal and transverse region of interest with Valsalva maneuver
4. Sagittal and transverse region of interest utilizing split-screen function, with and without compression

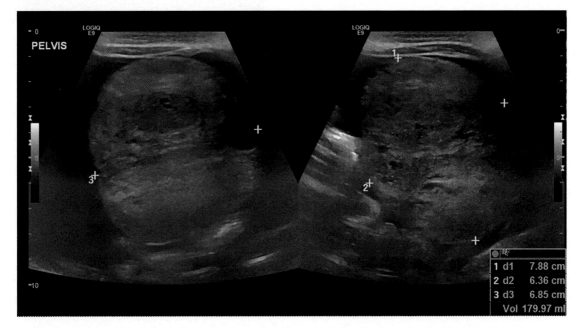

FIGURE 20-1. A 3-month-old female with omphalocele status post repair. Now presenting with umbilical hernia and abdominal distension.

Note: If a hernia is visualized and compresses, this provides information to the radiologist whether there is indication of obstruction or strangulation of herniated bowel, and if the hernia is reducible. It is helpful to note whether the neck or opening of the defect is wide or narrow, as this helps in determining risk for strangulation. If the patient experiences pain with compression, this should also be documented as it is a sign for a positive finding.

5. If unilateral, sagittal and transverse region of interest utilizing split-screen function demonstrating contralateral side for comparison.

Still images in upright position include:

1. Sagittal and transverse region of interest in grayscale
2. Sagittal and transverse region of interest with color Doppler
3. Sagittal and transverse region of interest with Valsalva maneuver
4. Sagittal and transverse region of interest utilizing split-screen function, with and without compression
5. If unilateral, sagittal and transverse region of interest utilizing split-screen function demonstrating contralateral side for comparison

INGUINAL HERNIA

An inguinal hernia is associated with a patent vaginal process, or processus vaginalis, and includes 75% of all hernias. Inguinal hernias are more commonly right-sided, since the right processus vaginalis closes following the left. Inguinal hernias can include bowel, omentum, surrounding structures, or solely fluid. Inguinal hernia in males may present as scrotal enlargement of unknown cause, and possible bowel incarceration or strangulation may be present. Valsalva maneuver performed during inguinal hernia sonogram can demonstrate fluid or air-filled bowel peristalsing within the scrotum. This technique is performed to rule out ischemic bowel changes. Sonographic appearance of inguinal hernia with omentum in the inguinal canal appears as a complex echogenic mass (Figs. 20-2 and 20-3). With inguinal hernia, the inguinal canal measures greater than 4 mm at internal ring level.

In boys, the incidence of inguinal hernia is highest during the first year of life and peaks during the first month. More than 80% of incarcerated inguinal hernias occur in babies younger than 1 year of age. Ultrasound plays a critical role in the identification of an incarcerated inguinal hernia, as strangulation can occur within 2 hours of onset. Imaging features of incarcerated hernia include lack of peristalsis, wall edema, fluid within the hernia sac as well as presence of air. Inguinal hernias in females

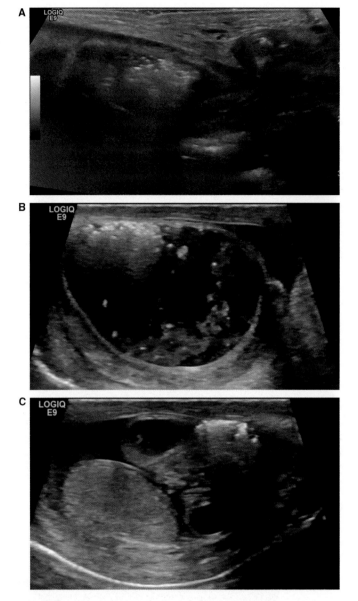

FIGURE 20-2. A 1-month-old male with firm, swollen right scrotal sac. Air is seen along with non-peristalsing bowel in the scrotal sac. Exploratory laparoscopy confirmed incarcerated inguinal hernia, as well as intestinal perforation.

are caused by the persistence of the diverticulum of Nuck. These hernias typically contain the ovaries and fallopian tubes (Fig. 20-4(a) and (b)).

UMBILICAL HERNIA

An umbilical hernia is a ventral hernia involving anterior bulging of bowel structures into the umbilical region near the umbilical ring. Umbilical hernias are the most common ventral hernia and may be acquired or congenital. Sonographic appearance includes a wide umbilical ring with bulging noted near the umbilical region, particularly when the patient is straining or crying (Fig. 20-5(a) to (c)).

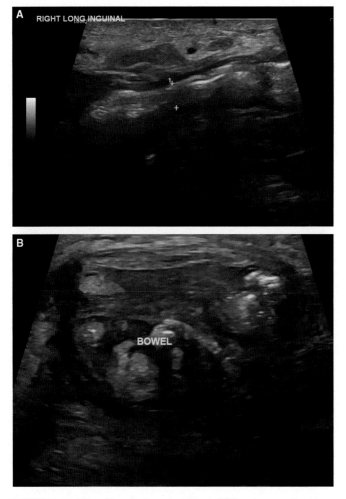

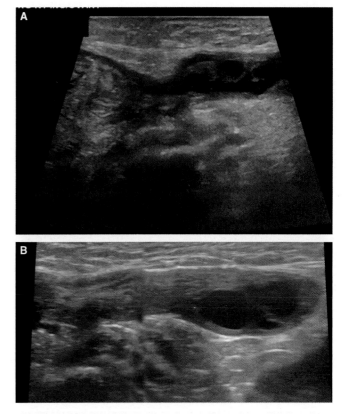

FIGURE 20-4. A 4-month-old (25-week) infant. Right inguinal hernia containing the right ovary.

FIGURE 20-3. Dilated inguinal canal with bowel filling the scrotal sac in a 3-month-old male with swollen scrotum.

PARAUMBILICAL HERNIA

A paraumbilical hernia is a ventral hernia involving anterolateral bulging of bowel structures into the paraumbilical region, due to linea alba defect. Paraumbilical hernias are common in premature female patients. Sonographic appearance includes a wide linea alba with swelling noted superior or inferior to the umbilicus.

EPIGASTRIC HERNIA

An epigastric hernia is a bulging of the abdominal contents through the anterior abdominal wall, along the linea alba. This hernia is located in the epigastric region, halfway between the umbilicus and xiphoid process. Sonographic appearance includes a wide linea alba with echogenic, fatty mass noted in the epigastric region.

INCISIONAL HERNIA

An incisional hernial occurs at the region of a surgical scar following abdominal surgery.

SPIGELIAN HERNIA

A Spiegelian hernia occurs along the spigelian fascia near the inguinal ring, involving defect in the rectus sheath and transverse abdominal muscles. These hernias are best visualized in upright position.

CONGENITAL (BOCHDALEK) HERNIA

Congenital diaphragmatic hernia defect results from incomplete closure of the embryonic pleuroperitoneal membrane. The 5 "Bs" that describe features of this hernia are: Bochdalek, back and lateral (usually left-sided), big, baby, and bad (associated with pulmonary hypoplasia). These large hernias typically present in infancy and are often left-sided. The left posterior diaphragm opening closes later in fetal life in comparison to the right, which may also contribute to asymmetry. In 80% of patients, this congenital hernia is unilateral, posterolateral left-sided, and often diagnosed prenatally. When visualized in utero, asymmetric chest and scaphoid abdomen is seen. Left-sided defects may contain anomalies including the left lobe of liver, spleen, stomach, large bowel, small bowel, or the kidney. Right-sided defects are associated with hydrothorax, ascites, and Budd-Chiari syndrome due to compression or occlusion of the hepatic veins and lymphatic vessels. Complications

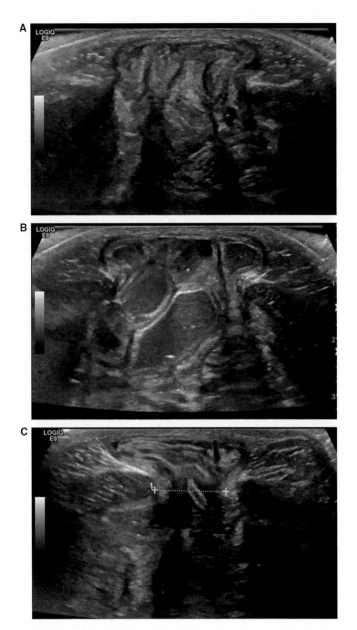

associated with congenital Bochdalek hernia include pulmonary hypoplasia and persistent fetal circulation. Sonographic findings include discontinuity of the normal linear diaphragmatic echoes and presence of abdominal contents in the ipsilateral hemithorax.

FIGURE 20-5. Umbilical hernia.

21

Pathologic Processes of the Urinary Tract

KIDNEYS

Horseshoe Kidney

Horseshoe kidney is the most common renal anomaly, occurring in approximately one out of every 400 births. Horseshoe kidney has a 2:1 male predominance, with the most common fusion site being at the kidney's lower poles connected by a midline isthmus. The isthmus of the horseshoe kidney may have fibrous tissue or functioning renal parenchyma, with the ureters crossing in front of the isthmus. Arterial supply varies and may arise from the common iliac arteries or from the lower aorta. Genitourinary anomalies associated with horseshoe kidney include vesicoureteral reflux, ureteropelvic junction obstruction, pelvicaliectasis, stone formation, duplicated collecting system, and renal dysplasia. Horseshoe kidney has a slightly increased risk for incidence of Wilms tumor and renal cell carcinoma. Sonographic findings include abnormal kidney axis, isthmus tissue crossing midline anterior to the spine and great vessels, and an anterior renal pelvis (see Figs. 21-1 to 21-3).

BILATERAL RENAL CYSTIC DISEASE

Autosomal Recessive Polycystic Kidney Disease

Autosomal Recessive Polycystic Kidney Disease (ARPKD) is also known as "infantile polycystic kidney disease." ARPKD is inherited as a recessive characteristic. With this disease, innumerable 1- to 2-millimeter cysts are seen throughout the medulla, representing dilated collecting tubules that extend into the cortex of the kidney. Sonographic findings in neonatal patients include bilateral renal enlargement, overall increase in parenchymal echogenicity with a hypoechoic peripheral rim,

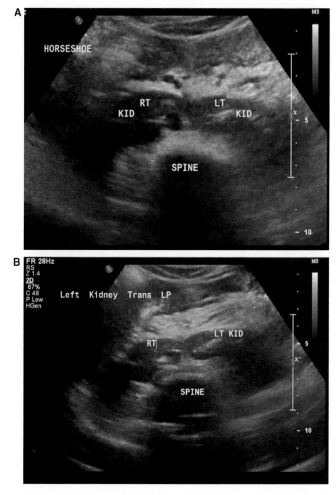

FIGURE 21-1. A 12-year-old pediatric patient with horseshoe kidney; transverse view.

153

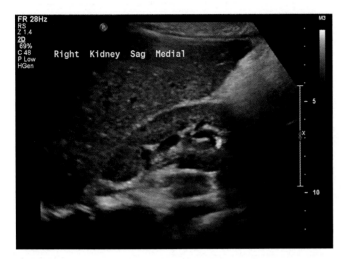

FIGURE 21-2. A 12-year-old pediatric patient with horseshoe kidney; sagittal right.

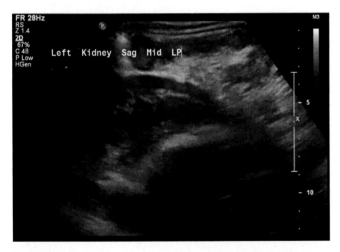

FIGURE 21-3. A 12-year-old pediatric patient with horseshoe kidney; sagittal left.

poor corticomedullary differentiation, and dilated bile ducts. In older children, the kidneys may only be mildly enlarged, have hyperechoic pyramids, small medullary cysts, and loss of corticomedullary differentiation.

Almost all patients with autosomal recessive polycystic disease have hepatic involvement in the form of congenital hepatic fibrosis, biliary ectasia, periportal hepatic fibrosis, and similar pathologies. The relationship between ARPKD and hepatic involvement is inverse. With worse presentation of ARPKD, there is less hepatic involvement and vice versa. Additionally, patients who present with renal disease early in life (i.e., perinatal, neonatal), renal involvement tends to dominate. However, patients presenting with renal disease later (i.e., infantile, juvenile), liver involvement tends to dominate.

Autosomal Dominant Polycystic Kidney Disease

Autosomal Dominant Polycystic Kidney Disease (ADPKD) is also known as "adult polycystic renal disease." Autosomal dominant polycystic kidney disease is a hereditary disorder arising from an abnormality on the short arm of chromosome 16 in 90% of cases, or from the long arm of chromosome 4 in 10% of cases. With ADPKD, cysts of varying size are seen within the renal cortex and medulla, with normal tissue located in between the cystic areas. Cysts may also develop within the liver, ovaries, pancreas, spleen, lungs, testes, and seminal vesicles. Clinical findings include a palpable abdominal mass in neonates, hypertension, flank pain, and hematuria. In neonates, the kidneys are diffusely echogenic with multiple small cysts. In older children, normal sized or enlarged kidneys may have multiple bilateral cortical cysts, calyceal distortion, hemorrhagic cysts containing internal low-level echoes, septations, thickened walls, and possible cysts within the liver.

Glomerulocystic Disease

Glomerulocystic disease is a rare renal disorder with cystic dilation of collecting tubules and Bowman spaces. This disorder is associated with other malformations including Zellweger syndrome, trisomy-13, and renal-retinal dysplasia. Sonographic findings include enlarged hyperechoic kidneys, poor corticomedullary differentiation, small cortical cysts measuring less than 1 centimeter, correlating hepatic adenomas, and hepatic cysts. Neonates may have large palpable kidneys with renal failure. Although rare, this etiology may be encountered as a distractor on the registry exam.

Medullary Sponge Kidney Disease

Medullary sponge kidney disease, also known as medullary tubular ectasia, is a sporadic, non-inherited disorder involving cystic dilation of the renal pyramid collecting tubules. This disorder is usually asymptomatic, but when urolithiasis or infection is present symptoms such as flank pain, renal colic, or hematuria may occur. If nephrocalcinosis occurs alongside medullary sponge kidney disease, sonographic findings may include hyperechoic pyramids with acoustic shadowing (Fig. 21-4 (a) to (c)).

NEPHRONOPHTHISIS

Nephronophthisis is an autosomal recessive hereditary disease. Over time this disease becomes an end-stage renal disease and is characterized by symptoms including polyuria, salt wasting, polydipsia, severe anemia, and renal failure. These symptoms generally become present during childhood into the adolescent years. Infantile nephronophthisis begins around 1 year of age. Juvenile nephronophthisis begins around 13 years of age. Adolescent nephronophthisis begins around 19 years of age. Sonographic findings include small-to-normal sized kidneys, containing small cysts in the medullary and corticomedullary junctions.

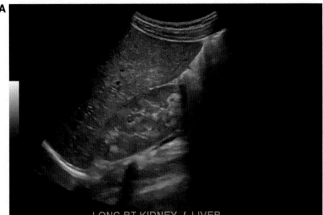

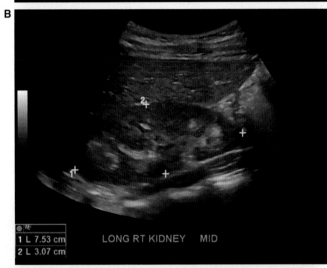

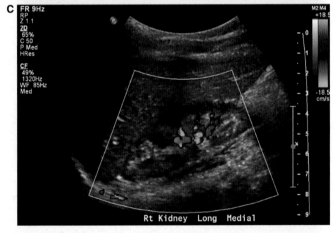

FIGURE 21-4. Hyperechogenicity of the renal pyramids consistent with medullary nephrocalcinosis in a 6-year-old pediatric patient with medullary sponge kidney disease.

UREMIC MEDULLARY CYSTIC DISEASE

Uremic medullary cystic disease is an autosomal dominant hereditary disease that usually presents in the second decade of life. This disease is characterized by polyuria, salt wasting, polydipsia, severe anemia, and renal failure. Sonographic findings include small kidney size, increased corticomedullary echogenicity, and medullary or corticomedullary cysts.

Tuberous Sclerosis

Tuberous sclerosis is an inherited autosomal dominant multisystem disorder that arises from a defect on chromosome 9. Many symptoms are associated with tuberous sclerosis including seizures, mental retardation, adenoma sebaceum, as well as cardiac, central nervous system, renal, and pulmonary lesions. When renal cysts occur with this disease, they are more commonly seen in infants and young children. Sonographic findings include multiple tiny bilateral hypoechoic or anechoic renal cystic lesions, and hyperechoic angiomyolipomas within the renal parenchyma (Fig. 21-5(a) and (b)).

VON HIPPEL-LINDAU DISEASE

Von Hippel-Lindau (vHL) disease in an inherited autosomal dominant multisystem disorder that arises from an error on the short arm of chromosome 3. This disease is associated with retinal and central nervous system hemangioblastomas, pancreatic cysts, islet cell tumors, renal cell carcinoma, and adrenal pheochromocytoma. Renal cysts occur in 60% of patients with vHL disease and may range from 0.5 to 3.0 centimeters in diameter.

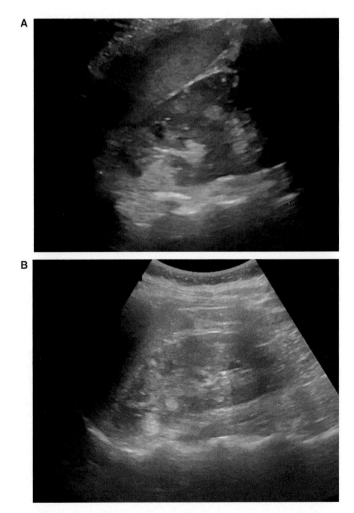

FIGURE 21-5. Multiple echogenic lesions in a kidney in an 11-year-old with tuberous sclerosis.

Acquired Cystic Renal Disease

Acquired renal cystic disease is typically seen in chronic renal failure patients on hemodialysis. Incidence of this disease increases with the number of years the patient is on dialysis. This is due to hyperplasia of the tubular epithelium with resulting nephron dilatation. Multiple small renal cysts are visualized in the medulla and cortex of the kidney, with bilateral small echogenic kidneys, possible cystic hemorrhage, and development of renal cell carcinoma. Other organs are not involved in this condition.

Miscellaneous Multisystem Disorders with Bilateral Renal Cysts

Other multisystem disorders involving bilateral simple renal cysts include Turner syndrome, Meckel syndrome, Jeune asphyxiating thoracic dystrophy, oral-facial-digital syndrome, and Zellweger syndrome, also known as cerebrohepatorenal syndrome. Meckel syndrome is also characterized by microcephaly, polydactyly, and posterior encephalocele. Jeune asphyxiating thoracic dystrophy patients may also have symptoms of respiratory failure, renal dysplasia, and an anatomically small thorax.

UNILATERAL RENAL CYSTIC DISEASES

Simple Renal Cysts

Simple renal cysts (Fig. 21-6) are rare in children, occurring in less than 1% of the pediatric population. When occurring, they are typically unilocular with clear serous fluid arising in renal cortex, noncommunicating with the collecting system, and usually solitary. Lesions that may mimic a simple renal cyst include aneurysm, pseudoaneurysm, lymphoma, or upper pole duplication.

Multicystic Dysplastic Kidney Disease

Multicystic dysplastic kidney disease (MCDKD) is a nonhereditary developmental anomaly due to early in-utero urinary tract obstruction that occurs within the first 10 weeks of gestation. Multiple non-communicating renal cysts of various sizes separated by fibrous tissue contain primitive dysplastic elements in the affected kidney. Most cases of multicystic dysplastic kidney disease are diagnosed during prenatal ultrasound. Sonographic findings of MCDKD include nondiscernable interface between the renal pelvis and sinus, absent renal parenchyma (Fig. 21-7(a) and (b)), and multiple cysts of varying sizes with random distribution (Fig. 21-8(a) to (c)). Multicystic dysplastic kidney disease is treated non-operatively, the affected kidney will spontaneously decrease in size during the first year of life and will be resorbed until it is eventually nonvisible upon ultrasound examination. Renal anomalies associated with MCDKD may include vesicoureteral reflux, uretero-pelvic junction obstruction, primary megaureter, and obstructed and/or duplex systems in the contralateral kidney (Fig. 21-9).

Cystic Nephroma

Multilocular cystic renal tumor was previously thought to be a tumor that occurred in both pediatrics and adults. This tumor is now thought to be two separate entities. In 2016, the World Health Organization classified the pediatric-specific multilocular cystic renal tumor as distinct, and it is now referred to as pediatric cystic nephroma. The adult-specific entity is multilocular cystic renal neoplasm of low malignant potential (previously multilocular cystic renal cell carcinoma). It was

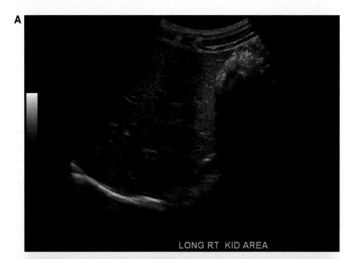
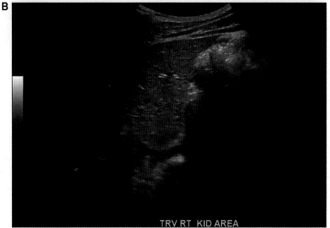

FIGURE 21-7. Right involuted multicystic dysplastic kidney.

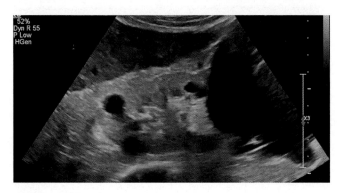

FIGURE 21-6. Simple renal cysts.

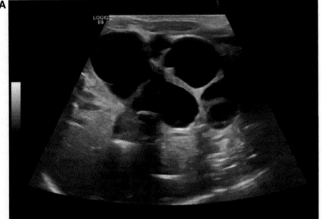

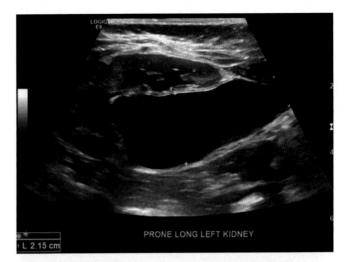

FIGURE 21-9. Absent renal parenchyma in a 3-year-old pediatric patient with history of right involuted multicystic dysplastic kidney, and ureteropelvic junction obstruction with severe pelvic dilatation in the contralateral kidney.

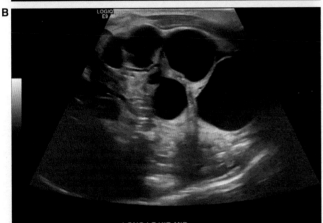

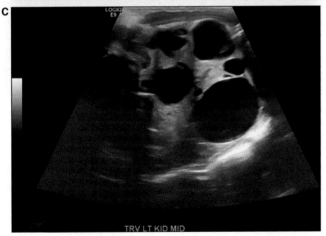

FIGURE 21-8. Musticystic dysplastic left kidney in a 3-day old pediatric patient, diagnosed on fetal MRI prior to birth. No normal renal tissue visualized; multiple non-communicating cysts are demonstrated in the left renal bed.

multiloculated, unifocal mass with a thick surrounding fibrous capsule compressing the renal parenchyma. The sonographic "claw sign" may be observed, where the renal parenchyma takes on a claw-shape adjacent to the mass, confirming the mass originates from the renal tissue. These lesions are generally treated by radical nephrectomy or heminephrectomy, with excision of the lymph nodes.

DUPLICATION ANOMALIES

Partial Renal Duplication

Duplication of the renal collecting system can be partial or complete and is the most common congenital anomaly of the urinary tract. Partial duplication can involve a bifid renal pelvis, Y-shaped ureters, or two ureters fusing along their course, producing a single distal ureter. Partial duplication anomalies are not clinically significant. A partially duplicated kidney (duplex kidney) is larger than a single-collecting system kidney with two separate echogenic renal sinuses (Fig. 21-10(a) and (b)).

Complete Renal Duplication

With complete ureteropelvic duplication, kidneys have two distinct pelvicaliceal systems and two ureters, with each its own insertion point into the kidney. The ureter at the lower pole is generally located at the normal insertion point, but not in the usual oblique lie, therefore prone to reflux. The ureter at the upper pole has an ectopic insertion and is prone to obstruction. This ureter can appear echogenic with small cysts due to dysplasia or may be hypoplastic rather than dilated. The distal portion of this ureter may insert below the trigone of the bladder and into the vagina, urethra, vestibule, uterus, cervix, or rectum in female patients. In males, the distal portion of this ureter can insert below the trigone and into the posterior urethra, bladder neck, ejaculation ducts, seminal vesicles, or rectum. These

determined that features between pediatric specific nephroma and adult cystic nephroma were genetically, morphologically, and immunohistochemically unique.

These tumors are rare, but most often occur in young children between 3 months and 5 years of age with a 75% male predominance. Pediatric cystic nephromas present as a non-painful palpable abdominal mass with possible urinary tract infections and/or hematuria. The tumor appears as a

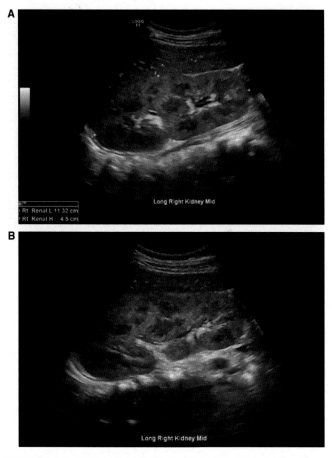

FIGURE 21-10. Enlarged right kidney in a 19-month-old pediatric patient consistent with partially duplex collecting system configuration.

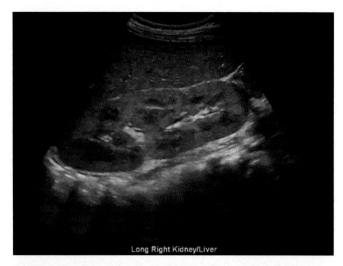

FIGURE 21-11. Enlarged right kidney with diffuse increase in cortical echogenicity in a 19-month-old pediatric patient consistent with pyelonephritis. This patient tested positive for urinary tract infection and has a history of vesicoureteral reflux.

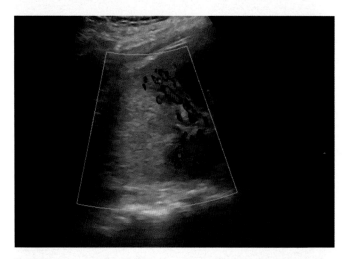

FIGURE 21-12. Pyelonephritis in the upper pole of the right kidney with increased echotexture and lack of vascularity.

anomalies are most common in females, presenting as urinary tract infections later in life with possible incontinence. A heminephrectomy may be performed in patients with severe upper pole hydronephrosis and poor renal function.

Complete duplication involves a kidney with two pelvicaliceal systems and two ureters that enter the bladder through separate orifices. Refractive duplication artifact can be easily confused with duplication of the renal collecting system. With refractive duplication artifact, refraction of sound at the interface between the kidney and spleen or liver and adjacent fat creates an image appearing similar to duplication of the superior aspect on the kidney or simulates a suprarenal mass. Renal duplication artifact occurs more frequently in the left kidney than in the right.

RENAL INFECTIONS

Acute Bacterial Pyelonephritis

Acute bacterial pyelonephritis is an infection of the collecting system and renal parenchyma. Bacterial pyelonephritis results most commonly from vesicoureteral reflux (ascending infection). Uncommonly, acute bacterial pyelonephritis can result from hematogenous spread (i.e., Escherichia coli bacteria). This bacterial infection causes global or focal kidney enlargement

with increased echogenicity, renal pelvic and ureter wall thickening, loss of corticomedullary differentiation, and decreased blood flow to varied renal tissues (Figs. 21-11 and 21-12). Clinical findings may include fever, vomiting, irritability, failure to gain weight, flank pain, and costovertebral tenderness.

Complicated Acute Pyelonephritis with Abscess

Complicated acute pyelonephritis includes a necrotic renal cavity filled with purulent material. This may result from an inadequately treated interstitial infection that liquefies. Clinical findings in patients with complicated acute pyelonephritis with abscess include fever, abdominal and flank pain, and pyuria. Sonographic findings include a hypoechoic renal mass with thick irregular walls, septations, mobile debris, echogenic foci with dirty shadowing due to gas-forming organisms, and hypoechoic perinephric fat resulting from edema. Treatment includes antibiotics and percutaneous or surgical drainage.

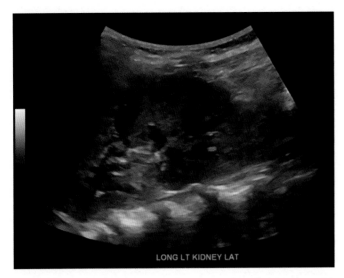

FIGURE 21-13. Lobular renal contour in a 5-year-old pediatric patient with recurrent pyelonephritis.

Chronic Pyelonephritis

Chronic pyelonephritis is defined as parenchymal scarring that results from single or multiple episodes of acute pyelonephritis. Sonographic findings include renal hypoplasia with cortical atrophy, cortical scarring, loss of corticomedullary differentiation, and irregular lobulated renal contour (Fig. 21-13).

Xanthogranulomatous Pyelonephritis

Xanthogranulomatous pyelonephritis is identified as a chronic granulomatous process due to recurrent urinary tract infection and obstruction. Clinical findings include renal parenchyma destruction replaced by necrotic inflammatory debris with macrophages (xanthoma cells) bordered by fibrous tissue. Fever, flank pain, and hematuria may result due to organisms Proteus and Escherichia coli retrograde entering the kidneys. Sonographic appearance includes nephromegaly, a hypoechoic cortical mass with shadowing stones in the adjacent calyx and renal sinus, areas of parenchymal destruction, and perinephric fluid collections, with the remainder of the kidney appearing normal. Treatment typically includes nephrectomy or partial nephrectomy.

Glomerulonephritis

Glomerulonephritis is an immune complex mediated condition with cellular infiltrate in the glomerular tufts, and interstitial edema. Clinical symptoms include hematuria and hypertension. Sonographic findings may include bilaterally enlarged kidneys with increased cortical echogenicity. Chronic glomerulonephritis may lead to small, diffusely echogenic kidneys with absent corticomedullary differentiation.

Acute Interstitial Nephritis

Acute interstitial nephritis is a reversible form of renal failure secondary to an acute hypersensitivity reaction to medication.

Acute interstitial nephritis resolves with termination of drug therapy. Sonographic findings include enlarged echogenic kidneys.

Pyonephritis

Pyonephrosis is an accumulation of purulent exudate within the hydronephrotic kidney. This accumulation of exudate occurs due to an obstructive uropathy, ureteral calculi, or ureteral stricture. The most common cause is Escherichia coli retrograde entering the kidney. Pyonephrosis is a urologic emergency that requires urgent percutaneous or surgical drainage. Left untreated, pyonephrosis can lead to gram-negative bacteremia, septic shock, and loss of renal function. Sonographic findings include dilated collecting system with mobile debris and debris in urine, bright echoes with dirty shadowing due to gas, and a fluid-debris level.

Renal Fungal Infection

Renal fungal infections usually occur due to indwelling catheters, prolonged immune-suppressing medication, or AIDS. Fungal infections result from hematogenous seeding of Candida albicans causing micro abscesses and fungal ball formation. Other fungal infections that may occur include renal cortex inflammatory infiltrate and necrotizing papillitis. Candidiasis is the most common renal fungal disease. Sonographic findings include enlarged kidneys, increased parenchymal echogenicity, abscess, non-shadowing echogenic masses representing fungal balls in the pelvis, calyces, or urinary bladder that may obstruct the collecting system, and pyonephrosis.

Acute Tubular Necrosis

Acute tubular necrosis is nephrotoxic or ischemic injury to renal tubules following medication administration. Acute tubular necrosis is accompanied by acute renal failure. Sonographic findings include renal enlargement, hyperechoic cortex, enlarged hypoechoic pyramids, reduced diastolic Doppler flow, and an elevated resistive index.

Acute Renal Cortical Necrosis

Acute renal cortical necrosis includes ischemic injury to the renal cortex, sparing the medullary pyramids. This form of necrosis is caused by severe dehydration, sepsis, blood loss, or sickle cell disease (see Figs. 21-14 and 21-15). Sonographic findings include increased cortical echogenicity and prominent pyramids, with cortical calcifications occurring in chronic forms of this disease.

BENIGN RENAL LESIONS

Mesoblastic Nephroma (Fetal Renal Hamartoma)

Mesoblastic nephroma, also known as "fetal renal hamartoma," is the most common renal tumor in the neonate. This benign process presents in the first 6 months of life and is associated

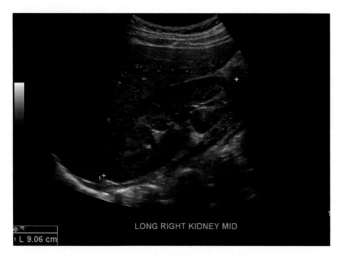

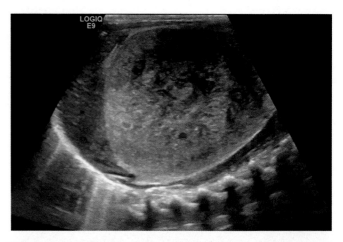

FIGURE 21-14. Hyperechogenicity and prominent renal pyramids in a 6-year-old pediatric patient with sickle-cell disease and mild renal artery stenosis

FIGURE 21-16. A 37-week neonate with a prenatal history of enlarged right kidney and palpable mass upon delivery.

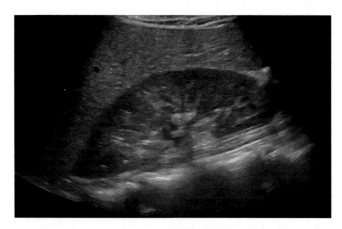

FIGURE 21-15. Prominent renal pyramids in a pediatric patient with sickle-cell disease.

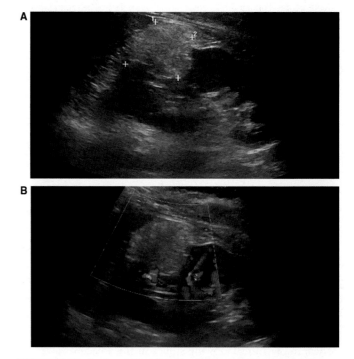

FIGURE 21-17. Angiomyolipoma arising in the superior renal cortex.

with cytogenic abnormalities on chromosome-11 and translocations. Clinical findings of mesoblastic nephroma include hypertension and a palpable abdominal mass. Sonographic appearance can include a large homogeneous or heterogeneous echogenic vascular mass with areas of necrosis and hemorrhage (Fig. 21-16). Concentric hypoechoic and hyperechoic rings surround the tumor and there are areas of highly reflective fat. Treatment options include nephrectomy or heminephrectomy with chemotherapy in patients with recurrent tumors.

Angiomyolipoma (Renal Hamartoma)

Angiomyolipoma, also referred to as "renal hamartoma," is a benign renal neoplasm with a varying amount of mature adipose tissue, smooth muscle, and blood vessels. Angiomyolipoma is the most common benign, solid lesion of the kidney which contains fat, although angiomyolipoma tends to be fat-poor in pediatrics. Usually an incidental finding, angiomyolipoma is a small bilateral hyperechoic neoplasm (Fig. 21-17(a) and (b)) in the renal cortex that causes hematuria, abdominal pain, and anemia secondary to hemorrhage. Angiomyolipoma

is often associated with tuberous sclerosis or other phakomatosis, such as neurofibromatosis type 1 (NF1, von Recklinghausen disease) or vHL syndrome. Angiomyolipoma is also associated with lymphangioleiomyomatosis, a type of low-grade metastasizing perivascular epithelioid cell tumor.

In cases of NF1 and vHL, angiomyolipoma generally presents by 10 years of age. In this setting, angiomyolipomas may be numerous, increased in size, and fat poor. Renal failure occurs once the tumor replaces the majority of normal renal parenchyma. An angiomyolipoma measuring greater than 3.5 centimeters has a higher risk of hemorrhage occurrence.

Metanephric Adenoma

Metanephric adenoma, also known as embryonal adenoma and metanephric adenofibroma, is a renal neoplasm consisting of epithelial and stromal cells. Clinical findings associated with metanephric adenoma include palpable flank mass, flank pain, hematuria, hypertension, hypercalcemia, and polycythemia from increased erythropoietin secretion. Sonographic appearance includes small well-defined, hypovascular, round, solid masses of varying echogenicity, containing echogenic psammomatous calcification and necrotic areas of hypoechoic foci.

Ossifying Renal Tumor of Infancy

Ossifying renal tumor of infancy is a rare neoplasm occurring in the first year after birth. This tumor presents as a palpable abdominal mass containing osteoid, osteoblasts, and spindle cells with gross hematuria. This tumor generally measures less than 2 to 3 centimeters in size. Sonographic appearance includes intense reflective echogenic foci with shadowing and hydronephrosis due to collecting system extension. Treatment options include nephrectomy or heminephrectomy. Although rare, this etiology may be encountered as a distractor on the registry exam.

Inflammatory Pseudotumor

Inflammatory pseudotumor is a benign tumor-like condition created from spindle-shaped cells and inflammatory lymphocytes, histiocytes, and plasma cells. Inflammatory pseudotumor is also referred to as inflammatory myoblastic tumor and plasma cell granuloma. Clinical findings include hematuria and abdominal pain. Sonographic findings may include a nonspecific homogeneous or heterogeneous mass in the renal parenchyma or pelvis.

MALIGNANT RENAL LESIONS

Wilms Tumor (Nephroblastoma)

Wilms tumor, or nephroblastoma, is the most common renal malignancy in children. This pathologic process accounts for 90% of all pediatric renal malignancies and presents before 5 years of age. Clinical findings include a palpable abdominal mass, abdominal pain, fever, microscopic or gross hematuria, and hypertension due to compression of the hilar vessels. Sonographic findings include a homogeneous or heterogeneous mass containing areas of necrosis, fat, and calcification (Fig. 21-18(a) to (e)). This mass is contained within the renal tissue. These masses can get large in size and may be seen greater than 12 centimeters. Wilms tumor is categorized in stages I-V (Table 21-1). With stage I, the tumor is limited to the kidney alone and can be resected. With stage II, Wilms tumor extends beyond the kidney; however, may still be resected. In stage III, the Wilms tumor is confined to the abdomen without hematogenous spread. With stage IV, hematogenous metastasis may be seen in the lung, liver, bone, and brain tissues. Lastly, stage V consists of bilateral renal involvement at the time of diagnosis.

Syndromes associated with Wilms tumor include Beckwith-Wiedemann syndrome, congenital hemihypertrophy, WAGR syndrome, Drash syndrome, and Perlman syndrome. WAGR syndrome is comprised of *W*ilms tumor, sporadic *A*niridia, *G*enital malformations, and mental *R*etardation (currently referred to as intellectual disability). Drash syndrome consists of male pesuedohermaphroditism and nephritis. Perlman syndrome is a compilation of fetal overgrowth, neonatal macrosomia, macrocephaly, dysmorphic facial features, visceromegaly, nephroblastomatosis.

Nephroblastomatosis

Nephroblastomatosis is a multifocal or diffuse renal involvement with nephrogenic rests. Nephrogenic rests are clusters of embryonal cells that prevail during renal development, representing microscopic abnormalities. Nephroblastomatosis is a malignant nephrogenesis abnormality and potentially a precursor to Wilms tumor. In 30 to 40% of cases, nephrogenic rests induce Wilms tumor, and are found in 99% of bilateral Wilms tumors. This process is characterized by fetal renal blastema and nephrogenic rests persisting beyond 36 weeks gestational age. Nephrogenic rests may be intralobar, perilobar, or mixed renal lobules with tumor development. Clinical findings include flank mass or bilateral nephromegaly during high-risk obstetrical screening examination. Sonographic appearance is variable, but most commonly seen are multiple hypoechoic tissue masses in enlarged reniform-shape kidneys with absent corticomedullary differentiation (Fig. 21-19). Treatment for nephroblastomatosis includes chemotherapy.

Renal Cell Carcinoma

Renal cell carcinoma is a rare neoplasm in pediatric patients arising from epithelial cells of the renal tubule. Although rare in pediatrics, this etiology may be encountered as a distractor on the registry exam. This malignant process has a 2:1 male predominance ratio, most commonly occurring around 10 years

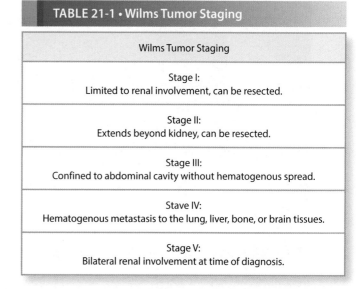

TABLE 21-1 • Wilms Tumor Staging
Wilms Tumor Staging
Stage I: Limited to renal involvement, can be resected.
Stage II: Extends beyond kidney, can be resected.
Stage III: Confined to abdominal cavity without hematogenous spread.
Stave IV: Hematogenous metastasis to the lung, liver, bone, or brain tissues.
Stage V: Bilateral renal involvement at time of diagnosis.

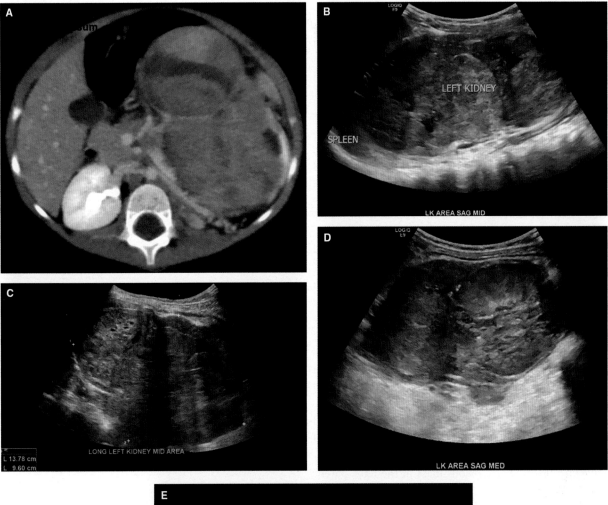

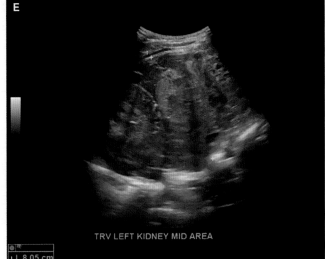

FIGURE 21-18. In a 3-year-old pediatric patient, the demonstrated left kidney is replaced by nodular masses with calcifications and whorling soft tissue bands. In this age group, Wilms tumor is the most likely cause and was confirmed by needle biopsy.

of age. Clinical findings include flank pain, palpable abdominal mass, fever, hematuria, hypertension, polycythemia, and dysuria. Metastasis to the lungs, liver, bone, renal vein, and invasion of the inferior vena cava are possible. Sonographic findings include a solid renal mass of varying echogenicity and size.

Areas of necrosis, hemorrhage, and calcification are commonly seen. Renal cell carcinoma is associated with vHL syndrome, urogenital malformations, tuberous sclerosis, and Beckwith-Wiedemann syndrome. Renal cell carcinoma presents in 2 to 4% of patients with tuberous sclerosis.

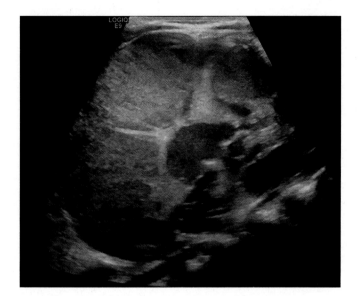

FIGURE 21-19. Nephroblastomatosis in a 2-year-old.

Lymphoma

Renal lymphoma most commonly presents as multiple bilateral infiltrative or hypodense renal cortical masses. Sonographically, multiple hypoechoic lesions are seen within the renal parenchyma with minimal internal vascularity and absent distal acoustic enhancement. Alternatively, renal lymphoma can appear as a solitary hypoechoic renal mass due to direct invasion via the lymph nodes. Renal involvement occurs because of hematogenous spread or by direct extension of retroperitoneal tumor. It is also pondered primary renal lymphoma originates from the renal capsule or lymphoid-rich peri-renal fat, extending into the renal parenchyma. If retroperitoneal lymph nodes compress the ureter, ureteral dilatation and hydronephrosis can occur. The kidneys are more commonly affected by lymphoma in non-Hodgkin pediatric patients greater than 5 years of age. The most common clinical symptom occurring in 56% of renal lymphoma patients less than 18 years of age is fever. The most common clinical symptom occurring in 62% of renal lymphoma patients greater than 18 years of age is flank pain. Additional clinical symptoms include palpable mass, hematuria, weight loss, and with infiltrative disease, acute renal failure.

Leukemia

Acute lymphoblastic leukemia is the most common general malignancy of childhood, most prevalent in children 3 to 5 years of age. Clinical findings may include abdominal pain, hypertension, hematuria, and renal failure. Sonographic findings for diffuse leukemia include nephromegaly with smooth renal contour, overall maintained reniform shape, normal to decreased echogenicity, and loss of corticomedullary differentiation. Sonographic findings related to the kidneys include solitary or multiple renal masses and hydronephrosis due to ureteral obstruction by enlarged retroperitoneal lymph nodes.

Rhabdoid Tumor (Medullary)

Rhabdoid tumor is a rare aggressive malignant neoplasm of the renal medulla. This medullary tumor accounts for only 2% of malignancies and occurs around 18 months of age. Clinical findings include abdominal mass, fever, hypertension, and hypercalcemia. Sonographic findings involve a large heterogeneous intrarenal mass with indistinct margins, infiltration of the renal hilum, and possible extension into the renal vein and inferior vena cava. Although rare, this etiology may be encountered as a distractor on the registry exam.

Clear Cell Sarcoma (Medullary)

Clear cell sarcoma is a malignancy arising from the renal medulla in pediatric patients between 1 to 4 years of age. Occasionally clear cell sarcoma can present in-utero or in neonatal patients. Sonographic findings include a poorly defined heterogeneous mass with cystic changes, infiltration of renal medulla and pelvis, and metastasis.

Renal Medullary Carcinoma

Renal medullary carcinoma is an aggressive neoplasm of epithelial origin within the renal medulla. This malignant process is commonly found in patients with sickle cell trait and hemoglobin sickle cell disease. The right kidney is most susceptible to renal medullary carcinoma, usually occurring in the second to third decade of life. Clinical findings include flank and abdominal pain, gross hematuria, occasional palpable mass, weight loss, and fever. Sonographic findings include a heterogeneous hypovascular mass containing hemorrhage and necrosis in the parenchyma (Fig. 21-20). This mass can invade the renal pelvis causing caliectasis, and generally has a poor prognosis.

Primitive Neuroectodermal Tumor

Primitive neuroectodermal tumor is a rare, highly malignant neoplasm associated with translocation of tissue between chromosomes 11 and 21. Sonographic findings include nonspecific poorly defined, solid, infiltrative mass with calcifications, necrosis, and hemorrhage. Primitive neuroectodermal tumor can extend into the renal vein and inferior vena cava. Although rare, this etiology may be encountered as a distractor on the registry exam.

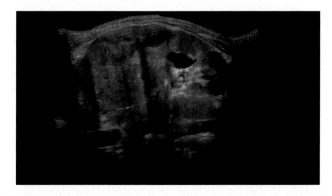

FIGURE 21-20. Renal medullary carcinoma in a 13-year-old with sickle cell trait with distended abdomen.

Primary Sarcoma

Rare sarcoma subtypes include leiomyosarcoma, angiosarcoma, hemangiopericytoma, rhabdomyosarcoma, fibrosarcoma, and osteosarcoma which are indistinguishable from renal tumors. Sarcomas appear as well defined or diffuse neoplasms with systemic metastasis. Although rare, these etiologies may be encountered as distractors on the registry exam.

RENAL TRANSPLANTS AND FAILURE

Normal Renal Allograft

In young pediatric patients, the transplant kidney is anastomosed to the distal aorta and inferior vena cava within the intraperitoneal cavity. In older pediatric patients, the transplant kidney is anastomosed to the iliac vessels in the retroperitoneum. The normal sonographic appearance of a transplant kidney should be like that of the native kidney. The resistive index (RI) should fall between 0.4 and 0.8, with a mean RI of 0.6.

Please see information related to renal transplant protocol in Chapter 11, "Pediatric Renal Vasculature."

Transplant Rejection

Rejection is the most common cause of allograft failure. Acute rejection occurs within the first 3 months. Clinical findings of acute rejection include oliguria, fever, graft enlargement, tenderness, and elevated creatinine. Chronic rejection occurs 3 months to years after the transplant. With chronic rejection, scarring and cortical thinning of the transplant kidney occurs. Clinical findings of chronic rejection include azotemia (elevated blood urea nitrogen [BUN] and creatinine), proteinuria, and hypertension.

Interstitial Transplant Rejection

Interstitial transplant rejection is characterized by cellular infiltration of the cortex, interstitial edema, and tubular necrosis. Sonographic findings of interstitial transplant rejection include a normal RI and no increase in vascular impedance.

Vascular Transplant Rejection

Vascular transplant rejection is characterized by endovasculitis, endothelium swelling and inflammation, vessel wall damage, thrombus, and luminal obliteration. Sonographic findings of acute vascular rejection are increased vascular impedance with decreased or absent diastolic flow. Sonographic findings of chronic vascular rejection are a high resistance waveform, elevated peak systolic velocity, decreased or reversed diastolic flow, and elevated resistive indices between 0.7 and 1.0 (Fig. 21-21).

Transplant Acute Tubular Necrosis

Transplant acute tubular necrosis occurs in the first 24 hours after the transplant, resulting from prolonged ischemia. Sonographic findings include graft enlargement, increased cortical echogenicity, loss of corticomedullary differentiation, enlarged

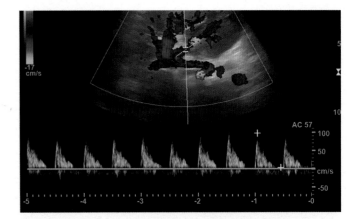

FIGURE 21-21. A 6-year-old female with elevated creatinine levels. Sonogram demonstrates abnormal arterial waveforms on all interrogated arteries, with increased resistive indices (1.0) and loss of diastolic flow. Rejection was present on renal allograft biopsy.

hypoechoic pyramids, reversed diastolic flow, and a high resistive index.

Drug Toxicity Transplant Failure

Drug toxicity transplant failure is cyclosporine-induced nephropathy producing tubular damage, glomerular thrombi, endothelial swelling, and interstitial nephritis. This form of transplant failure occurs 1 to 4 months following the transplant. Sonographic findings are nonspecific.

Transplant Perinephric Fluid Collections

Transplant perinephric fluid collections include lymphocele, urinoma, hematoma, and abscess.

Perinephric Lymphocele

Perinephric lymphocele is the most common perinephric fluid collection. This collection results from seepage of lymph from severed lymphatic vessels following transplant. Lymphocele typically develops 2 to 8 weeks following surgery. Clinical symptoms include decreased renal function secondary to ureteral compression, pelvic or inguinal mass, and ipsilateral lower extremity edema. Sonographic appearance includes a welldefined, complex, hypoechoic mass with septation inferomedial to the allograft between the bladder and transplant kidney with present hydronephrosis.

Perinephric Urinoma

Perinephric urinoma (Fig. 21-22) is less common in comparison to other perinephric fluid collections. Urinomas occur from ureteroneocystostomy defects causing urine leakage within the first 2 weeks following a transplant. Clinical findings include oliguria, pain, and swelling over allograft site.

Perinephric Hematoma

Perinephric hematoma occurs immediately post-op following allograft surgery and has varying clinical significance based on hematoma size. Potential adverse effects related to perinephric hematoma include a decrease in hematocrit, compression

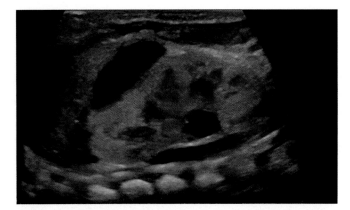

FIGURE 21-22. Perinephric urinoma in a 1-month-old patient with posterior urethral valves status post ablation.

of the kidney, ureter, or vessels, decreased urine output secondary to ureteral compression, and/or shock. Clinical findings include allograft and back pain. Sonographic appearance includes hyperechoic acute hemorrhage, complex subacute, or hypoechoic chronic hemorrhage. Perinephric hematoma is observed to resolution.

Perinephric Abscess

Perinephric abscess results from superimposed infection of lymphocele, hematoma, or urinoma. Abscess may also result as a complication of graft pyelonephritis. Clinical findings include fever, leukocytosis, and pain over the allograft site. Sonographic appearance includes a hypoechoic fluid collection containing debris or septations, with reflective echoes and dirty shadow due to gas-producing components (Figs. 21-23 and 21-24).

Renal Trauma

The kidneys are the third most frequently injured organ resulting from blunt abdominal trauma, following the liver and spleen. Symptoms and findings of renal trauma include marked hematuria, hematoma, laceration, contusion, and possible kidney shattering.

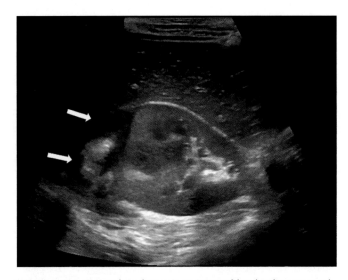

FIGURE 21-23. Perinephric abscess in an 8-year-old male who presented with fever of unknown origin.

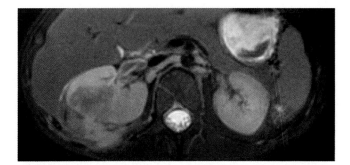

FIGURE 21-24. MRI showing perinephric abscess in an 8-year-old male who presented with fever of unknown origin.

RENAL VASCULAR DISEASE

Renal Artery Stenosis

In children, fibromuscular dysplasia is the most common cause of renal artery stenosis. Fibromuscular dysplasia is a non-inflammatory vascular disease that most commonly affects the renal arteries. Renal artery stenosis can cause hypertension and usually involves the mid to distal main renal artery. Sonographic findings of renal artery stenosis include a size discrepancy between kidneys due to ischemia. In children, a length differential of >1 centimeter between two kidneys when hypertension is present is considered abnormal. On ultrasound, the stenosed kidney generally atrophies while the contralateral, nonaffected kidney appears increased in size due to compensatory hypertrophy. Doppler evaluation in the affected kidney will show stenosis of the main renal artery, which is characterized by a >60% vessel diameter narrowing. The stenosed kidney will have an increased peak systolic velocity of >150 cm/s at the site of stenosis (Fig. 21-25), with post-stenotic turbulence, spectral broadening, tardus parvus waveforms, acceleration time of >0.07 seconds, and a renal-aortic ratio (RAR) of >3.5.

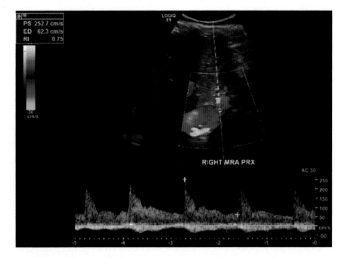

FIGURE 21-25. Throughout the right main renal artery in a 13-year-old pediatric patient there is increased peak systolic velocity, demonstrated up to 252.7 cm/s at origin. Velocities greater than 200 cm/s indicate underlying stenosis in an adult patient, and velocities greater than 150 cm/s demonstrate underlying stenosis in pediatrics.

The RAR can be calculated by dividing the renal artery peak systolic velocity by the aorta's peak systolic velocity.

$$RAR = \frac{HIGHEST\ RENAL\ ARTERY\ PSV}{AORTIC\ PSV}$$

If the aortic velocity is too high or low, the RAR may be inaccurate. An aortic velocity <40 cm/s can falsely increase the RAR (i.e., if the RAR is >3, the PSV should be >200 cm/s to document a 60-99% stenosis). An aortic velocity >100 cm/s may lead to an inaccurate, falsely low RAR.

Renal Artery Thrombosis

Renal artery thrombosis usually occurs in infants with sepsis, dehydration, hemoconcentration, indwelling umbilical artery catheter, or in infants with diabetic mothers. Clinical findings with renal artery thrombosis include acute flank pain and hematuria. In older children, renal artery thrombosis can occur due to vasculitis, emboli, or traumatic dissection. Sonographic findings include global kidney infarct, and an echogenic kidney followed by absent or reversed Doppler flow in the main segmental renal arteries suggesting occlusion. A chronic ischemic kidney appears atrophied with increased echogenicity.

Renal Vein Thrombosis

Predominantly a newborn disease, renal vein thrombosis usually occurs because of severe dehydration, hemoconcentration secondary to blood loss, sepsis, or diarrhea. Thrombus generally begins in the inferior vena cava and propagates into the renal vein. Clinical symptoms include palpable flank mass, flank pain, hematuria, and proteinuria. Sonographic findings of renal vein thrombosis include edema, hemorrhage, adrenal hemorrhage if the left renal vein is involved, acute enlarged kidney with increased echogenicity, absent corticomedullary differentiation, and absent venous signal around the thrombus in the main renal vein to the inferior vena cava junction. These findings are followed by chronic decreased echogenicity and an atrophied heterogeneous kidney if left untreated.

BLADDER AND URETERS

Ureterocele

A simple ureterocele in pediatrics is the abnormal dilation of the distal ureteral segment which balloons, or herniates, into the bladder (Figs. 21-26 and 21-27). This ballooning occurs secondary to an abnormal ureterovesical junction (UVJ), resulting from congenital stenosis or an inflammatory stricture. Ureterocele is a congenital anomaly that has a female and Caucasian predominance. Ureterocele may be intravesical (25%) or extravesical (75%) in location. Intravesical ureterocele occurs at the UVJ whereas extravesical, or ectopic, ureterocele occurs at the region of the bladder neck. In pediatric patients, ureteroceles can be associated with obstruction, renal dysplasia, hydroureter,

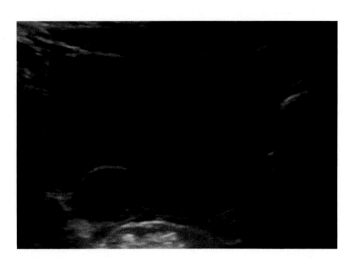

FIGURE 21-26. Ureterocele.

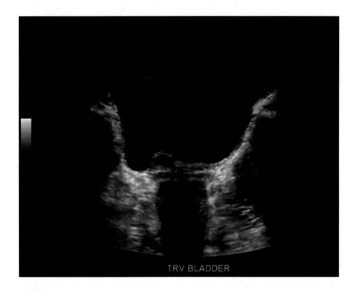

FIGURE 21-27. Right trigonal ureterocele in an 8-year-old pediatric patient.

hydronephrosis, and urinary infection. A ureterocele may be seen collapsing during peristalsis upon imaging.

Bladder Exstrophy

Bladder exstrophy occurs due to failure of midline infraumbilical abdominal wall closure, leading to exposure of the anterior bladder wall, neck, and urethra. Surgical correction of this condition consists of bladder and abdominal wall closure with bladder augmentation where the bowel segment is attached to the native bladder. This attachment acts as the bladder base and neck. With this procedure, the bladder wall may have the "bowel signature" with hypoechoic outer wall and echogenic inner mucosa.

Urachal Anomalies

During fetal development, the umbilicus and anterior bladder wall communicate via the urachus. This tubular channel normally closes during the fourth to fifth month of gestation, leaving a fibrous urachal remnant (Fig. 21-28(a) and (b)). If

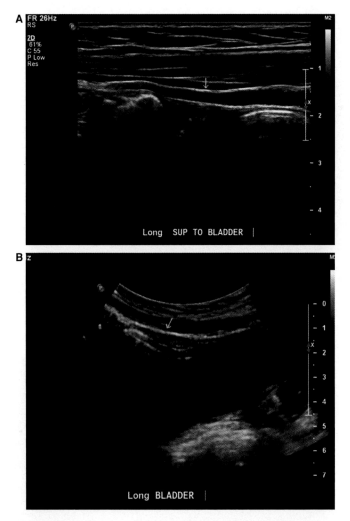

FIGURE 21-28. Fibrous urachal remnant without patent urachal tract visualized in an 11-year-old pediatric patient. A patent tract would appear anechoic, containing fluid.

the urachus does not completely close, it can result in a patent urachus, urachal sinus, urachal diverticulum, or urachal cyst. A patent urachus includes failed lumen closure with a patent channel, which can lead to umbilical drainage and infection. With a urachal sinus, the channel is present solely at the umbilicus with umbilical drainage and infection. Urachal diverticulum includes a channel present at the bladder alone. Urachal cysts may occur when the channel is closed at the umbilicus and bladder, but remains open in the center, resembling a cyst. Pyourachus is an infection of the urachal remnants with intraperitoneal abscess, ascites, and bladder wall thickening at the dome of the bladder.

Obstructive Processes

Ureteropelvic junction obstruction (UPJ) is also referred to as pelviureteric junction obstruction. UPJ can be acquired or congenital. Congenital UPJ is one of the most common causes of antenatal hydronephrosis. Congenital UPJ has a 2:1 male prevalence and occurs in 1 per 1,000 to 2,000 children.

Ureteral obstruction also occurs in 1 to 10% of transplants due to intrinsic lesions or extrinsic compression. Intrinsic

lesions may include ureteral stricture, clot, or calculi whereas extrinsic compression is caused by an external source such as hematoma, urinoma, or lymphocele. Compression may also be caused by vessels crossing at the UPJ. Most ureteral obstructive processes are located at or near the ureterovesical junction, and patients present with deteriorating renal function. A distended bladder is another obstructive process in which it increases resistance to ureteral emptying resulting in collecting system dilatation.

Vesicoureteral Reflux

Vesicoureteral reflux is the retrograde flow of urine from the bladder into the ureters or renal collecting system (Fig. 21-29(a) and (b)). Normal ureters enter the bladder at an oblique angle and most reflux is due to abnormal angle of ureter insertion into the bladder. This leads to incompetent anti-reflux flap-valve mechanism, which is the primary cause of vesicoureteral reflux. Secondary causes of reflux include bladder outlet obstruction, voiding dysfunction, neurogenic disease, and prune belly syndrome.

Guided cystography with microbubbles is a more recent technique to diagnose reflux, where the bladder is catheterized

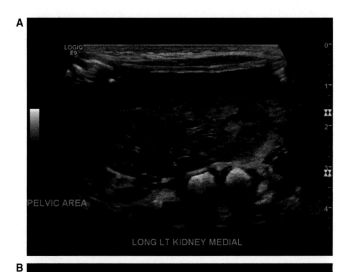

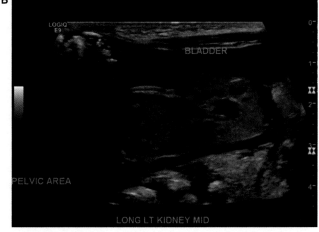

FIGURE 21-29. Left ectopic (pelvic) kidney in infant with vesicoureteral reflux.

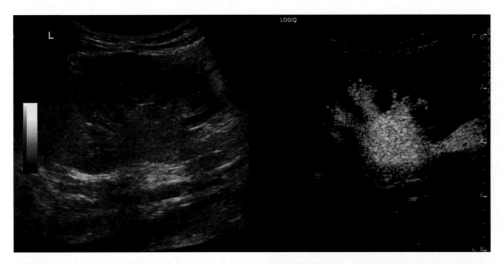

FIGURE 21-30. A 2-year-old female with multiple urinary tract infections being evaluated for reflux with voiding urosonogram. Grade 4 vesicoureteric reflux is present on the left during filling and voiding.

and saline or a contrast agent is injected to detect retrograde passage of microbubbles from the bladder into the ureters or renal pelvis (Fig. 21-30).

Alternative sonographic depiction includes color Doppler findings of reflux to include retrograde flow of urine from the bladder into the distal ureter. To properly demonstrate, this requires experience and meticulous technique.

Ultrasound alone is not considered dependable enough for routine clinical investigation of reflux but is a good accessory tool.

INFECTIONS

Infection is the most common disorder of the urinary tract in children, which can involve the kidneys and/or bladder. The kidneys are classified as part of the upper urinary tract, while the bladder (Figs. 21-31 and 21-32) is considered part of the lower urinary tract when describing area of infection. Hydronephrosis (Fig. 21-33(a) and (b)) and vesicoureteral reflux damage the urinary tract and can predispose children to urinary tract infections, pyonephrosis, or renal abscess.

Cystitis is inflammation of the urinary bladder due to bacteria, virus, fungal infection, or drug therapy. Patients with cystitis may have dysuria, hematuria, and diffuse bladder wall thickening greater than 3 millimeters. The bladder will have internal echogenic debris or fluid-fluid level with cystitis (Fig. 21-34). Occasionally, there may be a polypoid mass or focal thickening of the bladder wall with cystitis, in which case a biopsy may be needed to differentiate inflammation from a bladder wall tumor.

Cystitis cystica is an inflammatory process of the bladder mucosa localized to the trigone and ureteral orifices, which can mimic rhabdomyosarcoma.

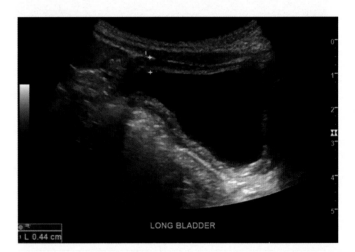

FIGURE 21-31. Mild bladder wall thickening in a 13-month-old pediatric patient with acute cystitis.

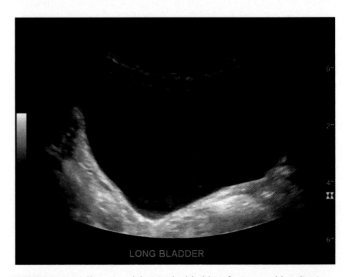

FIGURE 21-32. Clumping debris in the bladder of a 6-year-old pediatric patient.

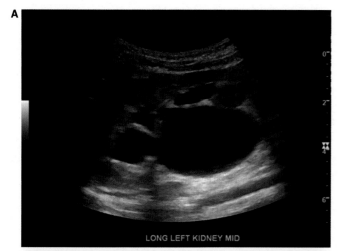

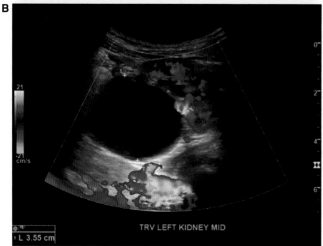

FIGURE 21-33. Moderate to severe hydronephrosis in a 13-month-old patient with urinary tract infection and acute cystitis.

BENIGN MASSES

Bladder masses in children are rare and usually malignant when occurring. Ultrasound alone may not definitively differentiate whether a bladder mass is benign versus malignant, therefore sonographic appearance should be an accessory to pathologic testing. Few benign bladder masses exist within the pediatric population which can include hemangioma, neurofibroma, paraganglioma (also known as pheochromocytoma), papilloma, nephrogenic adenoma, and leiomyomas. These masses are well-circumscribed, polypoid masses (Fig. 21-35) that arise in the bladder wall and project into the lumen of the bladder. Benign bladder masses are generally homogeneous or complex cystic lesions with possible hypervascularity.

MALIGNANT MASSES

Bladder Rhabdomyosarcoma

Rhabdomyosarcoma of the bladder is the most common childhood bladder tumor involving the submucosal trigone region. This malignant mass generally occurs between 2 to 6 years of age and 14 to 18 years of age. Clinical findings include urinary retention and painless gross hematuria. Sonographic findings include an echogenic pedunculated soft tissue mass that projects into the bladder lumen (Figs. 21-36 and 21-37). This mass occurs with a complex cystic appearance resembling bunches of grapes and focal wall thickening. Capacity for deep invasion of the bladder is diminished as the bladder wall becomes deformed and rigid. Hydronephrosis and perivesical invasion, as well as metastases to pelvic lymph nodes, can be seen. With bladder cystitis, there is uniform wall thickening, whereas with tumor infiltration such as seen with rhabdomyosarcoma, bladder wall thickening is irregular.

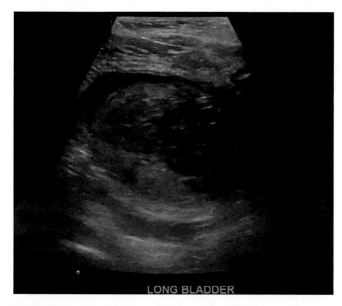

FIGURE 21-34. Hemorrhagic cystitis in a 10-year-old male status post bone marrow transplant, with low-level echo debris representing blood product.

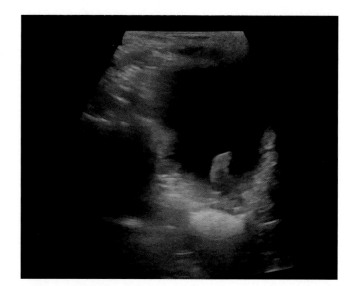

FIGURE 21-35. Epithelial polyp in the posterior urethra in a 2-year-old male with decreased urine output and dysuria.

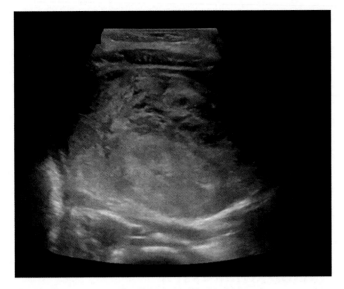

FIGURE 21-36. Arising from the dome of the bladder is a large, heterogeneous, predominantly solid tumor with lobulated margins and areas of cystic change due to necrosis, seen on ultrasound.

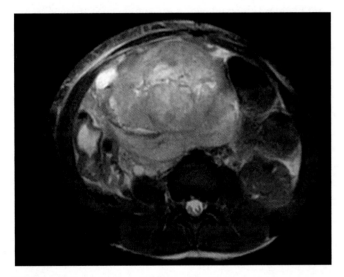

FIGURE 21-37. Arising from the dome of the bladder is a large, heterogeneous, predominantly solid tumor with lobulated margins and areas of cystic change due to necrosis, seen on MRI.

Transitional Cell Carcinoma

Transitional cell carcinoma is a rare bladder tumor in children. This malignancy can manifest as intraluminal polypoid masses or wall thickening. Although rare, this etiology may be encountered as a distractor on the registry exam.

Leiomyosarcoma

Leiomyosarcoma is a rare pediatric bladder tumor. Although rare, this etiology may be encountered as a distractor on the registry exam.

22

Pathology of the Male Genital Tract

HYDROCELE

Hydrocele is the presence of fluid surrounding the testis causing painless scrotal swelling. This fluid is located between the tunica vaginalis' parietal and visceral layers. In adolescents, hydrocele is typically acquired, resulting from inflammatory processes, trauma, or lesions. When seen in utero, neonates, or infants, hydrocele is generally congenital and results from a patent process vaginalis, leading to congenital hydrocele.

The sonographic appearance of hydrocele includes a thin-walled anechoic fluid collection (Fig. 22-1(a) and (b)). Chronic hydrocele may cause scrotal wall thickening or have associated scrotoliths. The testicle surrounded by hydrocele may have a larger volume than a contralateral teste not surrounded by hydrocele. A testicle surrounded by hydrocele may also have a higher resistive index due to venous congestion. Rarely, the hydrocele can communicate with the peritoneal cavity, or be due to ventriculoperitoneal shunts that may track into the scrotum via a patent process vaginalis.

HEMATOCELE

When blood is present in fluid surrounding the testis, it is referred to as hematocele. Hematocele consists of a blood collection in the tunica vaginalis, resulting from trauma or surgery. Sonographic appearance includes a fluid collection surrounding the testis. This may occur unilateral or bilaterally with possible low-level internal echoes from hemorrhage (Fig. 22-2).

Note: Hemat- is the prefix for blood.

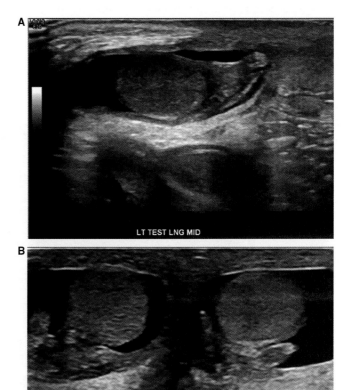

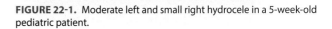

FIGURE 22-1. Moderate left and small right hydrocele in a 5-week-old pediatric patient.

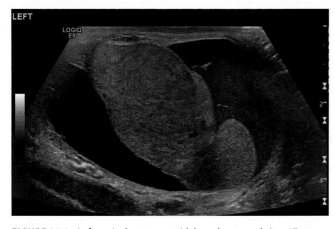

FIGURE 22-2. Left testicular rupture with large hematocele in a 17-year-old male status post trauma to scrotum.

PYOCELE

When pus is present in fluid surrounding the testis, it is called pyocele. Sonographic appearance includes a fluid collection with low-level echoes or a fluid-debris level surrounding the testis. This can occur unilateral or bilaterally from infection, calculi, and crystals. With pyocele, the patient may have elevated white blood cells. Abscess may result when there is much pus present due to infection. If abscess is visualized, there will be surrounding hyperemia with lack of color Doppler within the abscess.

> **Note:** Pyo- is the prefix for pus.

SCROTAL LYMPHOCELE

Scrotal lymphocele is associated with ipsilateral renal transplant and lymphatic disruption. Lymphatic fluid leaks into the tunica vaginalis via the inguinal canal, causing the scrotal lymphocele. Sonographic appearance includes a septated fluid collection surrounding the testicles.

VARICOCELE

Varicocele is a dilatation of veins in the spermatic cord's pampiniform plexus from incompetent vein valves, allowing for retrograde blood flow. Varicocele occurs more commonly on the left. Sonographic appearance consists of tortuous anechoic serpiginous structures adjacent to the testicles, measuring >3 millimeters (Fig. 22-3(a) and (b)). Varicocele size typically increases during Valsalva maneuver.

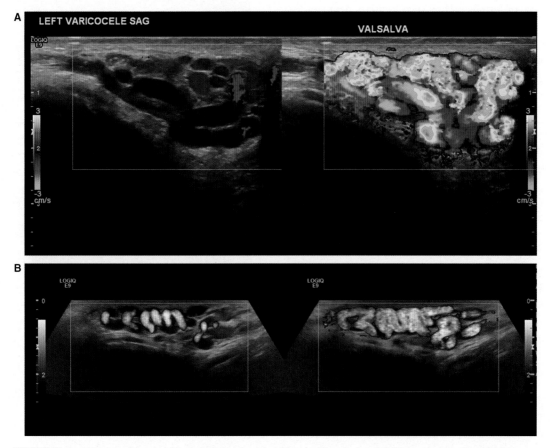

FIGURE 22-3. A 13-year-old male with grade 2-3 varicocele with color Doppler in exhibit (a) and power Doppler in exhibit (b).

SPERMATOCELE AND EPIDYMAL CYSTS

Spermatocele is a painless palpable mass resulting from cystic dilatation of the efferent tubules. Spermatocele is seen in the epididymis head and only occurs in post-pubertal patients, whereas an epididymal cyst (Fig. 22-4(a) to (c)) can arise anywhere within the epididymis and may occur at any age. Spermatocele also contains spermatozoa, where an epididymal cyst contains no spermatozoa.

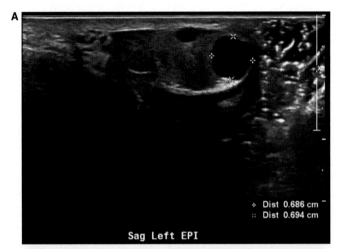

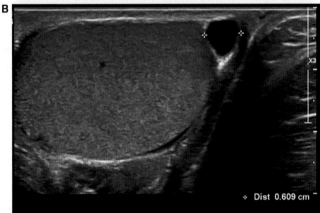

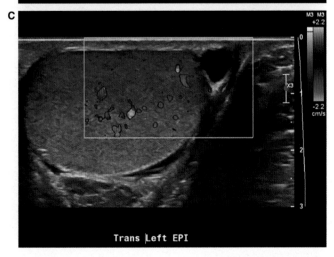

FIGURE 22-4. Left-sided epididymal cyst in a 15-year-old pediatric patient.

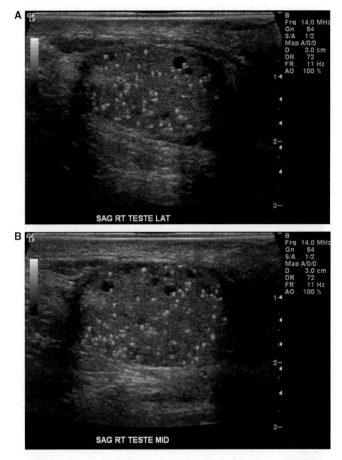

FIGURE 22-5. Patient with Trisomy-21 presents with testicular pain and swelling. Multiple small cysts along with microlithiasis are visualized within the right testicle.

TESTICULAR CYSTS

Simple testicular cysts are rare in pediatric patients. When occurring, they may be seen as painless scrotal enlargement. Sonographic findings consist of anechoic masses with posterior acoustic enhancement (Fig. 22-5(a) and (b)).

CRYPTORCHIDISM

Cryptorchidism is an incomplete descent of the testicle. Testicular descent is generally completed at birth but may continue postnatally and should be complete by 3 months of age. An undescended testis poses risk for infertility and malignancy. About 80% of undescended testicles are located within the inguinal canal (Fig. 22-6(a) to (c)). When visualized, the sonographer should notate whether the testicle is seen in the low, mid, or high inguinal region. The remaining 20% of undescended testicles are visualized within the peritoneal cavity. Orchiopexy, or the surgical moving of the undescended teste into the scrotal sac, does not relieve the risk for malignancy or infertility due to underlying testicular dysplasia. The gubernaculums testis is the cord-like structure that connects the testicle to the scrotum

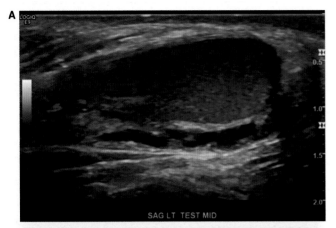

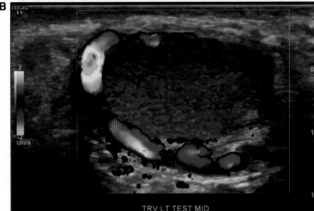

FIGURE 22-6. Left testicle demonstrated within inguinal canal and right testicle demonstrated within scrotum of 11-year-old patient.

during fetal development, and atrophies when descent is complete. If the descent is incomplete, the gubernaculums testis can become an ovoid remnant visualized with ultrasound.

POLYORCHIDISM

Polyorchidism is testicular duplication. This rare anomaly usually occurs with multiple testes on one side of the scrotum. Polyorchidism is most commonly left-sided, with the duplicated testicles sharing a common epididymis.

Note: Poly- is the prefix for many.

SCROTAL TORSION

Scrotal torsion occurs when the testis and spermatic cord twist 1 or more times, obstructing blood flow. Torsion knot is the term given to a twisted appearance of the radiating, congested spermatic cord and vessels, with or without epididymal involvement. A spiral twisting of the spermatic cord also gives rise to the sonographic whirlpool sign (Fig. 22-7). It is important that the sonographer evaluate with color Doppler to differentiate torsion knot from a pseudomass. Scrotal torsion can be extravaginal or more commonly intravaginal in nature. With intravaginal scrotal torsion, the tunica vaginalis surrounds the testis and inserts high on the spermatic cord. This prevents the testis from fixating on the scrotum and is called the "bell-clapper deformity." With intravaginal torsion, there is a sudden onset of pain with clinical symptoms such as nausea, vomiting, low-grade fever, and scrotal swelling. Sonographic findings of intravaginal torsion include an initially enlarged, hypoechoic testis (Fig. 22-8(a) to (c)) with skin thickening and hydrocele occurring within 4 to 6 hours. This appearance is followed by a heterogenous, hemorrhagic, nonviable testis with surrounding hydrocele after 24 hours of being left untreated. Extravaginal scrotal torsion can occur in neonatal patients at the level of the spermatic cord that is poorly fixed within the inguinal canal. With extravaginal torsion, the scrotal contents on the affected side are strangled, resulting in an acute swollen, red scrotum with a firm enlarged testis. Extravaginal torsion can occur unilaterally or bilaterally and is generally necrotic at birth, so salvage is unlikely. Chronic torsion may appear as a heterogeneous testicle, with complex debris-filled hydrocele, and calcifications within the tunica albuginea.

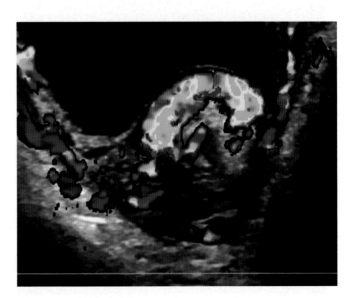

FIGURE 22-7. Whirlpool sign.

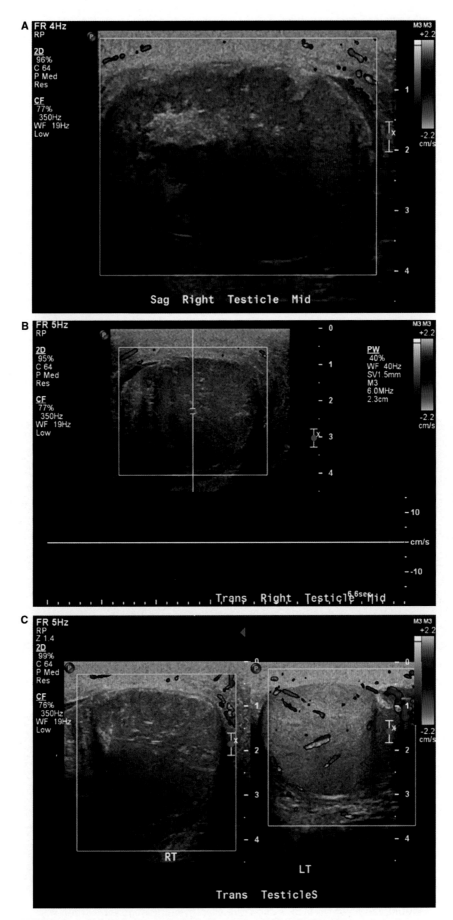

FIGURE 22-8. Right-sided testicular torsion in a 16-year-old pediatric patient.

TESTICULAR APPENDAGE TORSION

Two testicular appendages consist of the appendix epididymis and appendix testis. These appendages can torse, leading to acute scrotum. Torsion of the testicular appendages (Fig. 22-9) is one of the three most common causes of acute scrotal pain in prepubertal males, along with testicular torsion and epididymitis. The appendix epididymis is comprised of embryologic remnants of the blind-ending mesonephric (Wolffian) tubules. The appendix testis (hydatid of Morgagni) is a vestigial Mullerian duct remnant. The appendix testis most commonly torses among the two testicular appendages. Sonographic findings include a small hyper- or hypoechoic mass adjacent (superior) to the testis. This is usually seen along with testicular or epididymal enlargement, scrotal skin thickening, and reactive hydrocele.

ORCHITIS

Orchitis is testicular inflammation which can be a result of a bacterial infection, viral infection, or secondary to epididymitis. Sonographic appearance includes diffuse testicular hypervascularity or a focal hypoechoic area, dependent on whether the inflammation is diffuse or located within a single area (Fig. 22-10).

EPIDIDYMITIS

Epididymitis is an epididymal infection. This is commonly caused by a lower urinary tract infection. Epididymitis appears sonographically as an epididymis increased in size and vascularity. Epididymitis is one of the three most common reasons for acute scrotal pain in the male pediatric population, along with testicular torsion and torsion of a testicular appendage.

BENIGN MASSES

Testicular Teratoma

A teratoma is a benign primary germ cell tumor that mainly occurs in children less than 4 years of age. Testicular teratomas are the second most common pediatric germ cell tumor, following yolk sac carcinoma. These neoplasms make up 70 to 90% of all primary testicular neoplasms in childhood.

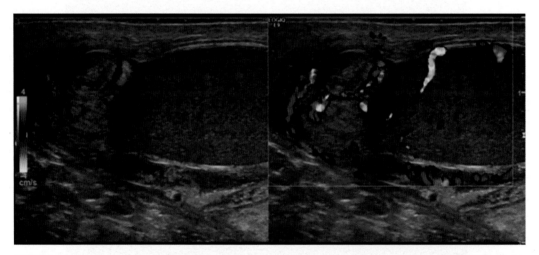

FIGURE 22-9. Gray scale and color Doppler demonstrating enlarged, avascular appendix testis in a 7-year-old boy with right scrotal pain.

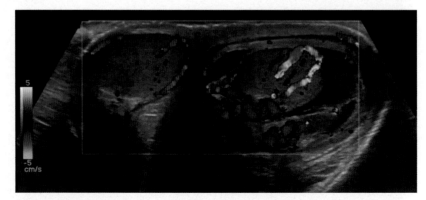

FIGURE 22-10. Asymmetric flow with a hyperemic left testicle in an 8-year-old male with acute pain and swelling.

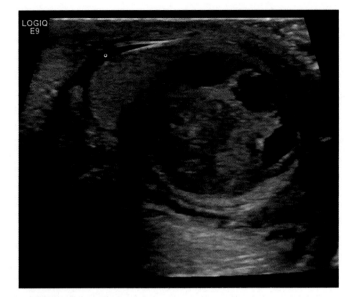

FIGURE 22-11. A 3-month-old with scrotal swelling.

Approximately 85% of teratomas contain elements from all three germ cell layers. If the teratoma contains any malignant elements in pubertal patients, aggressive tendencies may be seen, and typically the testicle is removed. Sonographic findings include a well-defined heterogeneous mass with hypoechoic areas of serous fluid and hyperechoic calcification components with shadowing (Fig. 22-11).

Stromal Tumor

Stromal tumors are made up of Sertoli cell, juvenile granulosa, and Leydig cell tumors. Approximately 40% of stromal tumors are Sertoli cell, 40% are juvenile granulosa, and the remaining 20% are Leydig cell. Most stromal tumors are benign, although malignant Sertoli tumors have been reported in older children.

Sertoli Cell Tumor

Sertoli cell tumors are most commonly benign stromal tumors but have potential for malignancy. These generally benign tumors present as painless masses within the first year of life. They produce estrogen, are hormonally active, and may result in gynecomastia. Sonographic findings include small, bilateral, well-defined, hypoechoic, homogeneous masses. These masses may have areas of necrosis, hemorrhage, and calcifications in larger tumors.

Juvenile Granulosa Cell Tumor

Juvenile granulosa cell tumor is a benign stromal tumor. These hormonally inactive tumors typically present within the first 6 months of life. Sonographic findings include solid or multiseptated, complex, cystic masses with vascular septations.

Leydig Cell Tumor

Leydig cell tumor is a benign stromal tumor most commonly found in prepubescent boys around 7 years of age. This tumor

is associated with Klinefelter syndrome, a chromosomal condition affecting male physical and cognitive development. Sonographic findings include small, well-defined, hypoechoic homogeneous masses. These masses may have necrosis and hemorrhagic areas, especially within larger tumors.

Leydig Cell Hyperplasia

Leydig cell hyperplasia is a rare, benign condition. Leydig cell hyperplasia occurs in males presenting with precocious puberty, usually between 5 and 9 years of age. Sonographic findings include multiple small, bilateral, hyperechoic, or hypoechoic testicular nodules. Although rare, this etiology may be encountered as a distractor on the registry exam.

Epidermoid Cyst

An epidermoid cyst is a rare benign, painless testicular mass. These masses appear as true cysts but are surrounded by fibrous tissue and squamous epithelium with unclear origin. It is suggested epidermoid cysts may be a form of ectoderm-related teratoma, but this has not been confirmed. Sonographic findings include a well-defined, hypoechoic mass with an echogenic capsule resembling layers of an onion skin. This capsule may or may not contain calcifications. Although rare, this etiology may be encountered as a distractor on the registry exam.

Gonadoblastoma

Gonadoblastoma is a rare, benign germ cell tumor with a 10% potential for malignancy. Gonadoblastomas occur in phenotypic, hermaphrodite females with male karyotype. These patients have streak gonads, gonadal dysgenesis, or hypoplasia usually diagnosed at time of surgery. Sonographic findings include a solid hypoechoic tumor with multiple cystic areas. Although rare, this etiology may be encountered as a distractor on the registry exam.

Other Benign Miscellaneous Lesions

Other benign lesions include lipoma, hemangioma, true cyst, neurofibroma, fibroma, and hamartoma. These lesions are solid and hypoechoic but can also appear complex or hyperechoic.

MALIGNANT MASSES

Lab value markers that are used to detect testicular cancer include lactate dehydrogenase, alpha-fetoprotein (AFP), and human chorionic gonadotropin (HCG).

Yolk Sac Carcinoma (Endodermal Sinus Tumor)

Yolk sac tumor (Fig. 22-12(a) to (c)) is otherwise known as endodermal sinus tumor. This lesion presents in prepubescent boys around 2 years of age. Approximately 80% of these tumors are located in the scrotum and are associated with elevated serum AFP levels.

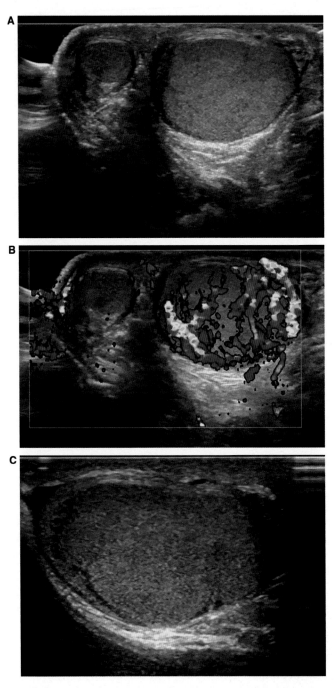

FIGURE 22-12. Pathology proven yolk sac tumor in a 5-month-old male presenting with enlarged left testis. The left testicle has a volume of 4.0 cc (compared to the right-sided volume of 0.3 cc). This volume is largely occupied by a circumscribed, lobulated isoechoic intratesticular mass which measures 2.2 × 1.3 × 1.9 cm and demonstrates pronounced internal vascularity.

Seminoma

Seminomas are malignant germ cell tumors that are rare in children, although the most common testicular tumor in adults. This neoplasm is commonly associated with cryptorchidism and is usually found later in adolescence if discovered during a pediatric age. Sonographic findings consist of a homogenous lesion with low-level echoes, typically hypoechoic to normal testicular echogenicity. Serum placental-like alkaline phosphatase may be associated with seminoma but is still being investigated. Although rare, this etiology may be encountered as a distractor on the registry exam.

Primary Germ Cell Neoplasms

Yolk sac carcinoma and mature teratoma are the two most common primary germ cell tumors, making up 70 to 90% of all primary testicular neoplasms in childhood. Testicular teratoma is a typically benign neoplasm with potential for malignancy, whereas yolk sac carcinoma is most commonly malignant. Other germ cell tumors include immature teratoma, embryonal carcinoma, teratocarcinoma, and choriocarcinoma. These primary germ cell tumors are aggressive and can metastasize via lymphatic and hematogenous routes in adolescents or young adults with elevated serum beta-HCG.

Secondary Testicular Neoplasms

Leukemia, lymphoma, and metastases account for secondary testicular neoplasms which are spread from a solid tumor elsewhere in the body.

Paratesticular Tumors

Paratesticular tumors can be categorized into benign and malignant neoplasms. Malignant paratesticular tumors arise most commonly from the spermatic cord, as well as from the epididymis in children less than 5 years of age or in adolescence. Rhabdomyosarcoma is the most common malignant pediatric paratesticular tumor. Benign paratesticular tumors are comprised of fluid-filled masses such as spermatoceles, epididymal cysts, and tunica albuginea cysts.

23

Pathology of the Female Genital Tract

VAGINAL ATRESIA

Vaginal atresia is an anomaly of the urogenital sinus or paramesonephric ducts, leading to absence of the vaginal canal. Sonographically, uterine or vaginal fluid collections may be visualized.

GARTNER'S DUCT CYST

Gartner's duct cysts are benign, fluid-filled vaginal lesions resulting from embryological duct remnants.

NABOTHIAN CYST

Nabothian cysts are benign, fluid-filled cervical lesions that appear anechoic on ultrasound.

HYDROMETROCOLPOS

Hydrometrocolpos is distention of the uterus and vagina with fluid due to obstruction from transverse membranes or septa (Table 23-1). Sonographically with hydrometrocolpos appears anechoic.

TABLE 23-1 • Helpful Prefixes and Suffixes
Hydro-Water/Fluid
Hemat-Blood
Colpos-Vagina
Metro-Uterus

HEMATOMETROCOLPOS

Hematometrocolpos is defined as distention of the uterus and vagina with blood product due to obstruction from transverse membranes or septa. Sonographically, blood product appears as fluid containing low-level echoes. Hematocolpos is blood product in the vaginal canal (Figs. 23-1 and 23-2). With hematometrocolpos, blood product would be seen within the uterus as well as the vaginal canal.

PRECOCIOUS PUBERTY

Precocious puberty is the onset of physical pubertal characteristics and hormone levels prior to 8 years of age. This may be caused by dysfunction of the ovaries or adrenal glands and can cause a premature onset of menses. Sonographically, the uterus and ovaries may appear like that of a pubertal patient. With precocious pseudopuberty, the uterus and unilateral ovary may appear prepubescent, however, a single ovary may be enlarged in the presence of an ovarian mass.

MULLERIAN DUCT ANOMALIES

Congenital anomalies of the Mullerian ducts (paramesonephric ducts) arise when the Mullerian ducts fail to develop properly. Some anomalies of the Mullerian ducts can be classified with ultrasound, particularly with the uterus well visualized in coronal plane. However, magnetic resonance imaging is often needed for a definitive diagnosis. To classify anomalies of the Mullerian ducts, a seven-class system was created as follows.

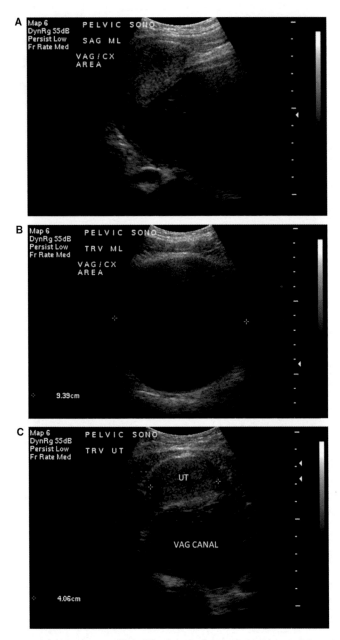

FIGURE 23-1. Hematocolpos (blood in vaginal canal) in a 13-year-old pediatric patient presenting with increasing pelvic pain and palpable mass. In this case, the patient had not yet had their first menstrual cycle.

Uterine Agenesis to Hypoplasia (Class I)

This is a severe anomaly of the Mullerian ducts leading to an absent or underdeveloped uterus. Uterine agenesis involves a complete absence of the uterus because of a lack of primordial tissue during embryonic development. Uterine aplasia refers to the presence of primordial tissue which does not develop after the early embryologic stage. With uterine hypoplasia, the uterus is histologically normal but is underdeveloped because of a failure of primordial tissue progression. Sonographically, the uterus, cervix, and/or vagina may not be visualized. This can be subclassified depending on severity as agenesis or hypoplasia of the vagina (Ia), cervix (Ib), uterine fundus (Ic), tubal region (Id), or a combination of the prior mentioned (Ie).

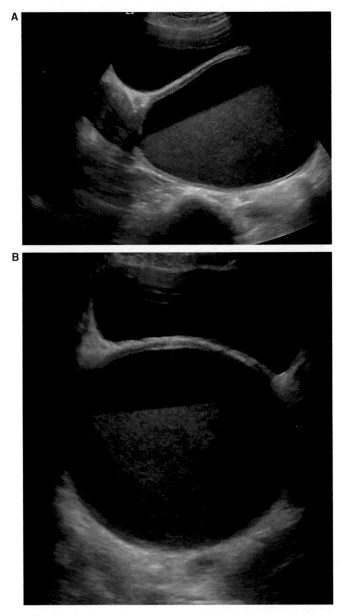

FIGURE 23-2. A 14-year-old with increasing pelvic pain and no menarche.

Mayer-Rokitansky-Kuster-Hauser (MRKH) syndrome is the total absence of the Mullerian ducts. MRKH syndrome can be further subclassified as types A and B. Type A involves lack of a uterus and superior two-thirds of the vaginal canal while the anomalous type B further involves fallopian tube, ovarian, and renal abnormalities.

Unicornuate Uterus (Unicornis Unicollis) (Class II)

This class involves a single horned uterus which exhibits tapered, banana-like shape and empties into a single Fallopian tube (Fig. 23-3). This anomaly occurs when one Mullerian duct develops properly while the other fails to adequately elongate. This can be further subclassified as a contralateral rudimentary horn which communicates and contains an endometrium (IIa), a contralateral rudimentary horn which does not communicate and contains an endometrium (IIb), a contralateral

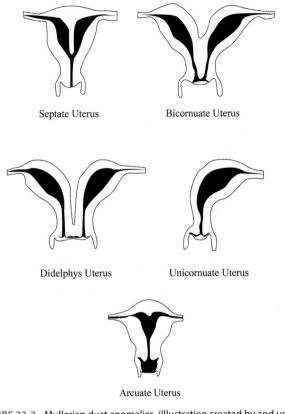

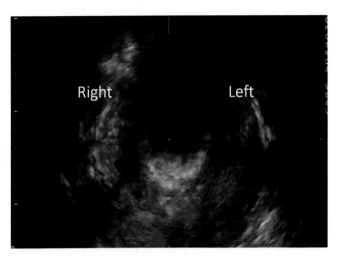

FIGURE 23-3. Mullerian duct anomalies. (Illustration created by and used with permission from Isaiah Forestier.)

FIGURE 23-5. 3D reconstruction of a didelphys uterus in a 17-year-old patient with OHVIRA (obstructed hemivagina and ipsilateral renal anomaly).

rudimentary horn which does not contain an endometrium (IIc), or the absence of a rudimentary horn (IId).

Didelphys Uterus (Class III)

When the Mullerian ducts completely fail to fuse, didelphys uterus results. Sonographically, a duplicated vaginal canal, cervix, and uterus is seen (Figs. 23-4 and 23-5). Didelphys uterus is greatly associated with reproductive complications. If a vaginal septum exists, one-sided hydro- or hematocolpos can occur.

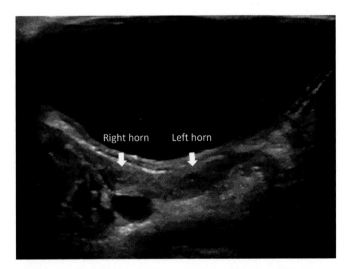

FIGURE 23-4. Didelphys uterus demonstrated in a 5-month-old patient with Mullerian duct abnormality.

Bicornuate Uterus (Class IV)

This occurs when the Mullerian ducts partially fuse, and the uterus separates into two horns. Bicornuate uterus can be further subclassified as bicornuate bicollis which involves a full division to the external os (Class IVa) or bicornuate unicollis which involves a partial extension towards the internal os (IVb). Sonographically, bicornuate bicollis is the presence of a single vaginal canal with duplicated cervixes and uterine cavities. Uterus bicornuate unicollis is the presence of a single vaginal canal and cervix with duplicated uterine cavities. Bicornuate uterus is associated with obstetric complications in reproductive years including recurrent spontaneous abortion and preterm labor. Menstrual ailments in adolescence should be investigated for potential treatment of surgical unification or high-level obstetric monitoring during the child-bearing period of life.

Septate Uterus (Class V)

This occurs when the Mullerian ducts begin to fuse and there is lack of resorption of the fibrous median septum. This septum persists and extends into the uterine cavity, dividing it into two distinct cavities. Septate uterus can be further subclassified as a full division to the internal or external os (Class Va) or partial division with endometrial involvement only (Class Vb). Sonographically, this appears as two endometrial canals within a single uterus. Depending on severity, the septation may extend to the external cervical os or vaginal canal. It is important for the sonographer to recognize septate uterus as it can be a cause of recurrent spontaneous miscarriage in the reproductive years. The fibrous uterine septum is poorly vascularized. It is speculated recurrent pregnancy loss is associated with embryo implantation in the septal region.

Arcuate Uterus (Class VI)

This involves a minor indentation of the endometrium at the fundus of the uterus and is widely considered a normal variant. Arcuate uterus occurs because of partial resorption of the uterine-vaginal septum. In the transverse imaging plane the uterine diamater can be increased with the fundal endometrium indenting less than 1 centimeter. Arcuate uterus is typically an incidental finding and has the lowest association with reproductive complications.

T-Shaped Uterus (Class VII)

Between 1940 and 1971 the synthetic non-steroidal estrogen medication Diethylstilbestrol (DES) was prescribed to pregnant mothers for the prevention of early spontaneous miscarriage, pregnancy-related complications, and premature birth. It was later discovered that exposure to this medication put fetuses at a higher risk for developing vaginal and cervical clear cell adenocarcinoma later in life. It also led to a maldeveloped T-shaped uterine configuration in female fetuses born to the exposed mothers. In the year 2000, the FDA deemed DES a carcinogen, and this medication was removed from the market. T-shaped uterus occurs because of the exposure to DES in utero.

> **Hint:** The most common anomaly consists of septate uterus, with a 45% prevalence. The second most common Mullerian duct anomaly is bicornuate uterus, with a 25% prevalence.

OVARIAN TORSION

Ovarian torsion is a partial or complete rotation of an ovary on its vascular pedicle. Ovarian torsion is seen in all age groups but is more common among adolescents and young women. Torsion can occur in a nonpathological ovary or due to an underlying mass. When torsion occurs in the presence of a mass, typically the mass acts as a fulcrum leading to rotation of the ovary. Ovarian torsion due to a mass is more common in infants. Sonographic findings include an enlarged ovary with multiple small peripheral cysts, abnormal echogenicity, increased acoustic enhancement, fluid within the cul-de-sac, displacement of the affected ovary, and absence of Doppler flow (Figs. 23-6 and 23-7). In the absence of Doppler flow, initially the arterial

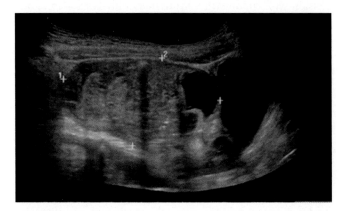

FIGURE 23-6. Edematous right ovary with a 11.9-cm dermoid cyst, torsed 360 degrees.

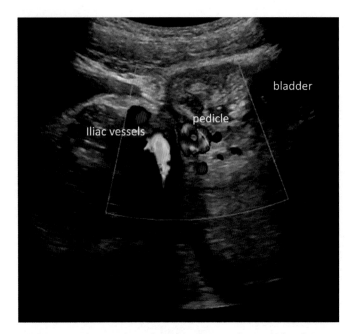

FIGURE 23-7. The vascular pedicle is displaying a classic whirlpool sign.

waveform can still be present, whereas venous occlusion produces symptoms before arterial occlusion occurs.

PELVIC INFLAMMATORY DISEASE

Pelvic inflammatory disease involves inflammation of one or more pelvic structures, including the peritoneum, cervix, uterus, ovaries, and fallopian tubes. This may occur as a result of microorganism introduction through the vaginal canal.

PERITONITIS

Peritonitis is an inflammation of the peritoneum. Sonographic findings include hypervascularity of the adnexal regions.

SALPINGITIS

Salpingitis is inflammation of the fallopian tubes. Sonographic findings include fluid-filled, thickened fallopian tubes. Infection may be in the form of hydro- or pyosalpinx. Hydrosalpinx refers to fluid-filled fallopian tubes and pyosalpinx is pus-filled nodules within the fallopian tubes (Figs. 23-8(a) and (b)).

ENDOMETRITIS

Endometritis is inflammation of the endometrial lining (Fig. 23-9).

OVARIAN NEOPLASMS

In the pediatric population two-thirds of ovarian neoplasms are benign with one-third of ovarian neoplasms having potential for malignancy. All ovarian masses arise from the germ cells,

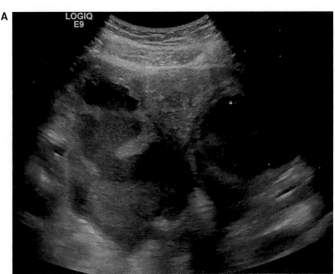

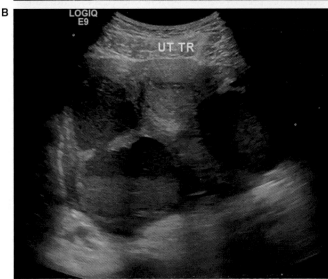

FIGURE 23-8. Transverse view of the pelvis in a 17-year-old female with exquisite lower abdominal pain. Findings consistent with bilateral tubo-ovarian abscesses.

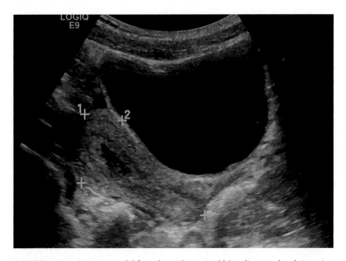

FIGURE 23-9. A 16-year-old female with vaginal bleeding and pelvic pain. There is an enlarged endometrial cavity containing complex, heterogenous fluid. Findings represent inflammation and blood products in the setting of recent IUD removal.

stroma, or surface epithelium, usually in the second decade of life. The majority of malignant germ-cell tumors arise in post-menarchal girls as asymptomatic pelvic or abdominal masses.

BENIGN MASSES

Mature Teratoma (Cystic Teratoma, Dermoid Cyst)

Mature teratoma, a benign ovarian tumor, is also referred to as cystic teratoma or dermoid cyst (Fig. 23-10). This typically unilateral neoplasm is the most common benign ovarian tumor, accounting for approximately 90% of all benign ovarian tumors. Mature teratomas contain all three germ-cell layers, the ectoderm, mesoderm, and endoderm. These masses range anywhere between 5 millimeters and 30 centimeters in size. Clinical findings include a palpable asymptomatic abdominal mass that may cause secondary pain related to hemorrhage, torsion, or tumor rupture. Sonographic appearance is complex and variable. Mature teratoma may appear as a hypoechoic mass with echogenic and anechoic components, to a solid appearance with calcification. This calcification is referred to as "tip of the iceberg" sign. Mature teratomas may have a fluid-fluid level if sebum, serous fluid, calcium, hair, or fat is involved. When hair is an internal component, it is referred to as a "dermoid mesh" sign.

Serous Cystadenoma

Serous cystadenoma is a rare, benign ovarian neoplasm seen in patients less than 20 years of age. Serous cystadenoma occurs more frequently than mucinous cystadenoma in childhood. This pelvic mass is filled with thin, watery fluid and can range

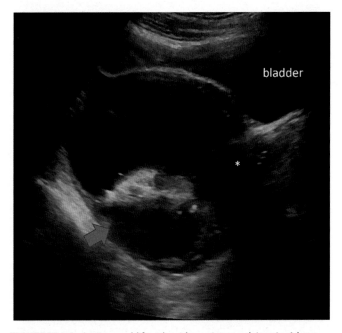

FIGURE 23-10. A 13-year-old female with persistent pelvic pain. A large, primarily cystic adnexal mass is seen, containing focal calcified components (arrow) and demonstrates posterior shadowing (asterisk).

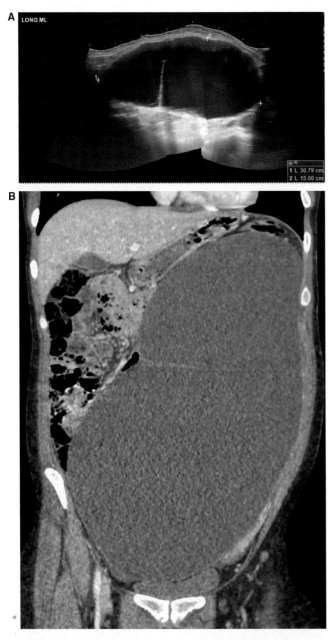

FIGURE 23-11. A 19-year-old female with distended abdomen. Massive primarily anechoic mass is visualized in the abdomen with septations and dependent debris. Pathology report is consistent with serous cystadenoma.

anywhere from 4 to 20 centimeters in size (Figs. 23-11(a) and (b)). Sonographic appearance includes a thin-walled unilocular cystic mass with possibility of thin septations and papillary projections. Although rare, this etiology may be encountered as a distractor on the registry exam.

Mucinous Cystadenoma

Mucinous cystadenoma is a rare, benign ovarian neoplasm seen in patients less than 20 years of age. Mucinous cystadenoma occurs less frequently than serous cystadenoma in childhood. This pelvic mass is filled with thick, viscous fluid and can range anywhere from 4 to 20 centimeters in size (Fig. 23-12). Sonographic appearance includes a multiloculated cystic lesion

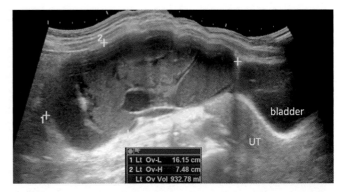

FIGURE 23-12. A 16-year-old female presents with pelvic pain. A complex cystic lesion is seen within the left ovary. Pathology report is consistent with mucinous cystadenoma.

with thin septations, low-level internal echoes, and papillary projections. The low-level internal echoes represent mucinoid material within the mass. Although rare, this etiology may be encountered as a distractor on the registry exam.

MALIGNANT MASSES

Dysgerminoma

Dysgerminoma is a malignant germ cell tumor comprised of undifferentiated germ cells (Figs. 23-13(a) and (b)). Dysgerminoma is the most common malignant pediatric ovarian tumor. Dysgerminoma is histologically indistinguishable from the testicular seminoma. This neoplasm occurs most frequently around 16 years of age.

Yolk Sac Carcinoma (Endodermal Sinus Tumor)

Yolk sac tumor is a malignant neoplasm also referred to as endodermal sinus tumor. Yolk sac tumors are germ cell tumors involving derivatives of all three germ cell layers, including the ectoderm, mesoderm, and endoderm. Sonographic appearance includes a solid echogenic or cystic-solid mass with irregular walls, thick septations, and papillary projections with calcifications throughout. Clinically, increased human chorionic gonadotropin (beta-HCG) and alpha-fetoprotein (AFP) levels are noted.

Immature Teratoma

Immature teratoma is a malignant neoplasm containing immature fetal tissue, primitive neuroectoderm, and mature tissue elements (Fig. 23-14). Sonographic appearance includes a solid echogenic mass with fine scattered calcifications. Increased AFP levels are seen clinically with immature teratoma.

Granulosa Cell Tumor

Granulosa cell tumor is a malignant sex-cord stromal tumor arising from sex-cords, or granulosa cells, of the embryonic gonad. Granulosa cell tumor is more common among premenarchal girls. Clinical findings include precocious puberty

A

B

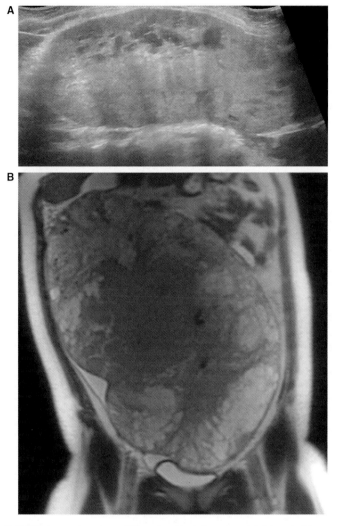

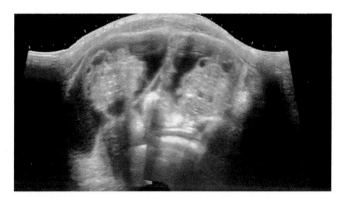

FIGURE 23-14. Panoramic image of the midline, depicting a mixed cystic and solid mass. Pathology report is consistent with metastatic immature teratoma.

due to excess estrogen production. Sonographic appearance includes a heterogeneous mass with cystic areas, solid components, and thick irregular septations with peripheral or central Doppler flow.

Sertoli-Leydig Tumor

Sertoli Leydig tumor is a malignant sex-cord stromal tumor arising from sex-cords, or Sertoli cells, of the embryonic gonad. Sertoli Leydig tumor is more common among premenarchal girls. Clinical findings include isosexual precocity due to excess androgen production. Sonographic appearance includes a heterogeneous mass with cystic areas, solid components, and thick irregular septations with peripheral or central Doppler flow (Fig. 23-15).

FIGURE 23-13. A 12-year-old female with abdomen and pelvic pain. There is a large cystic and solid intraperitoneal mass measuring approximately 33.5 × 25.2 × 12.2 cm. Pathology report is consistent with dysgerminoma.

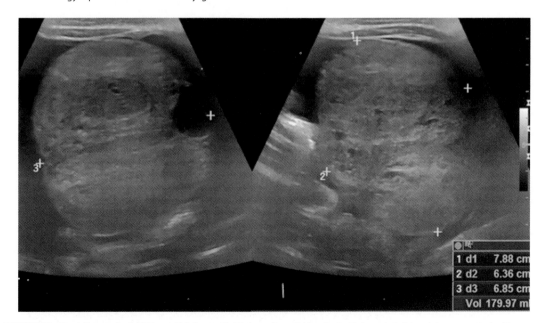

1 d1	7.88 cm
2 d2	6.36 cm
3 d3	6.85 cm
Vol	179.97 m

FIGURE 23-15. A 4-month-old (32-week) infant with history of omphalocele repair in early infancy, who presented with umbilical hernia and concern for intestinal obstruction. Ultrasound demonstrates a large right adnexal mass and significant ascites. The mass was surgically removed and pathology results indicated a sex-cord stromal tumor with Sertoli-Leydig histology.

Nonfunctioning Stromal Tumors

Nonfunctioning stromal tumors are malignant and include fibromas and sclerosing stromal tumor. Nonfunctioning stromal fibroma is associated with Meigs syndrome, which includes fibroma, ascites, and pleural effusion triad. Sonographic findings for fibroma and sclerosing stromal tumor are a heterogeneous or homogeneous solid mass with acoustic shadowing and small cystic components.

24

The Adrenal Glands and Associated Syndromes

ADRENAL RESTS

Adrenal rests are also called "accessory adrenal glands." These glands consist of separated fragments of adrenal tissue, containing cortical and medullary tissues found near the celiac plexus and along spermatic or ovarian veins. Sonographic appearance of adrenal rests includes round hypervascular, hypoechoic, nodular masses, most commonly near the mediastinum testis.

CUSHING SYNDROME

Cushing disease exclusively refers to excess glucocorticoid related to an adrenocorticotropic pituitary adenoma, which secretes hormones including cortisol. Comparatively, Cushing syndrome accounts for effects of various etiologies involving excess glucocorticoid. These may be endogenous or exogenous. Excess cortisol production from endogenous sources involves overproduction of cortisol and adrenocorticotropic hormone (ACTH) by ACTH-secreting tumors (i.e., pituitary adenoma) in 80% of cases. Adrenal adenomas make up the remaining 20%. Rare, endogenous sources include primary pigmented nodular adrenal dysplasia, corticotropin-releasing hormone-secreting tumor, and ACTH-independent macronodular adrenocortical hyperplasia. Clinical features include generalized or truncal obesity, muscle wasting, hypertension, and abdominal striae. Female patients specifically may develop signs of excess androgen (i.e., hirsutism). Sonographic findings include homogeneous round or oval echogenic masses between 2 to 5 centimeters with varying echogenicity and peripheral or central vascularity.

CONN SYNDROME

Conn Syndrome is also known as primary aldosteronism. Conn syndrome involves overproduction of mineralocorticoid aldosterone, resulting from an autonomous aldosterone-secreting adenoma, adrenal hyperplasia, or adrenal carcinoma. Clinical findings include hypertension, muscle weakness, tetany, reduced plasma rennin levels, hypokalemia, and inability to suppress aldosterone secretion with saline infusion. Sonographic appearance of Conn syndrome includes a small <2 centimeter round or oval lesion.

ADRENOGENITAL SYNDROME

Adrenogenital syndrome, otherwise known as congenital adrenal hyperplasia (CAH), is an autosomal recessive disorder and the most common inherited cause for adrenal insufficiency. This disorder most commonly occurs due to a 21-hydroxylase deficiency in up to 90% of cases. CAH leads to excessive pituitary ACTH production, chronic adrenal gland stimulation, and cortical hyperplasia. Sonographic appearance includes enlarged adrenal glands with increased cortical thickness and irregular margins.

WOLMAN DISEASE

Wolman disease is an autosomal recessive inborn error of lipid metabolism due to lysosomal acid lipase deficiency and massive cholesterol accumulation throughout the body. Clinical findings include hepatosplenomegaly, vomiting, diarrhea, steatorrhea, thickened bowel walls, and anemia. Sonographic appearance includes bilaterally enlarged echogenic adrenal glands with prominent necrotic areas and shadowing calcifications in the adrenal cortex.

BENIGN MASSES

Ganglioneuroma

Ganglioneuroma is a benign neural crest tumor made up of differentiated mature ganglion cells. Sonographic appearance includes a nonspecific solid echogenic mass with areas of calcification.

Adrenal Cysts

Cysts of the adrenal glands are rare, occurring in less than 1% of patients with a 3:1 female prevalence. Although rare, this etiology may be encountered as a distractor on the registry exam. Adrenal cysts are typically visualized as an incidental finding. Pathologic classification categorizes adrenal cysts as endothelial, epithelial, parasitic, or as posttraumatic (hemorrhagic) pseudocysts. Of these categories, endothelial is the most common with a 45% occurrence in adrenal cyst cases. One source describes adrenal endothelial, epithelial, and pseudocysts as pure. Adrenal cysts may also occur as a cystic tumor component, most frequently pheochromocytoma, neuroblastoma, teratoma, and ganglioneuroma. Additionally, parasitic adrenal cysts are usually Echinococcal (hydatid) in nature. Echinococcus of the adrenal gland is notably rare, occurring in only 0.5% of adrenal cyst cases. Sonographic appearance includes a well-defined round, anechoic mass with thin walls and through transmission within the adrenal space. Large >8 centimeter multilocular cystic masses may also form in the adrenal glands with Beckwith-Wiedemann syndrome.

Adrenal Myelolipoma

Adrenal myelolipoma is a rare, benign, nonfunctioning echogenic neoplasm with cystic changes created from fat and bone marrow elements. Although rare, this etiology may be encountered as a distractor on the registry exam.

Adrenal Hemangioendothelioma

Adrenal hemangioendothelioma is the most common rare stromal adrenal tumor. The sonographic appearance of this benign lesion includes a hypoechoic, suprarenal, hypervascular mass. Although rare, this etiology may be encountered as a distractor on the registry exam.

MALIGNANT MASSES

Ganglioneuroblastoma

Ganglioneuroblastoma is a primitive and differentiated ganglion cell neoplasm. This malignant neural crest tumor has a sonographic appearance of nonspecific solid echogenic mass with areas of calcification.

Adrenal Neuroblastoma

Adrenal neuroblastoma is the most common solid extracranial malignant tumor in children, arising in the adrenal medulla or ganglion chain. This adrenal medullary neoplasm has an autosomal dominant inheritance pattern related to an abnormality in the short arm of chromosome 16. Neuroblastoma can present with findings of metastases and has multiple stages. The treatment for neuroblastoma depends on the stage of the tumor. Sonographic appearance includes a suprarenal or paraspinal hyperechoic mass with areas of calcification, necrosis, cystic change, and fluctuating vascularity. This mass may appear hypoechoic in neonatal patients (Fig. 24-1(a) to (g)).

Pheochromocytoma

Pheochromocytoma is a malignant catecholamine-secreting tumor arising from chromaffin cells of the sympathetic nervous system in the adrenal medulla. Clinical findings include episodes of hypertension, headache, tachycardia, palpitation, and pallor. The sonographic appearance includes a large > 2 centimeter well-marginated lesion with solid heterogeneous appearance due to necrosis, hemorrhage, and calcification (Fig. 24-2(a) to (c)). These lesions are typically surrounded by enlarged lymph nodes. Increased incidence of pheochromocytoma is noted in patients with tuberous sclerosis, von Hippel Lindau disease, Sturge-Weber syndrome, neurofibromatosis, and multiple endocrine neoplasia (MEN) syndrome type 2.

Adrenal Carcinoma

Adrenal carcinoma is a rare malignant, hormonally active adrenal cortex neoplasm. Clinical findings include virilism in females and pseudoprecocious puberty in boys, feminization, and hyperaldosteronism. Sonographic appearance includes large >5 centimeter heterogeneous mass of varying echogenicity, necrosis, hemorrhage, calcification, with inferior vena cava, liver, and lymph node invasion. Adrenal carcinoma is associated with Beckwith-Wiedemann syndrome and hemihypertrophy.

ADRENAL HEMORRHAGE

Neonatal Adrenal Hemorrhage

Neonatal adrenal hemorrhage occurs secondary to birth trauma, perinatal anoxia, or anticoagulation therapy. The right adrenal gland is more commonly affected than the left. Clinical findings include palpable mass, anemia, and jaundice. Sonographic appearance includes round, oval, or triangular suprarenal mass replacing the entire adrenal gland (Fig. 24-3).

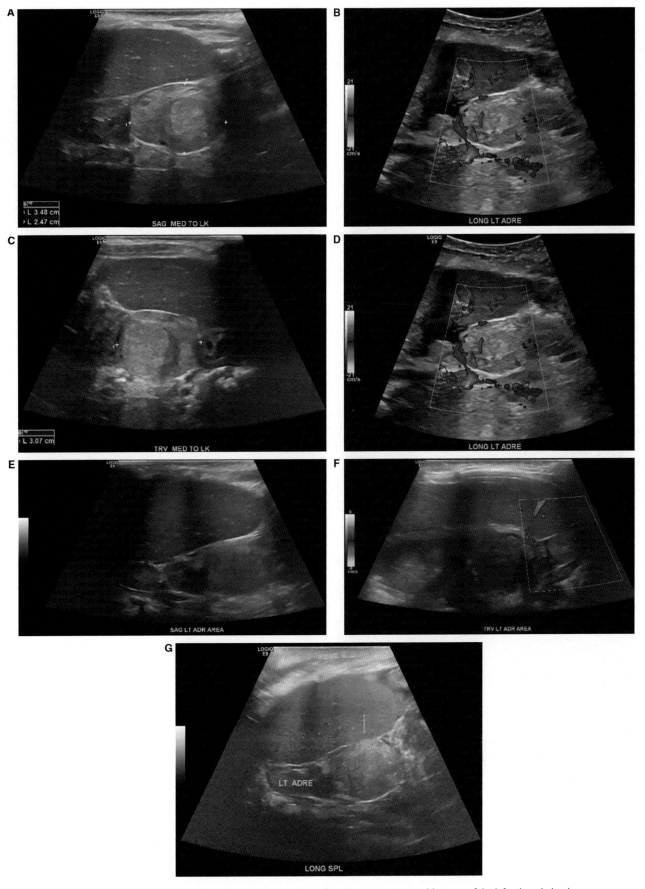

FIGURE 24-1. A 3-month-old pediatric patient with confirmed metastatic neuroblastoma of the left adrenal gland.

A

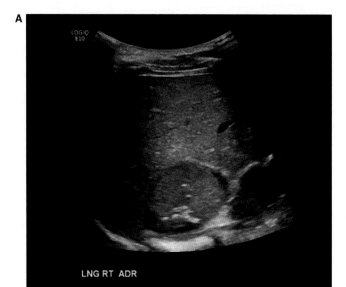

LNG RT ADR

B

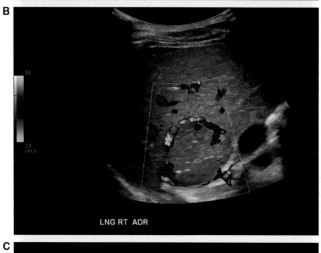

LNG RT ADR

C

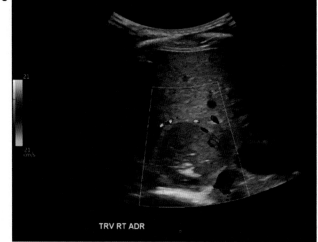

TRV RT ADR

FIGURE 24-2. Right adrenal mass in a 14-year-old pediatric patient. Favored as heterogeneous enhancing pheochromocytoma with central necrosis on follow-up MRI.

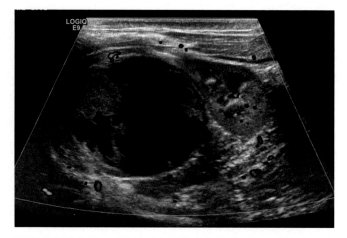

FIGURE 24-3. Incidentally detected left adrenal hemorrhage in a 66-day old female.

25

Neck Pathology

VASCULAR LESIONS OF THE NECK

Hemangioma

A hemangioma is a benign congenital vascular mass made up of endothelial cells. The sonographic appearance includes a homogeneous or heterogeneous well-defined hypoechoic mass with increased vascularity.

INFECTIONS AND INFLAMMATORY PROCESSES

Cervical Adenitis and Abscess

Cervical adenitis is an inflammatory neck mass caused by viral adenovirus, enterovirus, upper respiratory tract infection, staphylococcal or streptococcal bacterial infection, or recent dental work. Cervical adenitis includes the deep cervical jugular chain (Fig. 25-1) and submandibular lymph nodes. These lymph nodes can become enlarged and painful, appearing as well-defined hypoechoic oval structures with a hyperechoic vascular hilum. Enlarged nodes have the potential for abscess formation, which may need surgical or percutaneous draining. If abscess is present along with cervical adenitis, the sonographic appearance can include a thickened lymph node wall, through transmission, and absent central hilar stripe replaced by internal debris echoes.

Acquired Immunodeficiency Syndrome (AIDS)

When parotid lesions and cervical nodal enlargement are combined with decreased CD4 lymphocyte counts, possibility of human immunodeficiency virus infection should be suspected.

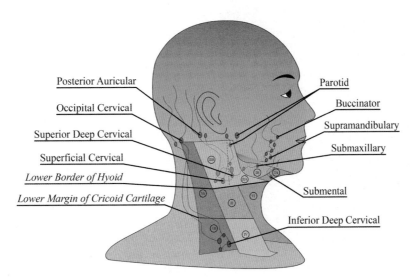

FIGURE 25-1. Lymph node chains correlating to zones of the neck. (Illustration created by and used with permission from Isaiah Forestier.)

Miscellaneous Inflammatory Nodal Diseases of the Neck

Inflammatory nodal diseases of the neck include mononucleosis, cat-scratch disease, sinus histiocytosis, Kawasaki disease, Langerhans histiocytosis, and sarcoidosis. Sonographic appearance of these diseases includes enlarged hypoechoic lymph nodes with a heterogeneous or homogeneous matrix.

AUTOIMMUNE DISORDERS

Hashimoto Thyroiditis

Hashimoto thyroiditis is an autoimmune disorder of the thyroid where antibodies attack the thyroid tissues. Hashimoto thyroiditis is the most common cause of acquired hypothyroidism and most common thyroid dysfunction in pediatrics. Sonographic appearance varies with stage and may initially appear as a swollen, heterogeneous gland with poorly defined nodules (Fig. 25-2(a) and (b)). As the patient ages, the thyroid becomes hyperechoic and decreases in size. It is not uncommon for cervical adenopathy to be visualized adjacent to the thyroid gland. Lab values associated with Hashimoto thyroiditis include a decrease in T3 and T4 and an increase in TSH.

Graves Disease

Graves disease is an autoimmune disorder associated with hyperthyroidism and involves an excess release of T3, T4, and

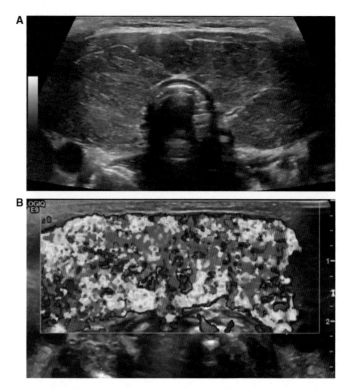

FIGURE 25-3. The thyroid gland demonstrates diffusely coarse echotexture with increased vascularity in a 15-year-old female with Grave's disease.

thyroid-stimulating immunoglobulins. Clinically, patients with Graves disease present with weight loss, intolerance to heat, excessive sweating, tachycardia, and exophthalmos. Sonographically, the thyroid gland appears increased in vascularity (Fig. 25-3(a) and (b)). "Thyroid inferno" is the term given to the depiction of diffuse increased color Doppler flow throughout the thyroid gland in patients with Graves disease, indicating hypervascularity. Graves disease has a maternal history prevalence and is most common in adolescent females.

BENIGN MASSES

Parathyroid Adenoma

Parathyroid adenoma is a benign growth of one or more of the parathyroid glands and is the most common cause of primary hyperparathyroidism in pediatric patients. Hyperparathyroidism is overactivity of the parathyroid glands, which are four small glands that lie adjacent to the thyroid. In children, elevated levels of parathyroid hormone, called "parathormone," leads to hypercalcemia and in turn the occurrence of renal stones due to high calcium levels. Other consequences of calcium overabundance are osteomalacia and osteoporosis, which are a weakening of the developing bones. Common clinical symptoms specific to children include referred pain to the joints, pancreas, kidneys, and bones, and frequent urination. These primarily present due to the coinciding hypercalcemia that occurs from

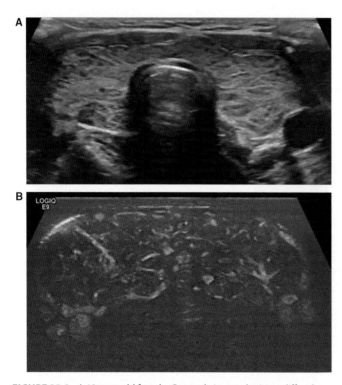

FIGURE 25-2. A 13-year-old female. Grayscale image depicts a diffusely enlarged thyroid gland with heterogeneous parenchyma. B-flow demonstrates hypervascularity. Sonographic features compatible with Hashimoto's thyroiditis.

presence of the adenoma. Sonographic appearance of parathyroid adenoma is a hypoechoic, homogeneous nodule compared to the thyroid gland's echogenicity. Most often parathyroid adenoma is only present on a single parathyroid gland, but it is possible for adenoma to be located on multiple parathyroid glands. Parathyroid nodules can be differentiated from thyroid nodules as the hyperechoic capsule of the thyroid can be seen separating thyroid tissue from the parathyroid growth. Use of color Doppler can demonstrate a small branch of the inferior thyroid artery perfusing the adenoma and peripheral vascularity may be present.

Branchial Cleft Cyst

Anomalies of the branchial cleft include a spectrum of head and neck defects. The branchial apparatus contains six arches and five clefts. The branchial cleft is a groove between the arches in the cervical region's branchial network, where branchial apparatus abnormalities may occur. In early development, between 3 and 5 weeks gestational age, the second arch begins to cover arches 3, 4, and 6. As the second arch fuses to the skin caudally, the cervical sinus forms. If the branchial cleft persists, cervical anomalies can ensue, and may include a cyst, fistula, or sinus depending on severity.

Benign branchial cleft cysts most commonly occur within this groove, with 90-95% originating in the second branchial cleft. Anomalies of the second branchial cleft are located deep to the superficial layer of deep cervical fascia and between the carotid bifurcation and mandibular angle. A branchial cleft cyst is a congenital epithelial cyst that presents as a non-tender neck mass and has no internal or external communication. In pediatric patients, branchial cleft cysts are the most common non-inflammatory masses located in the lateral neck region.

The sonographic appearance of a branchial cleft cyst includes a painless lateral anechoic neck mass near the common carotid artery that does not drain or communicate with the skin or pharynx. They are commonly seen near the inferior pole of the parotid gland or anterior to the sternocleidomastoid muscle.

Cervical Dermoid Cyst

A cervical dermoid cyst, also called "cervical teratoma," is an abnormal growth containing epidermis, hair follicles, and sebaceous glands, derived from residual embryonic cells. It is a benign, congenital, pluripotential, germ-cell mass inclusive of tissue from all three-germ cell layers, the ectoderm, mesoderm, and endoderm. Physical appearance involves a large neck lesion which can cause dyspnea, dysphagia, and stridor. While in-utero, cervical teratoma is associated with polyhydramnios. Sonographic appearance is variable and may include a well-defined, midline neck mass which ranges from heterogeneous and cystic to homogeneous and hypoechoic in echogenicity, with calcifications within the cyst wall (Fig. 25-4(a) and (b)).

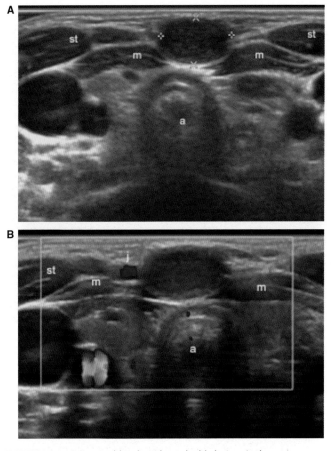

FIGURE 25-4. A 6-year-old male with a palpable lesion. At the region of interest, there is an echogenic nodule and absent blood flow on color imaging, consistent with dermoid.

Cervical Thymic Cyst

Cervical thymic cysts develop from thymopharyngeal ducts and areas of cystic degeneration within the thymus gland. These benign cysts present as non-tender, slowly enlarging masses in the lower one-third of the lateral neck, most commonly on the left (Figs. 25-5 and 25-6).

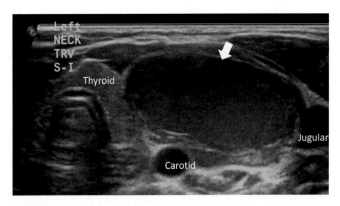

FIGURE 25-5. Ultrasound shows an elongated, bilobed 6 x 2 centimeter lesion in the left neck, filled with mobile internal echoes in a 6-year-old with localized swelling for 1 month.

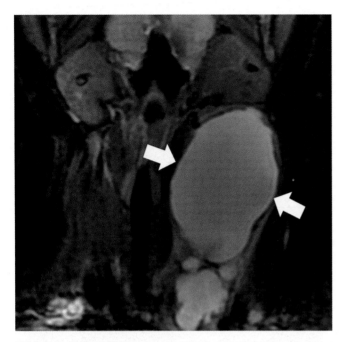

FIGURE 25-6. MRI shows an elongated, bilobed 6 x 2 centimeter lesion in the left neck, filled with mobile internal echoes in a 6-year-old with localized swelling for 1 month.

Esophageal Duplication Cyst

Esophageal duplication cysts are also known as "bronchogenic cysts." These benign lesions can cause stridor and tracheal compression in the lower neck. Esophageal duplication cysts have the typical appearance of anechoic, thin-walled masses with through transmission. Fluid-fluid levels may be present with thick walls if purulent or hemorrhagic material is within the cyst.

Ectopic Thymus

Ectopic thymus is a lateral neck mass caused by incomplete descent of the embryonic thymus, more commonly present on the right side. Cervical thymus and cervical extension of the thymus are often painless and may cause neck asymmetry. Sonographic findings include separate thymic tissue visualized anteromedial to the carotid artery and vein, with no connection to normal thymic tissue (Fig. 25-7(a) to (e)). Ectopic thymic tissue appears hypoechoic to muscle, with linear echogenic foci and mild to moderate vascularity.

Cervical Lymphangioma (Cystic Hygroma)

Cervical lymphangioma is also known as "cystic hygroma." This benign mass is a congenital lymphatic malformation that is comprised of an endothelial lined, dilated lymphatic space. This space is separated by connective tissue stroma, resulting from congenital blockage of lymphatic drainage canals. Clinical findings include a cervical mass in the first 2 years of life. These masses are usually painless unless they become infected, or inflammation/hemorrhage occurs. Cervical lymphangioma may cause esophageal or airway compression. Sonographic appearance includes a thin walled, loculated mass with increased echogenicity, acoustic enhancement, and low velocity Doppler flow within the masses' septations.

Fibromatosis Colli

Fibromatosis colli is an uncommon infantile fibromatosis occurring within the sternocleidomastoid muscle. The result of fibromatosis (pseudomass) is head tilt towards the mass with contralateral chin rotation. This mass is most often located on the right side of the neck and is found shortly after birth. Fibromatosis colli is related to use of forceps or in the instance of traumatic breech birth. The mass slowly regresses in 4 to 8 months with therapy. Sonographic appearance includes an enlarged, hypoechoic sternocleidomastoid muscle (Fig. 25-8(a) and (b)) with bright foci and posterior shadowing.

Aggressive Fibromatosis

Aggressive fibromatosis is a benign, aggressive fibrous tissue lesion that recurs locally after surgical excision. This form of fibromatosis usually occurs after puberty and presents as a firm, hypoechoic neck mass with low Doppler flow and possible areas of necrosis and calcification.

MALIGNANT MASSES

Cervical Lymphoma

Cervical lymphoma is the third most common malignant tumor in children, with cervical involvement more common in Hodgkin-type lymphoma. Clinical findings include painless, enlarged cervical adenopathy. Lymph nodes in the upper neck near the spinal and internal jugular veins are more commonly involved. Sonographic findings include bilateral enlarged, homogeneous, hypoechoic, round soft-tissue mass with central and peripheral Doppler flow.

Neck Neuroblastoma

Neck neuroblastoma is the most common neurogenic tumor of the neck, along with neurofibroma. Occurrence is very rare. Although rare, this etiology may be encountered as a distractor on the registry exam. This malignant mass is seen in children less than 5 years of age as a painless, firm, lateral neck mass. Clinical findings include airway obstruction, dysphagia, voice hoarseness, and paralysis of the lower cranial nerves. Sonographic appearance includes a paraspinal round or oval mass which is hyperechoic to the adjacent muscle. Echotexture can be homogeneous or heterogeneous, with mild to moderate Doppler flow and scattered calcifications. Age is the only indication to differentiate neuroblastoma from neurofibroma, tissue-sampling must be performed for definitive diagnosis.

Neck Neurofibroma

Neck neurofibroma is the most common neurogenic tumor of the neck, along with neuroblastoma. This disease is genetic and

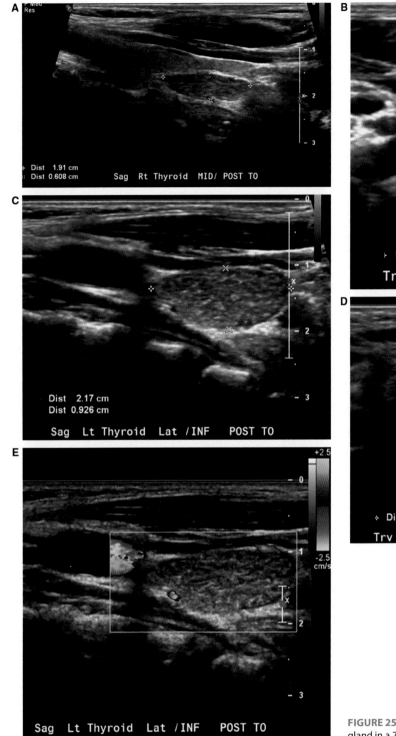

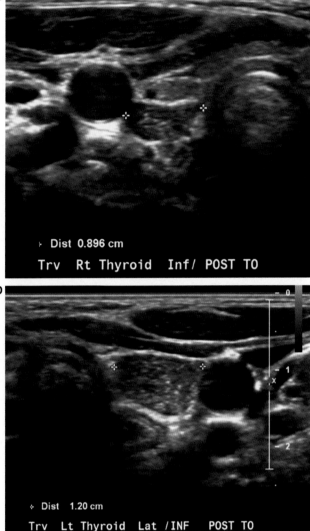

FIGURE 25-7. Bilateral ectopic thymus tissue noted adjacent to the thyroid gland in a 7-year-old pediatric patient.

can be inherited. Neurofibroma of the neck occurs due to a gene mutation in the protein that monitors growth of nerve tissues. Pediatrics with neurofibromatosis type 1 have a greater risk of developing plexiform neurofibroma, which can occur within soft tissues of the cervical region. Most often neurofibroma of the neck occurs in patients with neurofibromatosis, however a patient can develop sporadic neurofibroma for unknown

reasons. This malignant nerve root tumor is seen in the second decade of life as a painless, firm lateral neck mass. Clinical findings include airway obstruction, dysphagia, voice hoarseness, and paralysis of the lower cranial nerves. Sonographic appearance is the same as neuroblastoma, presenting as a round or oval echogenic paraspinal mass, hyperechoic to the adjacent muscle. Echotexture can be homogeneous or heterogeneous with mild

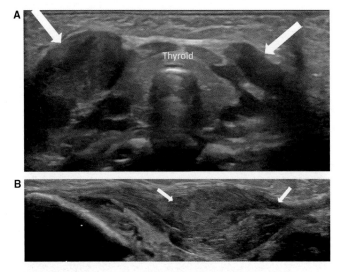

FIGURE 25-8. There is echogenic fusiform thickening of the right sternocleidomastoid muscle, consistent with fibromatosis colli.

to moderate Doppler flow and scattered calcifications. Age is the only indication to differentiate neuroblastoma from neurofibroma, tissue-sampling must be performed for definitive diagnosis.

Rhabdomyosarcoma

Rhabdomyosarcoma is the most common soft tissue sarcoma of childhood. Approximately, 35 to 40% of rhabdomyosarcomas arise in the head and neck region. The most common head and neck locations for rhabdomyosarcoma to form is the nasopharynx, orbits, sinus, ear, neck, and skull base. Clinical findings include an enlarging painless malignant mass in patients less than 10 years of age. Sonographic appearance includes a mass which appears hypoechoic to the adjacent muscle, with homogeneous or heterogeneous echotexture, calcifications, central and peripheral Doppler flow, and enlarged surrounding lymph nodes.

26

Pathology of the Chest

INTRALOBAR SEQUESTRATION (ILS)

Sequestration of the lung is a bundle of lung tissue that lacks appropriate function. Intralobar, or acquired-confined sequestration, is a congenital thoracic malformation of segmental lung tissue that has no connection to the bronchial tree or pulmonary arteries. This form of sequestration is also known as an "accessory lung" with abnormal vasculature, presenting late in childhood in 75 to 85% of cases. Sonographic appearance includes increased echogenicity in the sequestrated segment of lung. This is visualized as a triangular, echogenic, solid mass made of nonfunctioning primitive tissue that does not communicate with normal lung tissue and may be visualized antenatally beginning at 16 weeks gestational age. *ILS is surrounded by normal lung tissue and closely connected to the adjacent normal lung but does not have a separate pleura.* Blood supply to the mass occurs from systemic circulation rather than pulmonary circulation, with multiple feeding vessels present in 15 to 20% of cases. Venous drainage occurs via pulmonary veins, portal vein, inferior vena cava, right atrium, or azygous/hemi-azygous system. Arterial supply is fed from the descending thoracic aorta in 75% of cases. Clinical findings during physical exam mimic a lung infection, with frequent respiratory tract infections and possible high output cardiac failure in neonatal patients. The lung's lower lobes are most affected, with prevalence towards the left lower lobe.

EXTRALOBAR SEQUESTRATION

Extralobar, or congenital sequestration, is a congenital thoracic malformation of segmental lung tissue that has no connection to the bronchial tree or pulmonary arteries. ELS is also known as an "accessory lung" with abnormal vasculature and occurs less commonly than ILS. *ELS has its own pleura, separate from any surrounding lung tissue.* ELS can be visualized as early at 16 weeks gestational age and occurs more commonly in males than

females. Sonographic appearance is similar to that of ILS. Blood supply to the mass is from systemic circulation rather than the pulmonary circulation, with multiple feeding vessels present in 15 to 20% of cases. Venous drainage occurs via systemic veins into the right atrium. Arterial supply is from thoracoabdominal or upper abdominal aorta, spleen, gastric, or celiac arteries. Clinical findings during physical exam mimic a lung infection, with frequent respiratory tract infections and possible high output cardiac failure in neonatal patients. More often, ELS presents as respiratory distress, cyanosis, or infection in newborns. Alternatively, ILS appears as recurring pulmonary infections in late childhood into adolescence. The left lower lobe is most affected, making up 65 to 90% of cases.

> **Note:** The primary difference between ELS and ILS, is that ELS is pleura-covered.

CONGENITAL PULMONARY AIRWAY MALFORMATIONS

Congenital pulmonary airway malformation is a continuum of pulmonary parenchyma and vessel maldevelopment. Congenital pulmonary airway malformation may also be termed "congenital cystic adenomatoid malformation" (CCAM). CCAM is a vascular malformation consisting of disorganized pulmonary tissue with normal vascular supply and communication to the bronchial tree. This mass is caused by an overgrowth of distal bronchiolar structures. CCAM appears as a multicystic, benign lung mass comprised of abnormal bronchiolar and primitive lung tissues. CCAM is broken into three types depending on cyst size. Type I and II cystic adenomatoid malformations have a sonographic appearance of a complex fluid-filled mass with echogenic septations and acoustic shadowing where the cysts contain air. In type III cystic adenomatoid malformation, the sonographic appearance is a solid avascular mass. Congenital pulmonary airway malformations include congenital lobar overinflation, intrapulmonary bronchogenic cysts, cystic adenomatoid malformations, and sequestrations.

CONGENITAL LOBAR OVERINFLATION

Congenital lobar overinflation, previously termed "congenital lobar emphysema," is a vascular malformation consisting of lung lobe hyperinflation without alveolar septa destruction. One or more lobes distends with or without an excess of alveoli. Most cases are idiopathic. Congenital lobar overinflation causes bronchial obstruction due to cartilage deficiency, and the left upper lobe is the most commonly affected. Sonographic appearance in the neonate includes a fluid-filled lobe with enhanced through-transmission and atelectasis of the ipsilateral lobe. In pediatric patients greater than neonatal age, this is called "overinflated lung" on radiograph, usually imaged following fluid drainage of the lobe(s).

INTRAPULMONARY BRONCHOGENIC CYST

Intrapulmonary bronchogenic cyst is a normal vascular malformation that results from a fetal lung bud failing to incorporate into primitive lung tissue. Sonographic appearance includes a unilocular, hypoechoic, rounded mass with smooth walls containing Doppler flow. This mass may be filled with air or fluid containing serous or mucoid material.

SIMPLE PLEURAL EFFUSION

Simple pleural effusion is a completely anechoic collection of fluid within the pleural space. Simple pleural effusion is without septations, debris, and internal echoes (Fig. 26-1). For imaging protocol, please refer to Chapter 5, "Sonographic Anatomy of the Pediatric Chest."

COMPLICATED PLEURAL EFFUSION

A complicated pleural effusion may contain internal echoes, debris, or septations. Sonography is considered superior to computed tomography and radiography in determining whether pleural effusion contains loculated fluid pockets. Internal echoes within a complicated pleural effusion indicates possible hemothorax when associated with pleural fluid hematocrit ≥50% of the peripheral blood hematocrit. Debris within a pleural effusion can indicate exudate or purulent fluid. Septations within a loculated complex pleural effusion may not allow fluid to be drainable via chest tube or aspiration. For imaging protocol, please refer to Chapter 5, "Sonographic Anatomy of the Pediatric Chest."

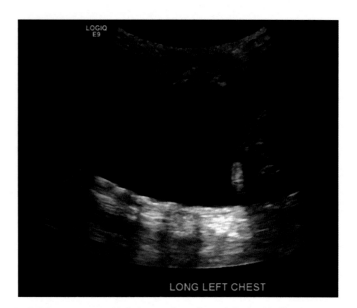

FIGURE 26-1. Coronal left chest with moderate left pleural effusion.

PNEUMOTHORAX

Pneumothorax is the presence of acquired or spontaneous air (gas) in the pleural space due to trauma or lung disease. Sonographic findings include air within the pleural space, usually seen as bright echogenic reflectors just deep to the parietal pleura. Visualized air may be mobile; however, structures underlying air may be nonvisualized due to artifact.

CONSOLIDATION

Consolidation occurs when lung tissue is airless, due to overabundance of solid or liquids in spaces that are normally air-filled due to infection (i.e., bacterial pneumonia, pus), water, or hemorrhage. Comparatively, atelectasis is the collapse of lung tissue, thus it does not contain air. The echogenicity of consolidated lung appears like the liver, referred to as hepatization (Fig. 26-2(a) and (b)). With hepatization, air filled bronchi appear as linear acoustic shadowing and are surrounded by fluid or mucoid-filled areas.

DIAPHRAGMATIC PARALYSIS (M-MODE)

Diaphragmatic paralysis results from phrenic nerve injury following cardiothoracic surgery, trauma, or injury during birth. With diaphragmatic paralysis, paradoxical diaphragmatic excursion during deep inspiration and expiration is absent. Ultrasound, which allows imaging in real-time, can be used as an alternative to fluoroscopy in the diagnosis of diaphragmatic paralysis. Ultrasound readily demonstrates spontaneous motion of the diaphragm during respiration. If the patient is on a ventilator, they may need to be temporarily disconnected by attending staff (i.e., physician, nurse, respiratory therapist). The diaphragm is demonstrated in axial, sagittal, or coronal plane

A

B

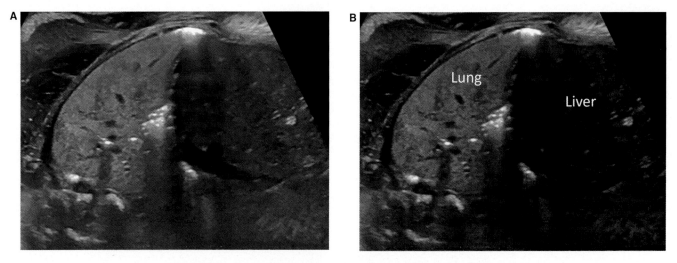

FIGURE 26-2. Consolidated lung parenchyma is seen, with a simple effusion.

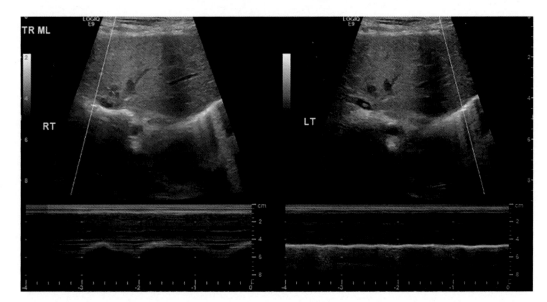

FIGURE 26-3. M-mode tracing shows diminished excursion on left (note lack of undulation), compared to robust hemidiaphragmatic movement on the right.

with M-mode. It is preferable to simultaneously demonstrate the two hemidiaphragms. To confirm diaphragmatic paralysis, there must be excursion <4 millimeters, paradoxical movement, and >50% difference between excursion of the bilateral hemidiaphragms (Fig. 26-3). Ultrasound is commonly used in the critical care setting and offers a high level of specificity. For imaging protocol, please refer to Chapter 5, "Sonographic Anatomy of the Pediatric Chest."

27

Pathology of the Joint, Tendon, and Synovium

DEVELOPMENTAL DYSPLASIA OF THE HIP (DDH)

DDH, formerly known as "congenital hip dislocation," is caused by abnormal ligamentous laxity which is accentuated by excessive circulating maternal estrogen levels. Risk factors for DDH include family history, breech birth, oligohydramnios during pregnancy, tight swaddling in infancy with the lower limbs extended, torticollis, foot deformities, and neuromuscular problems. DDH can range from mild acetabular dysplasia and reducible subluxation to irreducible subluxation and dislocation of the femoral head, which may develop anytime from birth until late infancy. If the femoral head subluxes or dislocates, the acetabulum becomes shallow during formation and fills with fibrofatty tissue as the labrum inverts. Normally, the acetabulum should become cup-shaped with the femoral head in place, providing stimulus.

Clinical signs showing possibility of DDH include asymmetric skin folds on the thigh, limited hip abduction, and abnormal Barlow and Ortolani maneuvers. The Barlow maneuver is a movement attempt for the femoral head to dislocate. With the Barlow maneuver, the thigh is pushed posteriorly with gentle adduction while the hip is flexed 90°. As the femoral head dislocates from the acetabulum, a palpable "clunk" can be felt. The Ortolani maneuver is a movement attempt for dislocated hip reduction. With the Ortolani maneuver, the thigh is lifted anteriorly with gently abduction while the hip is flexed 90°. As the dislocated femoral head reduces, a palpable "clunk" can be felt.

Sonography becomes less dependable for DDH evaluation when the femoral head ossifies, around 2 to 8 months of age. Evaluation of the hip with sonogram should be performed on patients at 6 months of age or less.

For evaluation with sonography, the highest frequency linear transducer that provides adequate soft tissue penetration should be used. Each hip should be evaluated in two perpendicular planes. Coronal (long-axis) and transverse (short-axis) images should be obtained (Figs. 27-1 and 27-2) in both neutral (15-20°) and flexion (90°) views. Short-axis stress views are obtained when allowable (i.e., not in Pavlik harness). On coronal neutral and flexion views, the proximal femoral epiphysis, or femoral head, should be covered in the acetabulum by at least 50% of the ilium.

DDH is diagnosed by findings of a shallow acetabulum or abnormal position of the femoral head at rest and with stress. With an abnormal acetabular roof, soft tissue may be visualized

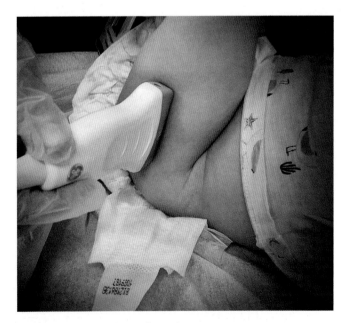

FIGURE 27-1. Long-axis transducer placement.

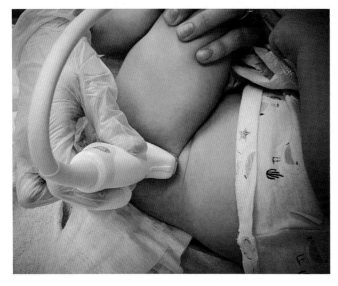

FIGURE 27-2. Short-axis transducer placement.

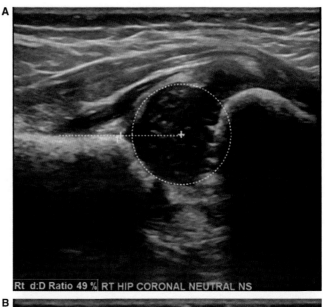

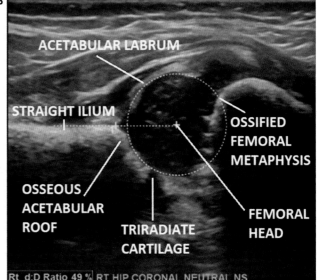

FIGURE 27-3. Coronal neutral view.

between the acetabulum and femoral head. With subluxation, the femoral head is partially covered by the acetabulum and can be moved. In cases of complete dislocation, the femoral head is not seen within the acetabulum and the labrum may be abnormally thickened.

> **Note:** Unless hip dislocation is obvious, ultrasound evaluation for developmental hip dysplasia should not be performed until the patient is at least 2 weeks of age to avoid unnecessary treatment in cases of transient laxity or instability due to hormones from the mother.

Positive finding of DDH is treated with a flexion-abduction external rotation harness known as the "Pavlik harness" to direct the femoral head toward the triradiate cartilage. This harness helps to stimulate acetabular development.

For patient cooperation, it may be helpful if the caregiver feeds the infant during examination as this can increase patient comfort and cooperation. The patient lies supine or in a right and left lateral decubitus position for the exam. The sonographer should not remove a Pavlik harness unless otherwise instructed by the orthopedic physician. Additionally, if the patient is in a harness, stress maneuvers should not be performed. The sonographer should always examine the hips bilaterally, using a high frequency linear (5-17 MHz) transducer.

Still images:

1. Right coronal hip, 15 to 20° neutral (Fig. 27-3(a) and (b)).

   Demonstrate a straight ilium, fibrocartilaginous tip of the labrum, echogenic medial lip of the acetabular roof, greater trochanter, and ischium. The imaging transducer is positioned 10 to 15° posterior (oblique) from the coronal imaging plane to produce a straight ilium. If the transducer is placed too far anterior, a false-positive finding can result.

The femoral head should appear round, centered on the image, and seated within the acetabulum (Fig. 27-3(b)).

2. Right coronal hip, 15 to 20° neutral with measurements. Measurements include alpha angle, beta angle, and femoral head coverage (Figs. 27-4 to 27-6). The alpha angle measures concavity of the acetabulum. The alpha angle is formed by the acetabular roof and ilium's vertical cortex. An alpha angle $\geq 60°$ is within normal limits. The beta angle demonstrates cartilaginous roof coverage of the acetabulum. It is produced by the labral fibrocartilage and vertical cortex of the ilium. In the normal hip, this measurement forms an angle of $<77°$. Femoral head coverage (Morin-Terjesen technique) calculates the percent of the femoral head covered in the acetabulum (Fig. 27-5 and 27-6). Coverage of the femoral epiphysis (d:D ratio) by the bony acetabular roof should be $>50\%$.

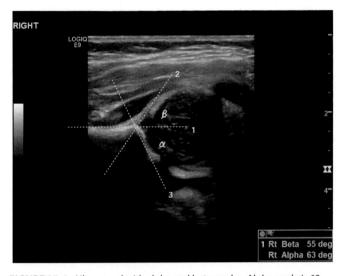

FIGURE 27-4. Ultrasound with alpha and beta angles. Alpha angle is 63 degrees (normal is greater than 60 degrees). The femoral head is well seated without subluxation on overall impression.

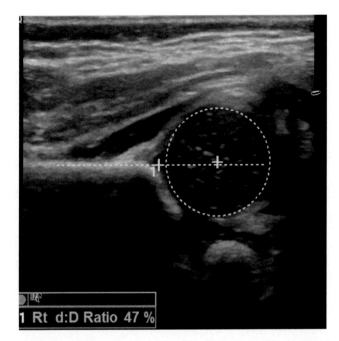

FIGURE 27-6. Mild acetabular undercoverage likely representing physiologic immaturity. Femoral head coverage is at 47% (normal is greater than 50%).

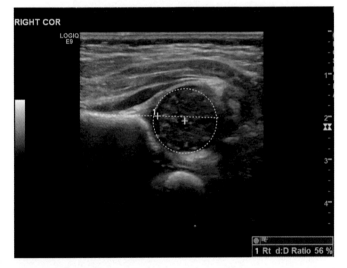

FIGURE 27-5. Femoral head appears well seated within the acetabulum at rest. Femoral head coverage is at 56% (normal is greater than 50%).

TABLE 27-1 • Patient Age and Alpha Angle	
Age (Weeks)	**Alpha Angle (Degrees)**
0	50
1	51
2	52
3	52
4	53
5	54
6	55
7	55
8	56
9	57
10	58
11	59
12	59
13	60

Robben S, Smithuis R. Developmental Dysplasia of the Hip - Ultrasound. The Radiology Assistant. https://radiologyassistant.nl/pediatrics/hip/developmental-dysplasia-of-the-hip -ultrasound. Published December 1, 2017.

Note: The alpha angle should be correlated to the infant's age (Table 27-1). In the neonatal period, it is within normal limits for the immature hip to produce an alpha angle between 50° to 59°. Reevaluation should be performed at ≥12 weeks postnatal age to ensure the alpha angle increases to ≥60°. Angle measurement is beginning to fall out of favor in many institutions. Coverage of the femoral head, acetabular morphology, and ability to sublux are of greater importance.

3. Right coronal hip, 90° flexion

    Demonstrate the coronal "egg in spoon" view with the hip flexed 90°. In this image, the femoral head is the "egg," the iliac line is the "spoon handle," and the acetabulum is the "scoop of the spoon" (Fig. 27-7).

Note: With unstable (dislocated) DDH, the "egg" (femoral head) comes completely out of the "spoon" (acetabulum); with stable (subluxated) dysplasia, the "spoon" (acetabulum) is too shallow for the "egg" (femoral head), and it rolls within the "spoon."

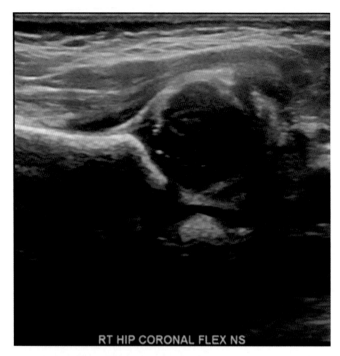

RT HIP CORONAL FLEX NS

FIGURE 27-7. Coronal flexion view.

4. Right transverse hip, 15 to 20° neutral

A "U-shaped" image is obtained, showing the femoral metaphysis anterior and the femoral head situated between the posterior ischium and anterior metaphysis. The femoral head is seated within the "U."

5. Right transverse hip, 90° flexion (Fig. 27-8)

Appearance is like the transverse neutral "U-shaped" view. This view has also been described as a "golf ball on a tee," "flower," or "ice cream cone" view. The femoral head is demonstrated lying over the triradiate cartilage. The "flower" is visualized with the femoral metaphysis anterior and femoral head situated between the posterior ischium and anterior metaphysis. In this image the triradiate cartilage is "flower stem," the pubis and ischium demonstrate the "flower leaves," and the femoral head is the "flower." (Fig. 27-9)

6. Right transverse hip, with stress (Fig. 27-10).

To "stress" the hip, the Barlow maneuver is performed (when allowable).

7. Left coronal hip, 15-20° neutral

8. Left coronal hip, 15-20° neutral with measurements

9. Left coronal hip, 90° flexion

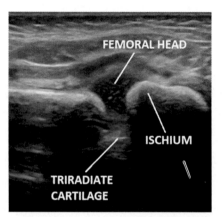

FIGURE 27-9. Short-axis (transverse) view without stress.

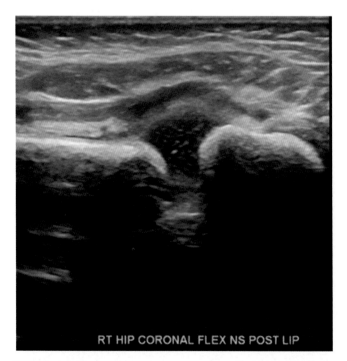

RT HIP CORONAL FLEX NS POST LIP

FIGURE 27-8. Short-axis (transverse) view without stress (NS, non-stress).

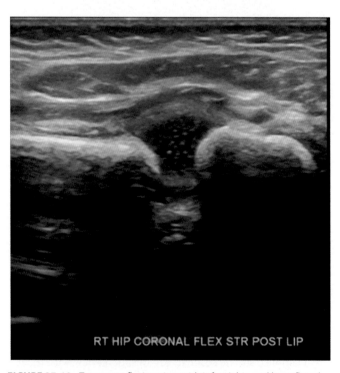

RT HIP CORONAL FLEX STR POST LIP

FIGURE 27-10. Transverse flexion view with infant's hip and knee flexed 90°, transducer is positioned perpendicular to the lateral portion of the infant's hip (coronal body plane).

10. Left transverse hip, 15-20° neutral

11. Left transverse hip, 90° flexion

12. Left transverse hip, with stress

13. Split-screen function demonstrating bilateral neutral hips, at 15-20° flexion

Cine-clips

1. Right transverse hip, dynamic with stress

   The Barlow maneuver involves abduction and posterior pistoning (push stress). Pistoning is a *gentle* posterior pressure that is applied to the femur with the hip flexed. A false positive exam can be produced if excessive pressure causes pelvic rotation.

2. Left transverse hip, dynamic with stress

> **Note:** This maneuver is performed only if the patient is not in a harness, cast, or brace. The metaphysis and ischium which create the "U" should become a deeper "U" with abduction and become and "V" shape with adduction. When an abnormal dislocation is present, the "U-shape" is not visualized. With subluxation, there will be an appearance of increased echogenicity between the acetabulum and femoral head because of interposition of pulvinar fibrofatty tissue. With dislocation, it is controversial whether the cartilaginous acetabular labrum is deformed or becomes inverted. In transverse plane the acetabular cartilage anterior to the triradiate cartilage on the pubic side is minimally thicker than it is posterior to the triradiate cartilage on the ischial side.

JOINT EFFUSION OF THE HIP

Joint effusion of the hip (Fig. 27-11(a) and (b)) may be caused by toxic synovitis or septic arthritis. Toxic synovitis, also known as "transient synovitis," is the most common cause of joint effusion. With joint effusion, fluid accumulates within the joint capsule. The patient may present with hip pain, limp, or inability to bear weight.

For evaluation of effusion of the hip joint, a high frequency (5-17 MHz) linear transducer should be used. No patient preparation is required.

Still images are obtained in sagittal view demonstrating the anterior hip joint bilaterally, providing a side-by-side comparison image using split-screen feature (Fig. 27-11(c)). Both joint capsules should be measured in split screen, evaluating for presence of joint effusion.

Bilateral joint appearance is significantly different in the presence of a unilateral effusion. A positive hip will contain an additional 2 to 3+ millimeters of fluid. On occasion, joint effusion of the hip is bilateral, but more commonly occurs unilaterally. Ultrasound can only determine presence of effusion, and

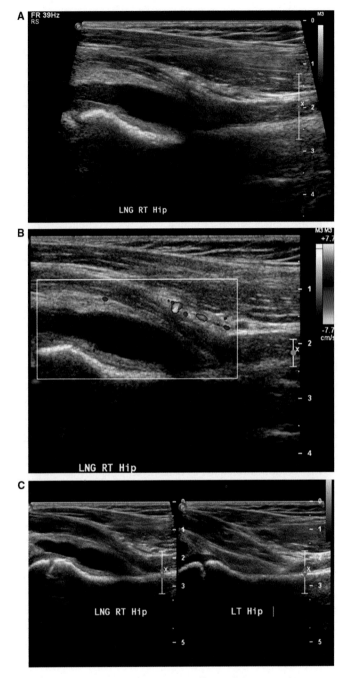

FIGURE 27-11. Moderate right-sided hip effusion demonstrated in a 4-year-old patient.

cannot differentiate between simple (i.e., viral, reactive) effusion and septic joint.

Still images:

1. Sagittal view of affected hip (anterior hip joint) in grayscale

2. Sagittal view of affected hip with capsule measurement

3. Sagittal view of affected hip with color Doppler

4. Sagittal split-screen of affected and contralateral hips in grayscale

5. Sagittal split-screen of affected and contralateral hips with capsule measurements

TOXIC SYNOVITIS

Toxic synovitis, otherwise known as "transient synovitis," is the most common cause of painful hip and joint effusion in children between 5 and 10 years of age. Clinical findings include hip or knee pain, limp, low grade fever, and mild leukocytosis. Sonographic appearance includes fluid within the hip joint capsule, increased capsule to bone distance, and convex capsule margin. Capsule to bone distance is considered increased when measuring greater than 3 millimeter, or 2 millimeter greater than the normal contralateral hip joint capsule. Sonographic images are taken with the transducer in sagittal plane, parallel to the long axis of the femoral neck, with comparison views obtained of the contralateral hip in split-screen function. The sensitivity of ultrasound detecting joint effusion ranges between 90 and 100% accuracy.

SEPTIC ARTHRITIS

Septic arthritis can arise as a hematogenous infection due to joint seeding from sepsis, direct implantation of organism from penetrating injury, or extension of osteomyelitis. With direct implantation streptococcal infection is most common among neonates, while staphylococcal infections are more prominent in infants and young children. Treatment for septic arthritis includes urgent arthrotomy and open drainage. This ensures further complication such as osteomyelitis, epiphyseal separation, joint destruction, fibrous and bony ankylosis, contracture, and femoral head osteonecrosis will not occur. Sonographic appearance includes fluid in the within the hip joint capsule, increased capsule to bone distance, and a convex capsule margin. Capsule to bone distance is considered increased when measuring greater than 3 mm, or 2 mm greater than the normal contralateral hip joint capsule. Sonographic images are taken with transducer in sagittal plane, parallel to the long axis of the femoral neck, with comparison views obtained of the contralateral hip in split-screen function. The sensitivity of ultrasound detecting joint effusion ranges between 90 and 100% accuracy; however, ultrasound cannot differentiate between a simple effusion and septic joint. For this determination, sampling of the joint fluid must be performed by a specialist such as an orthopedic physician.

KNEE EFFUSION

Effusion of the knee joint is very commonly encountered in pediatrics, particularly in a child presenting with limp. For evaluation of effusion of the knee joint, a 5-17 MHz linear transducer should be used. No patient preparation is required.

Still images are obtained in two planes demonstrating the knee joint bilaterally, providing a side-by-side comparison image using split-screen feature. Both joint capsules evaluated in split screen, observing for presence of joint effusion.

TENOSYNOVITIS

Tenosynovitis is inflammation of the tendon and synovium (Table 27-2). The most common cause of inflammatory tenosynovitis in pediatric patients is juvenile rheumatoid arthritis or overuse syndrome, which causes tendon and sheath microtrauma leading to secondary inflammation. The sonographic appearance of tenosynovitis includes an enlarged hyperemic tendon sheath containing fluid. With chronic inflammation tiny, scattered calcifications can be seen.

SYNOVIAL HYPERTROPHY

Synovial hypertrophy is an increase in synovium size resulting from irritation. This exam is very specialized, most relevant to diseases such as rheumatoid arthritis. Sonographic appearance includes an abnormal synovium hypoechoic to the subdermal fat and intra-articular non-displaceable, and poorly compressible tissue that may have a Doppler flow signal. Synovial hypertrophy may be a result of trauma or mild chondromalacia, but can be improved with arthroscopic debridement of the tissue. Synovial hypertrophy involves a grading system categorizing the synovium from normal to marked appearances. With Grade 0, or a normal appearance, this is no present thickening of the synovium. Mild thickening of the synovium is categorized as Grade I, where the angle begins to fill without top-of-bone line bulging. Grade II is a moderate synovial thickening where top-of-bone line bulging is present, but extension along the bone diaphysis has not occurred. Grade III includes a markedly thickened synovium with top-of-bone line bulging and extension along the bone diaphysis.

HEMARTHROSIS

Hemarthrosis occurs when there is bleeding into the joint cavity (Figs. 27-12 and 27-13). This may occur due to traumatic and nontraumatic injury, but is most commonly seen in patients with acquired and hereditary bleeding disorders, such as hemophilia. The typical presentation is decreased range of motion of the joint. Arthrocentesis may be required when indicated.

TABLE 27-2 • Inflammatory Musculoskeletal Processes		
Tendonitis	**Tenosynovitis**	**Synovitis**
Inflammation of the tendon.	Inflammation of the tendon and synovium.	Inflammation of the synovium

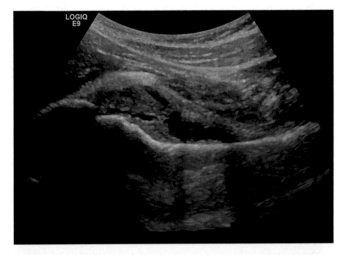

FIGURE 27-12. An 18-year-old with hemophilia and elbow joint swelling. Large hemarthrosis entering into adjacent muscle and tendon sheaths.

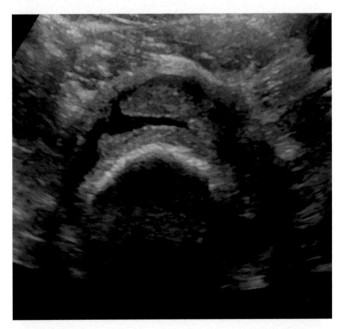

FIGURE 27-13. A 17-year-old with autoimmune hepatitis. Aspiration yielded 22 cc of hemorrhagic synovial fluid.

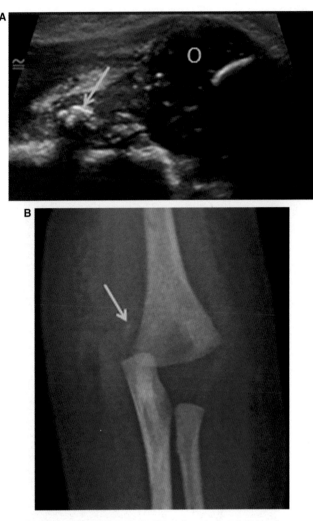

FIGURE 27-14. Posterior approach of the elbow in an infant less than one year of age, who is refusing to move the arm. The ultrasound and radiograph demonstrate a posteriorly displaced fracture through the humeral physis with fracture fragments (arrow).

ELBOW

Sonography is able to assist in suspected elbow injuries in patients with an inconclusive or negative x-ray, though radiographs are the preferred imaging modality. Typical indications include assessment for radiocapitellar dislocation (congenital or traumatic) (Fig. 27-14(a) and (b)), radiocapitellar subluxation (Fig. 27-15(a) and (b)), nursemaid elbow (Fig. 27-16), septic effusion, and osteomyelitis (Fig. 27-17(a) to (c)). Protocol images include anterior evaluation showing radiocapitellar alignment, the anterior fat pad, distal humerus and radial metaphysis. A lateral approach shows the capitellum and radial head, which is an important view for the assessment of nursemaid elbow. The posterior approach demonstrates the posterior fat pad, humerus, olecranon, and trochlea. From a medial approach the trochlea and ulna are visualized. Transverse images should be taken from the anterior and posterior approach. All images should be taken with the arm fully extended.

Still images:

1. Sagittal anterior of the elbow
2. Sagittal lateral image of the elbow
3. Sagittal posterior image of the elbow
4. Sagittal medial image of the elbow
5. Transverse anterior image of the elbow
6. Transverse posterior image of the elbow

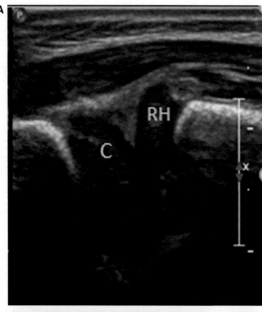

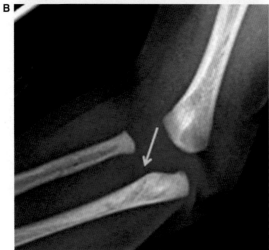

FIGURE 27-15. A 1-month-old female presenting with "popping" of the right elbow. Ultrasound and radiograph demonstrate subluxation of the radial head.

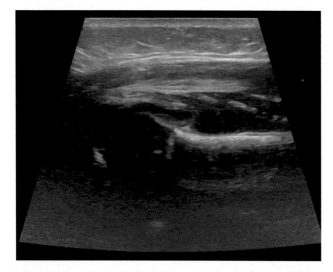

FIGURE 27-16. A 15-month-old female, not moving the left arm after a fall onto the left arm. No improvement in motion after attempted nursemaid reduction.

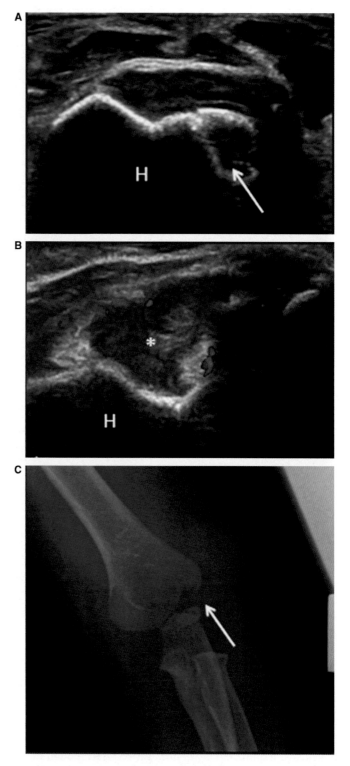

FIGURE 27-17. A 2-year-old with a swollen elbow and no history of trauma. Ultrasound demonstrates cortical erosion and complex joint effusion with surrounding hyperemia. The radiograph shows soft tissue swelling and a focal lytic lesion on the lateral humeral metaphysis. This patient had osteomyelitis and septic arthritis.

28

Pathology of Superficial Structures

A soft tissue ultrasound may be ordered for evaluation of superficial soft tissue abnormalities such as a palpable mass, cellulitis, abscess, or foreign body. Superficial imaging evaluation requires no preparation and is a straightforward examination. Superficial structures are best visualized using a high frequency (5-17 MHz) linear transducer. The area of interest should be surveyed, searching for abnormalities within the superficial soft tissues. Using the ultrasound unit's split-screen feature can be helpful in imaging the ipsilateral area of concern and normal contralateral side for visualization of discrete abnormalities. It can be helpful to document the relationship of findings to anatomic landmarks, including bones, vessels, or other superficial structures (i.e., the thyroid in soft-tissue neck imaging). In superficial findings, strain elastography can be used for further evaluation. Presence of central or peripheral vascularity should be documented with any positive findings by way of color and spectral Dopplers.

Still images include:

1. Sagittal area of concern in grayscale
2. Sagittal area of concern with color Doppler
3. Transverse area of concern in grayscale
4. Transverse area of concern with color Doppler
5. Sagittal split screen area of concern with compression
6. Transverse split screen area of concern with compression
7. Sagittal split screen area of concern and contralateral comparative anatomy in grayscale
8. Transverse split screen area of concern and contralateral comparative anatomy in grayscale
9. Measurements and interrogation of any findings

Cine-clips include:

1. Sagittal area of concern
2. Transverse area of concern

It is important to note that with sonographic imaging, superficial structure findings are commonly nonspecific and biopsy may be required for definitive diagnosis.

BENIGN MASSES

Soft Tissue Hemangioma

Soft tissue hemangioma is the most common vascular soft tissue tumor of infancy. Soft tissue hemangioma presents as a bluish skin discoloration. Sonographic appearance includes well-defined vascular, superficial soft tissue mass of varying echogenicity.

Soft Tissue Lipoma

Soft tissue lipoma is a benign fat-containing, subcutaneous tissue mass. Sonographic appearance includes a well-defined homogeneous lesion with minimal or absent color Doppler flow (Fig. 28-1(a) to (c)).

Lipoblastoma

Lipoblastoma is a lipomatous tumor containing multiple lobules of immature fatty tissue, separated by fibrous septa. Lipoblastoma most commonly occurs in children less than 3 years of age. Usually arising in the extremities, lipoblastoma has a sonographic appearance of a well-defined, complex echogenic mass.

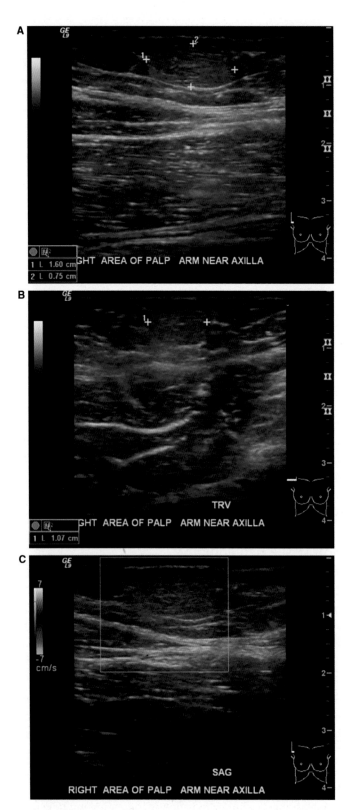

FIGURE 28-1. Lipoma demonstrated by ultrasound as a nonvascular, well-circumscribed, echogenic subcutaneous lesion.

Schwannoma

Schwannoma is the second most common benign nerve sheath tumor. This benign neoplasm grows at the nerve periphery.

Popliteal (Baker) Cyst

Popliteal cysts, or Baker cysts, consist of an abnormal fluid collection that accumulates within the gastrocnemius-semi-membranous bursa and communicates with the knee joint. Sonographic appearance is generally a well-defined anechoic collection, although septations or internal debris may be present (Figs. 28-2 (a) and (b)).

MALIGNANT MASSES

Rhabdomyosarcoma

Rhabdomyosarcoma is the most common malignant soft tissue tumor in children. Children less than 6 years of age are most commonly affected by rhabdomyosarcoma. The most common presenting symptom of rhabdomyosarcoma is a growing mass or swelling wherever the tumor forms. Sonographic appearance is a heterogeneous well-defined irregular mass of low to medium echogenicity with increased flow on color Doppler.

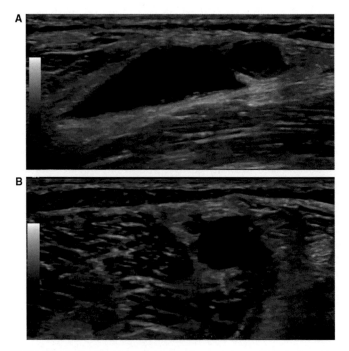

FIGURE 28-2. Popliteal fossa fluid collection correlates with Baker's cyst in (a) sagittal and (b) transverse plane.

29

Vascular Etiologies

ARTERIOVENOUS MALFORMATION

An arteriovenous malformation is a high flow direct connection between an artery and vein, in which there is absence of a capillary network. This leads to the formation of a pulsatile mass containing characteristics of bruit and thrill, pulsatile venous flow, and low-resistance arterial waveform due to a fistula between the two vessels.

ARTERIOVENOUS FISTULA

An arteriovenous fistula is a direct connection between an artery and vein without an intervening capillary network. This connection may be acquired from a biopsy, penetrating injury, or congenital anomaly. Large fistulas may lead to hypertension, hematuria, or high-output cardiac failure. Sonographic findings can include high velocity systolic flow and elevated diastolic flow in the feeding artery, turbulent flow at the shunt site, and arterialization of the draining vein upon Doppler evaluation.

VENOUS MALFORMATION

A venous malformation is a slow flow vascular lesion with abnormal venous and normal arterial components. This malformation is said to be an abnormally enlarged and tangled connection of veins. A venous vascular malformation will appear as a superficial compressible mass with blue skin discoloration. The sonographic appearance of a venous malformation includes a hypoechoic mass containing low-resistance monophasic flow or no flow within the venous component. A venous malformation may also contain calcified areas called "phleboliths."

CAPILLARY MALFORMATION (PORT-WINE STAIN)

A capillary vascular malformation is also known as a "port-wine stain," which is present at birth, grows in proportion with the patient, and does not resolve. A capillary vascular malformation appears as an irregular rosy-to-purple blotch on the skin and can occur anywhere on the body. These malformations are constructed of small vascular dermis channels. Prominent venous dermis channels throughout the body will contain an increased thickness of subcutaneous fat.

PSEUDOANEURYSM

A pseudoaneurysm is a confined hematoma that communicates with an artery. It occurs when the arterial wall is damaged. Arterial wall laceration can be related to percutaneous needle biopsy, femoral artery catheterization, and other penetrating or orthopedic injuries. A pseudoaneurysm is contained by the vessel's tunica adventitia layer, whereas a true aneurysm contains all layers of the vessel wall. Sonographic findings include a hypoechoic mass with a swirling disorganized Doppler flow pattern and mixed high-velocity arterial flow with a pulsatile venous waveform. Turbulent flow may be visualized on color Doppler as the "yin-yang" sign, signifying forward and backward flow. An established interventional treatment method for the correction of a reachable pseudoaneurysm whose diameter is too large to spontaneously thrombose is ultrasound duplex-guided compression. This can be performed with or without thrombin injection, depending on the diameter of the pseudoaneurysm. Ultrasound compression is aimed at the region of the pseudoaneurysm neck and is performed at 10-minute intervals. The entire procedure ranges from 10 minutes to 2.5 hours.

Following a favorable thrombosis, the patient is rescanned at 2 and 24-hour intervals. It is advantageous the patient remains on bed rest during this time frame. Surgical management is reserved for when this method of treatment is unsuccessful.

CENTRAL AND PERIPHERAL ARTERIAL PATHOLOGIES

Occlusive arterial disease involves complete absence of vessel patency, where blood is not able to flow through the vessel. Chronic arterial disease involves autoimmune-related disorders and atherosclerosis. Acute occlusive disease is usually a result of trauma or embolism. Arterial occlusion is associated with the five P's (5Ps): pain, pulselessness, pallor, paresthesia, and paralysis. Parasthesia and paralysis may trigger the possibility of acute limb ischemia. Examples of effects resulting from chronic arterial disease includes hair loss of the foot, shiny or smooth skin, thickened toenails, coolness of extremity, pallor during elevation and rubor during dependent limb positioning.

Miscellaneous arterial pathologies include thoracic outlet compression and entrapment syndromes, such as popliteal entrapment. With entrapment, muscles compress arterial supply. Entrapment is a congenital developmental defect, more frequently seen in the popliteus or gastrocnemius muscles of the leg. Thoracic outlet compression is a compression of the subclavian artery at the thoracic outlet by surrounding structures such as the clavicle, cervical rib, or muscles. With thoracic outlet compression syndrome abnormal Doppler waveforms are encountered in the subclavian artery of the affected arm. For confirmation, multiple tests can be performed including Wright's test (extremity hyperabduction), the Eden test (military brace, shoulders pulled down), or Adson's test (head rotation toward side affected). With these maneuvers, a waveform decrease is visualized.

CENTRAL AND PERIPHERAL VENOUS PATHOLOGIES

Venous pathologies primarily include various forms of venous thrombosis. This may include chronic deep vein thrombosis, superficial thrombus, thrombophlebitis, phlegmasia alba dolens, phlegmasia cerulea dolens, venous insufficiency, and venous thromboembolism (VTE). Acute thrombus refers to a thrombus which occurs in a time frame of less than 2 weeks (Fig. 29-1(a) and (b)). Following 1 month, or 28 days, thrombus is considered chronic, and exhibits a different sonographic appearance (Fig. 29-2).

Phlegmasia alba dolens is rare in pediatrics, but life-threatening when occurring. Phlegmasia alba dolens is an acute, extensive iliofemoral thrombus that does not allow blood to drain from the deep or superficial systems. Phlegmasia cerulea dolens is an extensive thrombus of the major or collateral veins.

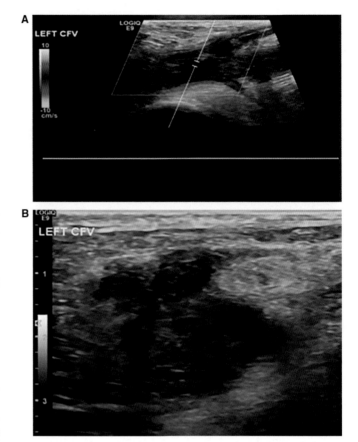

FIGURE 29-1. Acute thrombus of the left common femoral vein demonstrating lack of compressibility and echogenic material within the vessel lumen.

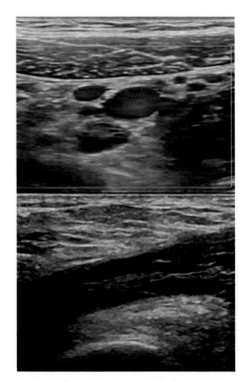

FIGURE 29-2. Chronic thrombus demonstrating thickened intima and irregular, echogenic material within the vessel lumen.

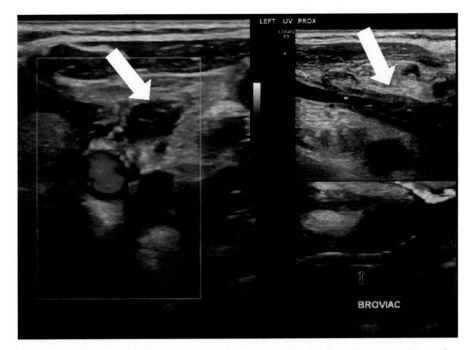

FIGURE 29-3. Extensive occlusive thrombosis in the central internal jugular vein with inflammatory change of surrounding tissues. A 16-year-old female patient presented with complaint of acute tenderness and left neck swelling, status post central catheter (Broviac) placement, with history of sickle cell disease, biliary atresia, and hepatorenal syndrome.

In the pediatric population, VTE most often occurs in the neonatal period, followed by the adolescent period. Central venous catheters (i.e., peripherally inserted central catheter line, Port-A-Cath, Broviac) contribute to 85% of pediatric VTE (Fig. 29-3). Clinical symptoms include chest pain, tachycardia, tachypnea, and swelling of the extremities. Other causes of venous thrombosis include blood clotting disorders, lack of mobility, sepsis, trauma, malignancy, other lesions which occupy space, and congenital anatomic variants (Fig. 29-4). Lab tests which may disclose abnormal values in the presence of thrombosis include D-dimer, fibrinogen, prothrombin time, and partial thromboplastin time.

Unrelated to venous thrombosis, but commonly visualized as an incidental finding during a lower extremity venous scan is a popliteal (Baker's) cyst, which is seen in the popliteal fossa as a dilated fluid-filled gastrocnemius-semimembranosus bursa. For additional information and imaging protocol, please refer to information in protocol in Chapter 28, "Pathology of Superficial Structures."

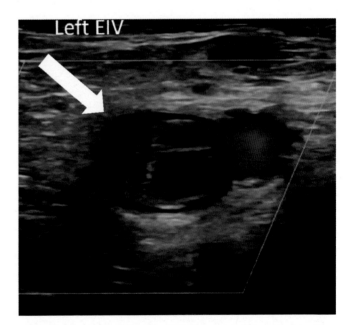

FIGURE 29-4. Extensive thrombus in the left external iliac vein extending from the left popliteal vein. A 17-year-old female patient presented with complaint of pain and swelling in the left lower extremity, with history of May-Thurner Syndrome and Factor V Leiden.

30

Neurocutaneous Syndromes

Neurocutaneous syndromes are a group of disorders which affect various parts of the body, including the central nervous system, kidneys, liver, lungs, skin, and bones, leading to complications such as tumor development, seizures, and developmental issues. The most commonly occurring neurocutaneous syndromes include tuberous sclerosis complex (TSC), Sturge-Weber syndrome, and neurofibromatosis (NF). Additional neurocutaneous syndromes include Von Hippel-Lindau syndrome, ataxia-telangiectasia, and cerebelloretinal hemangiomatosis.

TUBEROUS SCLEROSIS

This phakomatosis, or neurocutaneous, disorder is transmitted as an autosomal dominant trait with variable penetrance. The two genes in patients with TSC include TSC1 (TSC complex subunit 1) on chromosome 9q34 which codes protein hamartin, and TSC2 (TSC complex subunit 2) on chromosome 16p13.3 which codes protein tuberin. These two genes help with regulation of cell proliferation and differentiation. TSC is clinically characterized as a triad of adenoma sebaceum, mental retardation, and seizures. Only one-third of patients with TSC have this triad of symptoms. With TSC, 90% of patients will have skin lesions, 90% will have seizures, and 50% will have mental retardation. Although uncommon, a patient's ventricles may enlarge resulting from foramen obstruction. Cortical tubers in the frontal regions of the brain appear as hyperechoic foci or appear as cystic lesions within the white matter. TSC patients may also have lesions on the heart, kidneys, lung, spleen, brain, or cysts within the liver (Fig. 30-1). This syndrome can be the origin of pheochromocytoma, renal artery stenosis, renal cell carcinoma, and renal lipomyolipoma. Another name for TSC is Bourneville disease.

NEUROFIBROMATOSIS

NF is an autosomal dominant disorder. There are two types of NF. NF type 1 (NF1) results from a gene alteration on chromosome 17. NF type 2 (NF2) results from a gene alteration on

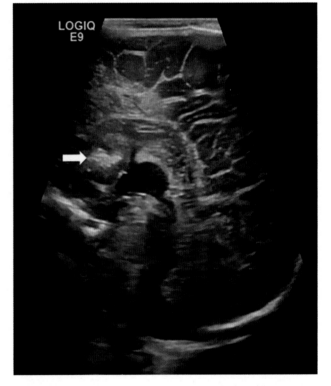

FIGURE 30-1. Giant cell tumor in a patient with tuberous sclerosis.

chromosome 22. NF is most often diagnosed amongst children and young adults, with NF1 being the most commonly occurring variation. NF1 occurs in approximately 1 out of every 3,000 births, whereas NF2 presents less frequently in 1 out of every 40,000 births. Complications of NF include anomalies of the skin, eyes (i.e., optic nerve), bone, nerves, heart, and brain. Etiologies often associated with NF that can be visualized sonographically include renal hamartoma (angiomyolipoma), adrenal pheochromocytoma, and neurofibroma of the neck. Pediatrics with NF1 have a greater risk of developing plexiform neurofibroma, which can occur within soft tissues of the cervical region. Schwannomatosis is a rare form of NF.

VON HIPPEL-LINDAU SYNDROME

Von-Hippel Lindau disease is an autosomal dominant disorder. This syndrome is characterized by pathologies due to an error on the short arm of chromosome 3. Some disease processes associated with Von-Hippel Lindau syndrome include retinal angiomatosis, cerebellar, medullary, and spinal hemangioblastomas, pheochromocytoma, and cysts within various organs. Cysts with this disease process can particularly be found within the pancreas, kidneys, liver, epididymis, and adrenal glands. Additional pathology associated with Von-Hippel Lindau syndrome may include epididymal cystadenoma which appears as complex cystic masses, multiple simple cysts in the liver, renal cell carcinoma arising from renal epithelial cells, and pheochromocytoma. With Von-Hippel Lindau syndrome, pheochromocytoma is a catecholamine-secreting tumor arising from chromaffin cells of the sympathetic nervous system, mainly originating in the adrenals. Pheochromocytoma is with increased incidence in patients having Von-Hippel Lindau syndrome, TSC, NF, and Sturge-Weber neurocutaneous syndromes.

STURGE-WEBER SYNDROME

Sturge-Weber syndrome is a neurocutaneous syndrome associated with vascular malformation lesions. Sturge-Weber patients may have nevus flammeus, which is a slow flow vascular lesion with abnormal venous spaces and normal arterial components. This is similar to what is visualized in patients with port-wine stains. There is an increased incidence of pheochromocytoma in patients with Sturge-Weber syndrome.

Section II Review: Pathologic Processes

1. In 2 to 4% of patients, tuberous sclerosis can be associated with
   a. Testicular carcinoma
   b. Breast carcinoma
   c. Renal cell carcinoma
   d. Brain carcinoma

2. Slow flow vascular lesions may be seen in patients with
   a. Sturge–Weber Syndrome
   b. Tuberous sclerosis
   c. Neurofibromatosis
   d. Turner malformation

3. Simple meningoceles will contain
   a. Fat
   b. Cerebrospinal fluid
   c. Cerebrospinal fluid and spinal cord
   d. Bone marrow

4. Extracorporeal oxygenation (ECMO) may cause the spleen to
   a. Become nonfunctioning
   b. Become smaller in size
   c. Become larger in size
   d. Form small nodules of splenic tissue

5. Splenic torsion may result in
   a. Necrosis of the pancreatic tail
   b. Necrosis of the pancreatic head
   c. Nonfunctional kidney
   d. Liver compromise

6. Cystic fibrosis will cause the pancreas to look
   a. Calcified
   b. Hypoechoic
   c. Hyperechoic
   d. Normal echogenicity

7. A large complex exocrine lesion arising from the pancreatic tail mostly likely is a
   a. Pancreaticoblastoma tumor
   b. Gastrinoma tumor
   c. Somatosatinoma tumor
   d. Pseudopapillary tumor

8. Extra-pancreatic fluid collections may be seen with
   a. Mild acute pancreatitis
   b. Severe acute pancreatitis
   c. Chronic pancreatitis
   d. Hereditary pancreatitis

9. Idiopathic fibrosing pancreatitis causes the pancreatic parenchyma to
   a. Become enlarged
   b. Be replaced with cysts
   c. Be replaced with fibrous tissue
   d. Become calcified

10. The pyloric channel is considered abnormal if it is greater than
    a. 3 to 4 millimeters
    b. 7 to 8 millimeters
    c. 12 to 13 millimeters
    d. 15 to 17 millimeters

11. In the transverse orientation pyloric stenosis appears as a
    a. Bull's eye sign
    b. Pseudokidney sign
    c. Ball of wool sign
    d. Lily pad sign

12. The peak occurrence of intussusception is
    a. 1 to 3 months
    b. 5 to 9 months
    c. 1 to 3 years
    d. 4 to 5 years

13. Duplication cysts are associated with the
    a. Pancreas
    b. Liver
    c. Urogenital system
    d. Gastrointestinal tract

14. The most common malignant gastrointestinal neoplasm in childhood is
    a. Gastric lymphoma
    b. Gastric carcinoma
    c. Gastrointestinal stromal tumor
    d. Gastric teratoma

15. The most common fusion site for a horseshoe kidney is

    a. Upper pole

    b. Mid pole

    c. Lower pole

    d. Posterior border

16. Autosomal recessive polycystic disease usually presents as

    a. Unilateral tiny cysts

    b. Bilateral tiny cysts

    c. Unilateral large cysts

    d. Bilateral large cysts

17. Medullary sponge kidney disease is a

    a. Autosomal recessive disease

    b. Autosomal dominant disease

    c. Non-inherited disease

    d. Non-classified disease

18. Angiomyolipomas are one of the common findings with

    a. Medullary sponge disease

    b. Tuberous sclerosis

    c. Turner syndrome

    d. Von Hippel-Lindau

19. Multiple cysts of various sizes seen on one kidney during a prenatal ultrasound exam is most likely

    a. Autosomal recessive polycystic kidney disease

    b. Medullary sponge kidney

    c. Tuberous sclerosis

    d. Multicystic dysplastic kidney disease

20. Renal duplication artifact occurs more frequently in the

    a. Left kidney

    b. Right kidney

    c. Both kidneys

    d. Renal ureters

21. A 4-month-old presents with abdominal pain, palpable mass, and red currant jelly-like stools. This most likely represents

    a. Bowel obstruction

    b. Pyloric stenosis

    c. Diverticulitis

    d. Intussusception

22. Echogenic debris in a dilated renal collecting system is suggestive of

    a. Glomerulonephritis

    b. Chronic pyelonephritis

    c. Xanthogranulomatous pyelonephritis

    d. Pyonephritis

23. In children a renal length difference of _____ raises suspicion for duplication

    a. > 1 millimeter

    b. > 5 millimeters

    c. > 1 centimeter

    d. > 2 centimeters

24. Renal artery ratio can be calculated by

    a. Dividing the renal artery peak systolic velocity by the aorta's peak systolic velocity

    b. Dividing the renal artery peak systolic velocity by the renal end diastolic velocity

    c. Subtracting the renal artery peak systolic by the end diastolic velocity then dividing the renal artery peak systolic velocity

    d. Subtracting the renal artery peak systolic by the end diastolic velocity then dividing the aorta's peak systolic velocity

25. Acute renal vein thrombus usually presents as

    a. A small kidney

    b. An enlarged kidney

    c. Increased venous signal

    d. Decreased echogenicity

26. The most common benign renal tumor in neonates is

    a. Metanephric adenoma

    b. Ossifying renal tumor

    c. Mesoblastic nephroma

    d. Angiomyolipoma

27. Renal angiomyolipoma usually occurs in what part of the kidney?

    a. Cortex

    b. Sinus

    c. Medulla

    d. Pelvis

28. **Wilms tumor accounts for what percentage of pediatric renal malignancies**

    a.   40%
    b.   60%
    c.   75%
    d.   90%

29. **The most prevalent age for acute lymphoblastic leukemia is**

    a.   3 to 5 months
    b.   1 to 2 years
    c.   3 to 5 years
    d.   7 to 10 years

30. **This malignant process is commonly found in patients with sickle cell trait and hemoglobin sickle cell disease**

    a.   Neuroectodermal tumor
    b.   Renal medullary carcinoma
    c.   Clear cell sarcoma
    d.   Rhabdoid tumor

31. **Rhabdoid neoplasm starts in the _____ part of the kidney.**

    a.   Medulla
    b.   Cortex
    c.   Sinus
    d.   Pelvic

32. **In the very young pediatric patient, the transplant kidney is anastomosed to the**

    a.   Iliac artery and vein
    b.   Iliac artery and IVC
    c.   Distal aorta and IVC
    d.   Distal aorta and iliac vein

33. **Sonographic findings of graft enlargement, increased cortical echogenicity, increased corticomedullary differentiation, and enlarged hypoechoic pyramids describe which type of renal transplant rejection?**

    a.   Drug toxicity transplant failure
    b.   Transplant acute tubular necrosis
    c.   Interstitial transplant rejection
    d.   Vascular transplant rejection

34. **A urachal cyst is a result of**

    a.   Channel is closed at the umbilicus and bladder, but remain open in the center
    b.   Failed lumen closure with present channel
    c.   Channel is present solely at the umbilicus
    d.   Channel present at the bladder alone

35. **The most common childhood bladder malignant mass is**

    a.   Transitional cell carcinoma
    b.   Leiomyosarcoma
    c.   Rhabdomyosarcoma
    d.   Nephroblastoma

36. **Bilateral enlarged echogenic adrenal glands with prominent necrotic areas and shadowing calcifications in the adrenal cortex is the usual sonographic features of**

    a.   Ganglioneuroma
    b.   Adrenogenital syndrome
    c.   Conn syndrome
    d.   Wolman disease

37. **Neuroblastoma most commonly arises in the**

    a.   Kidney
    b.   Bladder
    c.   Adrenal gland
    d.   Brain

38. **Spermatocele can occur in pediatric patients of which age group?**

    a.   Neonates
    b.   3 to 6 months
    c.   2 to 5 years
    d.   Postpubertal males

39. **Cryptorchidism increases the risk of**

    a.   Malignancy
    b.   Hydrocele
    c.   Varicocele
    d.   Epididymal cyst

40. **The most common infantile testicular tumor is**

    a.   Seminoma
    b.   Embryonal cell carcinoma
    c.   Mixed cell tumor
    d.   Teratoma

41. Mature teratoma accounts for approximately _____ of all benign ovarian tumors.

    a. 20%
    b. 45%
    c. 70%
    d. 90%

42. Yolk sac tumors cause an increase in

    a. AST
    b. Alpha-fetoprotein
    c. CA-125
    d. Lipase

43. In the cervical neck region, a thin-walled loculated mass with acoustic enhancement and low velocity Doppler flow within septations of the mass most likely describes

    a. Fibromatosis colli
    b. Cystic hygroma
    c. Dermoid cyst
    d. Thymic cyst

44. Which of the following is used to differentiate a neuroblastoma from neurofibroma?

    a. The size of the mass
    b. The echogenicity of the mass
    c. The patients gender
    d. The patients age

45. This pediatric pathology of the chest is more common in males than females

    a. Intralobar sequestration
    b. Extralobar sequestration
    c. Congenital lobar overinflation
    d. Cystic adenomatoid malformation

46. Most diaphragmatic hernias occur

    a. Unilateral on the left side
    b. Unilateral on the right side
    c. Bilaterally
    d. Midline

47. In normal pediatric hips, the proximal femoral head should be covered in the acetabulum by at least _____ of the ilium.

    a. 20%
    b. 35%
    c. 50%
    d. 75%

48. One of the most common causes of inflammatory tenosynovitis in pediatric patients is

    a. Lack of movement
    b. Juvenile rheumatoid arthritis
    c. Septic arthritis
    d. Synovial hypertrophy

49. The most common cause of painful hip and joint effusion in children between 5 and 10 years of age is

    a. Toxic synovitis
    b. Synovial hypertrophy
    c. Septic arthritis
    d. Synovial hypertrophy

50. Ventricular dilatation, thickened ependymal lining, intraventricular septations, and debris are sonographic findings of

    a. Hydrocephalus
    b. Meningitis
    c. Ventriculitis
    d. Arachnoid

51. The most common cause of congenital hydrocephalus is

    a. Hydranencephaly
    b. Aqueductal stenosis
    c. Ventriculitis
    d. Sickle-cell disease

52. Velocities greater than _____ cm/s are considered abnormal in a TCD exam.

    a. 75
    b. 100
    c. 150
    d. 200

53. **One of the most common complications of a liver transplant is**

    a. IVC thrombosis

    b. Abscess

    c. Hepatic artery thrombosis

    d. Portal vein thrombosis

54. **Van Gierke disease is a**

    a. Type I glycogen storage disease

    b. Type II glycogen storage disease

    c. Type III glycogen storage disease

    d. Type IV glycogen storage disease

55. **The "starry sky" sign is commonly associated with which of the following**

    a. Glycogen storage disease

    b. Acute hepatitis

    c. Polycystic disease

    d. Fatty infiltration

56. **This liver abscess can occur in immunocompromised children**

    a. Pyogenic abscess

    b. Fungal abscess

    c. Bartholin abscess

    d. Ascariasis

57. **The most common benign hepatic tumor of childhood is**

    a. Cavernous hemangioma

    b. Mesenchymal hamartoma

    c. Infantile hemangioendothelioma

    d. Hepatic adenoma

58. **This benign hepatic tumor is associated with type I glycogen storage disease**

    a. Cavernous hemangioma

    b. Mesenchymal hamartoma

    c. Infantile hemangioendothelioma

    d. Hepatic adenoma

59. **The second most common malignant pediatric liver tumor is**

    a. Hepatocellular carcinoma

    b. Hepatoblastoma

    c. Fibrolamellar hepatocellular carcinoma

    d. Hepatic leiomyosarcoma

60. **This is the most common vascular soft tissue tumor of infancy**

    a. Lipoblastoma

    b. Schwannoma

    c. Soft tissue hemangioma

    d. Soft tissue lipoma

61. **The sonographic appearance of rhabdomyosarcoma is**

    a. Heterogeneous well-defined irregular mass of low to medium echogenicity with increased flow

    b. Cystic mass with septations

    c. Irregular mass of low to medium echogenicity with no detectable flow

    d. Heterogeneous ill-defined mass of low echogenicity with decreased flow

62. **A clinical symptom of hypertrophic pyloric stenosis (HPS) is**

    a. Intermittent abdominal pain

    b. Projectile vomiting

    c. Currant jelly stools

    d. Right lower quadrant pain

63. **Distension of the uterus and vaginal canal with blood product is**

    a. Hematometrocolpos

    b. Hematocolpos

    c. Hydrometrocolpos

    d. Hydrocolpos

64. **A conus tip below which level is suggestive of a tethered cord?**

    a. L2-L3

    b. T12-L2

    c. T11-L1

    d. L1-L2

65. **The most common variant of the gallbladder is**

    a. Junctional fold

    b. Hartman's pouch

    c. Phrygian cap

    d. Septations

66. **What pathology is demonstrated in this image?**

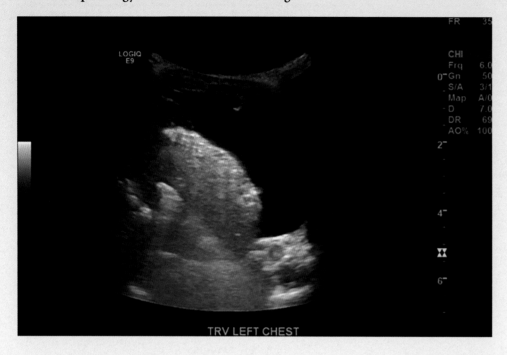

a. Ascites

b. Pericardial effusion

c. Pleural effusion

d. Distended gallbladder

67. **Postnatal hematopoiesis of the spleen can resume with which disorder?**

a. Osteoporosis

b. Thalassemia major

c. Hemochromatosis

d. Gaucher disease

68. **The most common pediatric congenital anomaly of the GI tract is**

a. Meckel's diverticulum

b. Duplication cyst

c. Gastric lymphadenopathy

d. Situs inversus

69. **Ultrasound of the chest is most performed to rule out**

a. Hiatal hernia

b. Mediastinal mass

c. Pleural effusion

d. Phrenic nerve palsy

70. **Which of the following is an autosomal dominant disorder?**

a. Cystic fibrosis

b. Wolman disease

c. Congenital adrenal hyperplasia

d. Tuberous sclerosis

71. **Which spinal defect is covered by the skin?**

a. Spina bifida aperta

b. Occult spinal dysraphism

c. Overt spinal dysraphism

d. Aperta spinal dysraphism

72. **What is being measured in this image?**

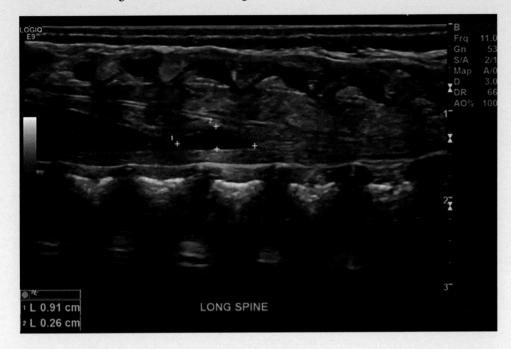

a. Meningocele

b. Myelocystocele

c. Filar cyst

d. Lipomyelocystocele

73. **Which of the following is an endocrine tumor?**

a. Gastrinoma

b. Pancreatic solid pseudopapillary tumor

c. Pancreatic adenocarcinoma

d. Pancreaticoblastoma

74. **Distension of the gallbladder without inflammation is known as**

a. Cholestasis

b. Hydrops

c. Cholelithiasis

d. Cholecystitis

75. **What is the most common renal anomaly?**

a. Ureterocele

b. Simple renal cysts

c. Nephrocalcinosis

d. Horseshoe kidney

76. **For confirmation of thoracic outlet compression syndrome, which test involves extremity hyperabduction?**

a. Adson's test

b. Eden test

c. Wright's test

d. Galeazzi's test

77. **The most common renal malignancy in children is**

a. Nephroblastoma

b. Metanephric adenoma

c. Renal cell carcinoma

d. Mesoblastic nephroma

78. **Which Wilms tumor staging involves confinement to the kidney and can be resected?**

a. I

b. II

c. III

d. IV

79. **Which of the following is a malignant nephrogenesis abnormality that is considered a precursor to Wilms tumor?**

    a. Renal hamartoma
    b. Nephroblastomatosis
    c. Leiomyosarcoma
    d. Renal medullary carcinoma

80. **What is the most common cause of allograft failure?**

    a. Edema
    b. Hematoma
    c. Rejection
    d. Lymphocele

81. **What is the most common perinephric fluid collection?**

    a. Urinoma
    b. Lymphocele
    c. Hematoma
    d. Abscess

82. **Which of the following involves overproduction of cortisol?**

    a. Wolman disease
    b. Conn syndrome
    c. Adrenogenital syndrome
    d. Cushing syndrome

83. **What is the prefix for blood?**

    a. Hemat-
    b. Hydro-
    c. Hypo-
    d. Pyo-

84. **The percent of undescended testicles located in the inguinal canal is**

    a. 20%
    b. 30%
    c. 70%
    d. 80%

85. **The most common cause of acute scrotal pain in prepubertal males is**

    a. Extravaginal scrotal torsion
    b. Intravaginal scrotal torsion
    c. Appendix testis torsion
    d. Orchitis

86. **Onset of physical pubertal characteristics and hormone levels prior to 8 years of age is**

    a. Pseudopuberty
    b. Precocious puberty
    c. Pubertal aplasia
    d. Pubertal atresia

87. **When Mullerian ducts completely fail to fuse this uterine variation results**

    a. Arcuate uterus
    b. Didelphys uterus
    c. Septate uterus
    d. Bicornuate uterus

88. **Inflammation of the fallopian tubes is**

    a. Peritonitis
    b. Epididymitis
    c. Endometritis
    d. Salpingitis

89. **What are the most common non-inflammatory masses located in the lateral neck?**

    a. Branchial cleft cyst
    b. Ectopic thymus
    c. Cervical dermoid cyst
    d. Cervical thymic cyst

90. **The most common cause of acquired hypothyroidism in pediatric is**

    a. Graves' disease
    b. Fibromatosis colli
    c. Hashimoto thyroiditis
    d. Toxic multinodular goiter

91. **Which of the following is a clinical sign for developmental hip dysplasia?**

    a. Limited hip adduction
    b. Limited hip abduction
    c. Normal Barlow maneuver
    d. Normal Ortolani maneuver

92. **The most common intracranial hemorrhage sit in premature infants is**

    a. Subdural hemorrhage
    b. Primary subarachnoid hemorrhage
    c. Subependymal germinal matrix hemorrhage
    d. Cerebellar hemorrhage

93. **Transcranial Doppler (TCD) studies are commonly performed to evaluate for stenosis or occlusion in patients with**

    a. Budd–Chiari malformation

    b. Ventriculomegaly

    c. Sickle-cell disease

    d. Caroli's disease

94. **A diffuse parenchymal disease involving increased iron storage in the liver is**

    a. Cirrhosis

    b. Hemochromatosis

    c. Hepatic fibrosis

    d. Cystic fibrosis

95. **A parasitic infection that causes complex cysts with internal daughter cysts in the liver, known as the *water lily sign*, is**

    a. Hydatid disease

    b. Amebic abscess

    c. Ascariasis

    d. Fungal abscess

96. **Which of the following would appear hyperechoic on ultrasound?**

    a. Ureterocele

    b. Lymphangioma

    c. Angiomyolipoma

    d. Perinephric lymphocele

31

Physics and Instrumentation

WHAT IS ULTRASOUND?

Ultrasound refers to sound waves within frequency ranges that are too high for humans to hear. Medical ultrasound procedures use ultrasound to generate images of structures within the body. Ultrasound is a useful diagnostic imaging tool for imaging pediatrics, as ultrasound does not utilize radiation to produce an image.

Sound waves are emitted from a transducer with piezoelectric properties in pulses. As the sound waves propagate through the body, they interact with the tissue, organs, and other structures, generating echoes that are received by the transducer and sent to the ultrasound machine to create an image. The higher the intensity, or amplitude, of the returning echo, the higher the voltage that is produced and the brighter the echo that is displayed on the monitor. The intensity, or amplitude, of this reflection determines the shade of gray which is displayed on the monitor. The returning echoes can be described as anechoic, hypoechoic, isoechoic, or hyperechoic. An area that is without echoes, or anechoic, appears black on the ultrasound display. Generally, fluid-filled structures such as the bladder, gallbladder or a cyst, appear anechoic. An area which is less bright, or darker, than its surrounding tissues is termed hypoechoic. On ultrasound, the majority of soft tissues exhibit a mid-level shade of gray. When two structures are very similar in echogenicity this is termed isoechoic. An area which is more bright, or brighter, than its surrounding tissues is described as hyperechoic.

TRANSDUCERS

Transducers are devices that convert one form of energy into another. An example of a transducer includes a light bulb, which converts electrical energy into light and heat energy.

In diagnostic ultrasound, transducers convert electricity into mechanical (sound) energy and vice versa.

There are different types of ultrasound imaging transducers, but all contain these essential parts (Fig. 31-1).

The case is comprised of metal or plastic and protects the integrity of the internal components, while the wire acts as the electrical connection between the ultrasound unit and transducer.

Insulating shields are made of a cork of rubber barrier which protects the sonographer and patient from electrical shock. Radio frequency shields are comprised of a metallic barrier which helps to keep outside interference or electrical noise from entering the transducer and causing artifacts (Fig. 31-2).

The backing or damping material is a material bonded to the back of the active element. Its purpose is to stop the active element from ringing to produce a short pulse. This helps to shorten the spatial pulse length, increase bandwidth, and improve axial resolution. The backing material is an epoxy resin impregnated with tungsten.

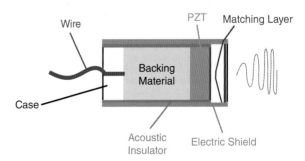

FIGURE 31-1. Components of a diagnostic sonographic imaging transducer.

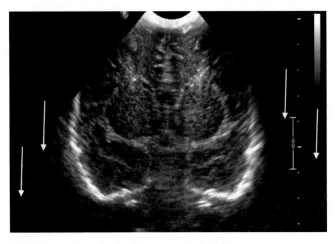

FIGURE 31-2. Example of artifact caused by interference.

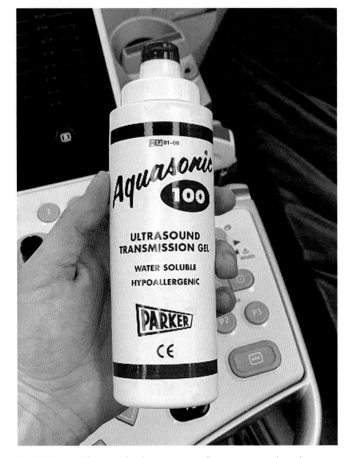

FIGURE 31-3. Ultrasound gel acts as a coupling agent to reduce the impedance mismatch between the transducer and the air between the skin and transducer.

The active elements within the transducer have piezoelectric properties. These piezoelectric elements emit the acoustic beam and receive the returning echoes. Piezoelectric elements within the ultrasound transducer are man-made, such as lead zirconate titanate, PZT, as they are less expensive, more rugged, and more efficient in converting mechanical energy to electrical energy. However, the active elements within imaging transducers are not naturally piezoelectric and must be made piezoelectric by heating the elements to what is called the "Curie temperature" (Curie point) while in the presence of a strong electrical field. Transducers must never be heated above the Curie temperature, or they will lose their piezoelectric capabilities. This is termed "depolarization."

Matching layers decrease the large acoustic mismatch between piezoelectric elements and the medium, thus transmitting more sound energy into the body. The matching layer has an acoustic impedance value between the PZT and the skin. Acoustic gel further reduces the impedance mismatch between the transducer and patient's skin by eliminating air (Fig. 31-3).

Modern Array Transducers

Current transducer technology uses multiple piezoelectric elements, where each element is attached to an individual electronic circuit. Element arrangements vary depending on the transducer type. Some examples of array transducers include phased or vector arrays, linear arrays, and curved linear arrays.

Transducers use electronic methods to create the image pattern. Delay lines inside the transducer are used to steer and focus the beam by delaying the electronic pulse to each element. Focusing is achieved by delaying the arriving pulse, so that the elements are pulsed in an outer to inner method. Time delays between the groupings will determine where the focal point will be. Electronic focusing allows moving the focal point or combining different focal zones on one image. Beam steering is achieved by delaying the arriving pulse so that there are tiny delays between each element. Most transducers will use a combination of both focusing and steering.

The thickness of the active element and the propagation speed of sound in the active element determines the frequency. The thicker the active element, the lower the frequency. Higher frequency transducers demonstrate less penetration when compared to low frequency transducers, but they have better spatial resolution (image detail). Transducers do not emit a single frequency but rather a range of frequencies above and below the main resonant frequency, termed "bandwidth." Transducers are marked with the bandwidth of the transducer. For example, a 5-9 MHz transducer emits frequencies between 5 and 9 MHz. Frequency and penetration are inversely related.

Linear array transducers (Fig. 31-4) have 256 or more active elements arranged in a row that are fired in groups, creating an image consisting of parallel scan lines to produce a rectangular image. The footprint of the transducer is also rectangular shaped. The linear array uses delay lines mostly for focusing but will apply steering to create a trapezoid-shaped image (Fig 31-5).

Curved Linear Array Transducers

Curved linear array transducers (Fig. 31-6) are linear arrays with the elements arranged in an arc pattern. These transducers are also termed "convex" or "curvilinear arrays." The beam pattern is created by the geometry of the transducer design, called

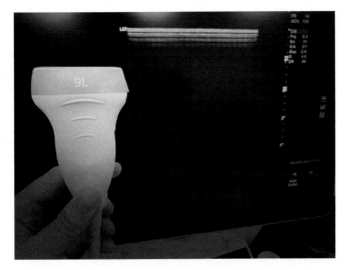

FIGURE 31-4. Linear sequential array transducer.

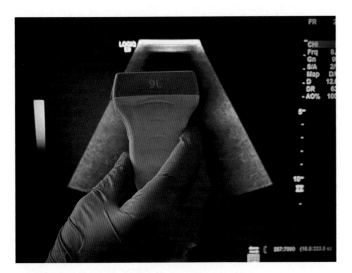

FIGURE 31-5. Linear sequential array transducer steered to create a trapezoidal image.

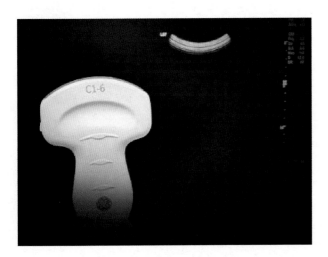

FIGURE 31-6. Curvilinear (curved linear array) transducer.

"geometric steering." The tighter the arc, the wider the field of view. These transducers use delay lines for focusing. Curved linear array transducers created a blunted-sector shaped image.

Phased Array Transducers

Phased array transducers (Figs. 31-7 and 31-8) have elements arranged in a matrix fashion like a checkerboard. All active elements are pulsed almost simultaneously to produce a sector shaped image. Delay lines are used to steer the beam into a sector format and are also used to focus the sound beam.

Vector Array Transducers

Vector array transducers (Figs. 31-9 and 31-10) are phased array transducers that incorporate linear array technology to produce

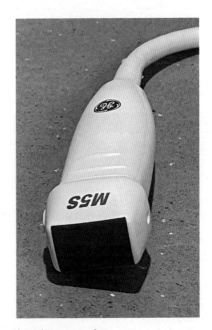

FIGURE 31-7. Phased array transducer.

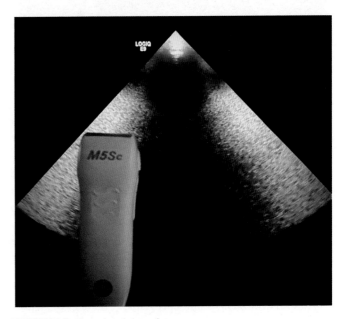

FIGURE 31-8 Phased array transducer.

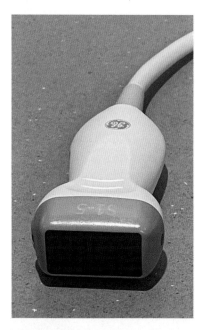

FIGURE 31-9. Vector array transducer.

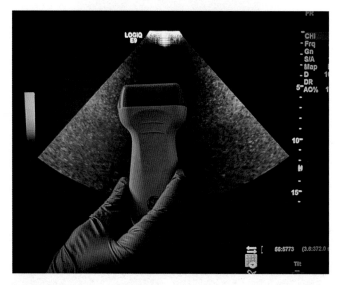

FIGURE 31-10 Vector array transducer.

a flat top sector. Instead of firing from the center of the transducer, as in a phased array, the beam is fired across the face of the transducer. This provides more of a near field and a wider sector angle. The image pattern is typically described as a flat top sector.

Frame rate is the number of frames displayed per second and is measured in frames per second. Temporal resolution is the ability to resolve two events related by time. The higher the frame rate, the better the temporal resolution. The human eye can see flickering at rates of less than 15 to 20 frames per second. Factors affecting frame rate are depth of field, sector angle, number of focal zones, and number of lines used to create the image. They are related by:

$$\text{Maximum depth (cm)} \times \text{lines per frame} \times \text{number of focuses} \times \text{frame rate} < 77{,}000$$

The sonographer can adjust the width of the image, the depth of the image, and the number of focal zones. Shallow images (i.e., thyroid or small-parts examination) allow multiple focal zones to be used whereas as deep structures (i.e., liver, pelvic structures) will have frame rate issues if more than one focal zone is used. Adding color Doppler increases the number of lines used to create the image by adding color lines to the gray scale imaging lines, thus decreasing the frame rate. Modern technology is eliminating the need for focal zones.

Because the pediatric population is considered to span multiple ages and development stages, transducer selection for the pediatric population is quite complex. The American Academy of Pediatrics defines pediatric ages to begin periconceptually and extend through age 21, unless the individual has special health care needs requiring pediatrician expertise. Moreover, examinations vary in body part and depth of structures.

Transducers are selected based on the principle that the highest frequency able to penetrate to the depth required will provide the best resolution. Sonographers may use low-frequency transducers such as convex C1-5 MHz to image the abdomen on an older pediatric patient, while needing a very high frequency transducer such as a linear array or hockey stick L6-15 MHz to image a superficial structure on a neonatal patient, such as the spine. A hockey stick transducer offers high resolution and a small transducer footprint, optimal for imaging small, superficial areas.

In addition, the footprint of the transducer (Fig. 31-11), which is the area of the transducer from which the beam is emitted, must be small enough to access the examination area. Some examples of small footprint transducers include a phased array transducer S8-3 MHz (Philips ultrasound) or 7V3c MHz

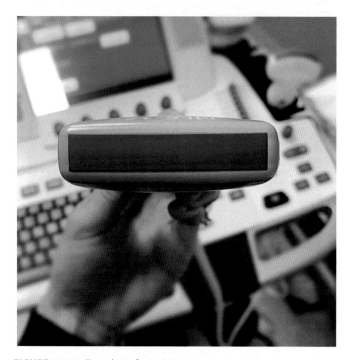

FIGURE 31-11. Transducer footprint.

(Acuson/Siemens ultrasound) for neonatal brain and cardiac studies, versus a convex or linear transducer used for abdominal exams. The footprint on the latter transducers would likely be too large to fit between thoracic ribs or cranial fontanelle for optimal cardiac imaging or visualization of the neonatal brain. Moreover, choices between the same types of transducers might also be factored in. For example, a linear 11L-D (GE Healthcare ultrasound) with a 38-mm footprint might be more suitable for imaging a smaller child rather than a 9L-D MHz (GE Healthcare ultrasound) with a 44-mm footprint. That said, the wider footprint will give a larger field of view; therefore, the wider footprint might be desired for older pediatric patients as it will cover a larger field of view in one image with areas not obstructed by artifacts such as rib shadowing.

Many specialty transducers are available to meet the various needs presented in the pediatric population, but one must always keep in mind the labeling of transducers is specific to the vendor. It is important to realize the numbers indicating the highest and lowest frequencies generated are ultimately the deciding factor to ensure proper penetration.

TRANSMISSION OF SOUND

Sound is a mechanical vibration transmitted through matter by a series of alternating compressions and rarefactions of the particles of the medium. Sound must have a medium to propagate its energy from the source to the receiver. It cannot travel in a vacuum.

The human range of hearing is from a low of 20 Hz to a high of 20,000 Hz or 20 kHz. (The "k" stands for kilo and is equal to 1,000). Hertz, abbreviated Hz, refers to the number of cycles per second. Ultrasound is any sound frequency above 20,000 Hz or 20 kHz. Diagnostic ultrasound uses frequencies above 1 MHz (megahertz), which is equal to 1,000,000 cycles per second.

Propagation speed (denoted by "c") is the speed at which a wave front travels through a medium. It is determined by the characteristics of the medium which include density and stiffness. Density is the concentration of molecules or mass/volume. Bone is dense, air is not. As density increases, the propagation speed decreases. Stiffness is the ability of a material to maintain its shape when pressure is applied to it. Bone is stiff, air is not. As stiffness increases, propagation speed increases. Stiffness differences between mediums dominate the effect of propagation. Propagation speed cannot be altered by the sonographer or the ultrasound unit. Disease processes can affect the velocity in a medium. All frequencies of sound will travel at the same velocity or speed through the same medium. Units include meters per second (m/s) and millimeters per microsecond (mm/μs).

The average propagation speed of soft tissue is 1,540 m/s or 1.54 mm/μs. Biologically, from the slowest to the fastest velocities is: gas, soft tissue, and bone, or more specifically: air, fat, soft tissue, blood, muscle, and bone. A ditty to remember this order is: All Frustrated Students Buy Many Books! Average propagation speed of sound includes the following: soft tissue 1,540 m/s; water 1,480 m/s; blood 1,575 m/s; bone 4080 m/s.

Frequency (denoted by "f") is the number of times the wave is repeated per second (cycles per second). It is determined by the transducer. Units include the Hertz (Hz) and megahertz (MHz).

Wavelength is the distance the sound wave travels in one cycle. It is determined by the transducer and medium. Units include the millimeter (mm) or any other unit of distance.

Velocity is equal to the product of frequency and wavelength. As frequency increases, the wavelength decreases. Higher frequencies have short wavelengths and lower frequencies have longer wavelengths. The following equation can be used to determine the wavelength of a particular frequency. Using a frequency in the MHz range, the answer is automatically in millimeters (mm).

$$\text{Wavelength} = 1.54/\text{Frequency}.$$

For example, a 5 MHz transducer is $1.54/5 = 0.3$ mm.

Amplitude (denoted by "A") is the maximum variation from normal resting or baseline level and represents the peak pressure, strength, or loudness. It is controlled by the overall gain control.

Intensity (denoted by "I") is the amount of energy flowing through a unit area. It is power of a beam divided by its cross-sectional area (cm^2). Power (denoted by "W") is the rate at which work is done, Units include watts per centimeter squared (W/cm^2) and milliwatts per centimeter squared (mW/cm^2). It is determined by the ultrasound system and can be varied by the sonographer with the acoustic power control.

As the sound beam travels through the body, it interacts with the tissue in a variety of ways and grows weaker with depth, which is termed attenuation. Attenuation is the progressive weakening of the amplitude of the sound beam. It is dependent on frequency, density of the medium, and number of interfaces. Rate of attenuation is high in air and bone, and low in water and biologic fluids such as blood and urine. Attenuation is caused by absorption, reflection, and scattering. Attenuation is directly related to frequency and distance. The higher the frequency or longer the distance, the higher the rate of attenuation.

Absorption is the process by which the sound beam imparts some of its energy into the medium through which it is propagating, by conversion of acoustic energy to heat. The higher the frequency, the higher the rate of absorption.

Scattering is the redirection of the sound beam in a random fashion and is caused by irregular surfaces and interfaces smaller than a wavelength. Scattering is the basis for nonspecular echoes, which are responsible for creating the echoes of anatomic parenchyma. Scattering increases with higher frequencies and are very weak in intensity.

Reflection is the redirection of a portion of the sound beam back toward the transducer. It is caused by the difference of acoustic impedance (denoted by "Z") between the two mediums. Acoustic impedance is equal to the product of the density (ρ) of the tissue and the propagation speed (Z = ρc). The greater the difference between the impedance of the two media, the greater the amount of reflection. The unit of acoustic impedance is the Rayl.

Types of reflections include specular reflections (Fig. 31-12), which result from large, smooth interfaces and nonspecular (diffuse) reflections (Fig. 31-13), or scattered echoes, which often occur from rough interfaces smaller than the sound beam. Examples of specular reflectors include the diaphragm, Glisson's capsule, and arterial walls. Specular reflectors are angle dependent and follow the rule: angle of incidence = angle of reflection. Normal incidence is when the sound beam strikes a boundary perpendicularly at 90°. Oblique incidence occurs when the sound beam strikes an interface at any angle other than 90°.

Refraction is a change in the sound wave's direction or bending of the sound wave while passing between tissues. The transmitted sound wave is the part of the beam that refracts, or bends. Refraction can only occur when there is a difference in velocity (propagation speed) between media and with an oblique angle of incidence.

There are also different types of resolution in ultrasound. Resolution is the ability to separate two closely spaced interfaces and is measured in millimeters. It is important for a sonographer to understand how to improve resolution.

Axial resolution is used to image structures one on top of the other. The closer the two structures are and can still be seen as two structures, the better the axial resolution. Axial resolution is along the path of the beam, parallel to the wave fronts and is determined by the spatial pulse length (SPL), which is determined by wavelength and pulse length. Axial resolution = 1/2 SPL. Axial resolution is improved with higher frequency transducers.

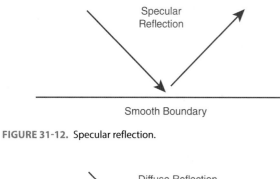

FIGURE 31-12. Specular reflection.

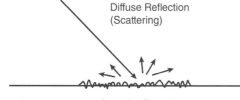

FIGURE 31-13. Nonspecular (diffuse) reflection.

Lateral resolution refers to the ability to image two structures side by side and still appear as two structures rather than one. Lateral resolution is perpendicular to the path of the beam. It is determined by beam width and varies along the path of the beam. It is improved with focusing as well as higher frequencies as higher frequencies produce thinner beams. Lateral resolution = beam width. The focal point is the point indicated on the screen by an arrow on the side of the monitor and is the point where lateral resolution is the best. The useful diagnostic range of transducer frequencies was chosen as a compromise between resolution and penetration.

Temporal resolution refers to time. The faster frames can be captured and displayed, the better the temporal resolution. There are many ways a sonographer can change the frame rate as described earlier. In addition, there are a few other types of resolution as well. Again, discussing all of these would be beyond the scope of this section. However, understanding these basic areas of ultrasound physics allows a sonographer to begin being able to use the concepts and adjustments to optimize images.

DOPPLER TECHNIQUES

A Doppler examination of the abdomen can be a very challenging examination. This is due in part to the depth of the vessels, overlying bowel gas, respiratory motion, and equipment sensitivity. Doppler allows evaluation of organs beyond the two-dimensional (2D) image by allowing physiologic information to be added to the anatomic information, thus enhancing the diagnosis. Color Doppler allows visualization and investigation of vessels that are not seen on the gray scale 2D image, as well as aiding in proper placement of the Doppler sample volume.

Doppler may be used to document the presence, direction, and velocity of flow, differentiate vascular structures from other tubular structures, demonstrate residual lumen, and evaluate the perfusion of flow within an organ.

To perform an adequate Doppler examination, it is necessary to understand the following concepts: normal direction of blood flow, expected wave form for the vessel being investigated, diagnostic criteria needed, limitations of the procedure and how to optimize the ultrasound machine.

Doppler Principles

The Doppler shift is used to determine how fast the blood is flowing and is determined by the Doppler equation:

$$f_D = f_t - f_r = \frac{2f_t v \cos(\theta)}{c}$$

where f_D is the Doppler shift, f_t is the transmitted frequency, f_r is the received frequency, v is the velocity of blood, $\cos \theta$ is the angle between the sound beam and blood flow and c is the average velocity of sound in soft tissue (1,540 m/s). The ultrasound unit knows all aspects of the equation excluding cos θ, which is determined by the angle correction control. Adjusting the angle correction is mandatory for determining the velocity of the blood flow. The most accurate velocity of the Doppler signal will come from angles that are parallel to blood flow, i.e., at 0°, as the cosine of 0 equals one. The angle correction indicator should be placed parallel to the walls of the vessel being investigated.·Doppler angles of less than 60° should be used. When an angle of greater than 60° is obtained, the transducer or patient needs to be repositioned so that an angle of less than 60° may be obtained.

As blood interacts with the sound beam, the direction of flow can be determined. If the Doppler shift created is a positive number, this indicates that the flow is toward the transducer. A negative number indicates flow away from the transducer. The velocity of the blood flow will determine the height of the signal, with faster flow having a taller signal.

Technically, the most difficult aspect of Doppler ultrasound is overcoming the scanning techniques used in gray scale imaging. A good Doppler signal will not always accompany an aesthetically appealing image. For imaging, perpendicular scan planes and high frequency transducers are used. Scanning planes of less than 60° to blood flow are required to obtain the best Doppler signal, and sometimes a lower frequency transducer is needed to elicit Doppler signals. This may require that two images be obtained: one for imaging and one for the Doppler waveform.

Because of the attenuation process, it may be necessary to image first and then change to a lower frequency transducer to obtain the weaker intensity Doppler signals. This is especially true in renal transplants and pediatrics, where a 5 MHz frequency is best for imaging but may not easily elicit good Doppler signals. However, taking advantage of the wide bandwidth, the frequency can be changed to a lower frequency by a control on the machine. Remember that lower frequencies provide greater penetration with a tradeoff for a decrease in detail (Fig. 31-14). Higher frequencies provide less penetration due to attenuation but have greater detail (Fig. 31-15).

To obtain the best Doppler signals, it is necessary to optimize the beam to vessel angle. To optimize this angle, it may be necessary to change the position of the patient and/or transducer. Doppler signals and color Doppler information can be obtained in sagittal (longitudinal), coronal, oblique or transverse planes. In vessels such as the aorta, where flow is perpendicular to the sound beam, it is necessary to create good Doppler angles, accomplished by using a "heel-toe" scanning technique. This is done by angling the transducer in a superior or inferior manner. This maneuver will cause the vessel to go from a parallel course across the screen to an oblique course, thus creating a 45 to 60° angle with the sound beam.

Optimizing the signal to noise ratio is important and is accomplished by using the correct transducer frequency, the proper power output, proper gain setting (color, spectral, and 2D image), and by placing the focal zone in the area of interest.

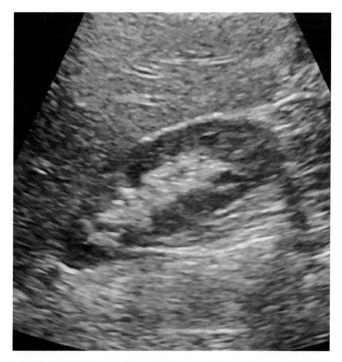

FIGURE 31-14. Imaging of the right kidney with lower frequency (4 MHz).

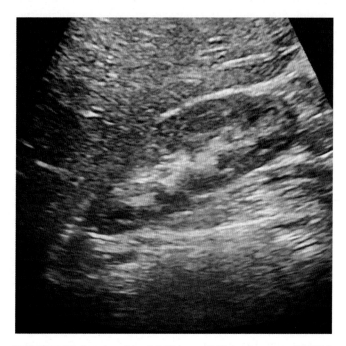

FIGURE 31-15. Imaging of the right kidney with higher frequency (5.5 MHz).

Increasing the output power will increase the intensity and sensitivity of the sound beam. The focal zone should be placed at or right below the area of interest.

To set the color gain properly, turn up the color gain until the background fills with color speckles, then decrease the color gain incrementally until these speckles disappear and areas of vasculature remain filled with color. If the 2D gain is too high or there is a lot of artifact in the lumen of the vessel, the machine may not overwrite the gray scale with color. If this happens, adjust the overall gray scale image gain, clean up the vessel utilizing the TGC function, use dynamic range control to make the image higher contrast (i.e., more black and white), or adjust the gray scale and color priority control if available. Adjust the Doppler gain to eliminate the background noise. Remember that small vessels have no systolic window. Sometimes to see a full spectrum from an especially weak signal, it may be necessary to display a "noisy" spectrum.

Vessel fill-in and color sensitivity can be improved by using the proper color velocity scale (pulse repetition frequency [PRF]) setting. The color velocity scale setting acts like a filter by concentrating on the velocities around the number of the color scale. For example, a color velocity scale set at 65 cm/s will be concentrating on faster velocities and may not display slower velocities, causing the vessel to appear as if there is no flow inside the vessel. High numbers for arterial flow, especially to reduce color aliasing, may cause venous flow to not be seen. A rule of thumb is to start at 10 to 20 cm/s for venous flow and between 20 and 30 cm/s for arterial flow. Please note that these values are a starting point and need to be adjusted according to the patient and their flow states. Slow flow settings of less than 6 to 7 cm/s should be used when looking for "trickle" flow or in low/slow flow states. If this control is set too high, color may not be displayed in a vessel thus leading to an incorrect diagnosis of vessel thrombosis. If this control is set too low, color aliasing will occur making the determination of flow direction difficult. A compromise between color velocity scale and aliasing may be required to have proper vessel fill-in. Minimizing the color sample box can help improve the color sensitivity as well as improve frame rates.

Color Doppler places a great demand on the machine, resulting in a sacrifice in frame rate. The frame rate can also be improved by using the smallest image scale size as possible. This will also help maximize your Doppler scale by improving the PRF. For example, when evaluating the hepatic veins, it is not necessary to see 4 to 5 centimeters beyond the diaphragm. By decreasing the image depth so that the diaphragm is at the bottom of the image, the PRF will be increased, therefore increasing the velocity before aliasing will occur.

On small vessels, like the hepatic artery, use zoom features to facilitate visualization. Place the Doppler sample volume on the zoomed or expanded image, then obtain the Doppler spectrum.

If the Doppler spectrum is weak or noisy, freeze the 2D image. This will improve the appearance of the spectrum by allowing the machine to concentrate on obtaining the Doppler information.

When evaluating arteries with high velocities, increase the Doppler filter. This allows the machine to concentrate on the higher velocities and improve visualization of the peak of the Doppler waveform.

Since patients will need to hold their breath during the actual exam, do not tire them out while setting the controls:

image scale size, color maps, baseline shift, filters, Doppler scale, color velocity scale, and 2D, color and Doppler gains (Figs. 31-16 to 31-18). Set these parameters with the patient breathing normally. If a patient has difficulty holding their breath, only a small amount of signal, one or two beats, needs to be obtained. One or two beats can be just as diagnostic as a full screen of five or more beats. Only one beat is needed to determine flow presence, type, direction of flow and to measure peak systolic velocity, end diastolic velocity and obtain the resistance index.

Power Doppler is an extension of the autocorrelation process of color Doppler and evaluates the power or intensity of the Doppler signal as opposed to its mean velocity. Benefits of power Doppler include increased flow sensitivity, quick evaluation of flow, angle independency, organ perfusion, increased spatial resolution meaning that the color does not bleed outside the vessel's wall and detection of low flow. The main disadvantage is that it does not provide flow direction information on all systems.

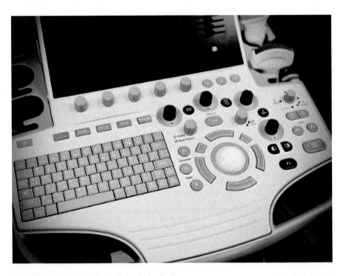

FIGURE 31-16. Keyboard and knobology.

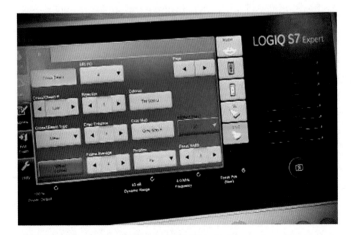

FIGURE 31-17. Touch screen panel (left), time gain compensation knobs (right), also demonstrated in Fig. 31-15.

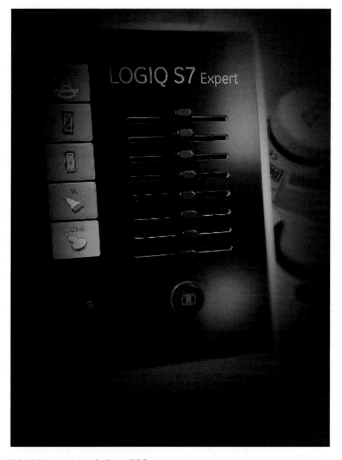

FIGURE 31-18. Knobology, TGC.

BIOEFFECTS

Ultrasound energy has the potential to cause biological effects, or bioeffects, and are created by either thermal or mechanical interactions with the tissue. The potential for bioeffects have been studied in-vivo, in-vitro, and with epidemiological studies. The biggest concerns for bioeffects with diagnostic ultrasound are exams of the fetus, the neonate, and the eye.

Ultrasound can be used for diagnostic or therapeutic reasons. Therapeutic ultrasound depends on producing bioeffects for treating certain types of pathology. Lithotripsy uses focused sound waves at a high intensity to cause mechanical interactions with kidney stones, causing fractures of the stone and breaking it into tiny fragments that can easily pass down the ureter and into the bladder. Therapeutic ultrasound is used to treat musculoskeletal issues by using absorption properties of the sound beam, causing thermal interactions, to heat up the tissue beneath the transducer. This ultrasound unit uses a continuous wave beam at higher intensities and low frequencies. This helps to heal the muscles and tendons that are too deep for superficial heating. This application of ultrasound is used primarily by physical therapists.

In diagnostic ultrasound, the type of bioeffect is determined by the type of tissue, the acoustic power (intensity) of the acoustic beam, how long the patient is exposed to the sound beam, how long the transducer stays in one place without moving (dwell time), and if continuous or pulsed ultrasound is used. High acoustic output or power as well as long scan times can increase the possibility of a bioeffect, with the scanning time having the greatest effect on patient exposure. Most ultrasound modes are pulsed modes except for M-mode, pulsed, and continuous wave Doppler which are called "continuous modes." With continuous mode imaging, the ultrasound beam generally stays in one location for a period of time, and since the sound beam does not move, the risk of a thermal effect is increased. Pulsed ultrasound modalities have low thermal and high mechanical risks, and continuous modalities have high thermal and low mechanical risks.

Diagnostic ultrasound machines have default intensity settings that have been determined to have a very low risk of producing a bioeffect. The intensity of the sound beam is set through the preset, which will be less than the maximum output of the machine. The maximum intensity for each exam type have been approved by the United States Food and Drug Administration (FDA) for patient safety. The intensity of the sound beam can be changed as needed by the sonographer with the power, output or transmit control but the intensity of the ultrasound beam will still be below FDA guidelines. Obstetrical presets will have the lowest intensity levels to protect the fetus, and transcranial Doppler setting will have the highest. Some pediatric presets may also have low intensity settings. To reduce the possibility of a bioeffect the sonographer should always follow the ALARA (As Low As Reasonably Achievable) principle. It is important not to sacrifice image quality just to have a low intensity setting. This means that the controls that affect the acoustic output should be at the lowest possible setting without compromising the ultrasound exam. To further reduce acoustic exposure, the sonographer should be conscious of transducer dwell and overall scanning time. Other controls that can affect the intensity of the sound beam include the mode selected such as grayscale versus pulsed Doppler, and the PRF. Changing these controls may increase or decrease the intensity of the sound beam.

The following statement is from the American Institute of Ultrasound in Medicine (AIUM): No independently confirmed adverse effects caused by exposure from present diagnostic ultrasound instruments have been reported in human patients in the absence of contrast agents. The AIUM further states that diagnostic ultrasound has an excellent safety record, but the hypothetical possibility of tissue damage on a microscopic scale cannot be completely ruled out under all ultrasound conditions (www.aium.org).

To document the patient's exposure there are two indices at the top of the image: the Mechanical Index, MI, and the Thermal Index, TI. It is important to understand that the MI and TI do not indicate that a biological effect is occurring but informs the sonographer that a mechanical or thermal bioeffect is possible.

A thermal effect is caused by the absorption of the ultrasound wave, causing heating of the tissue being insonated. It is affected by the acoustic output power. TI is used to determine the potential risk of a thermal bioeffect and does not indicate an actual increase of the temperature of the tissue. There are three thermal indices that can be displayed and are based on the preset used. TI_S (TI for soft tissue) provides information about the estimated temperature rise within homogeneous soft tissue. TI_B (TI for bone) provides information about the estimated temperature rise in bone. TI_C (TI for the cranial bone) provides information about the estimated temperature increase of the cranial bone. Even though there are three subcategories, only one value can be displayed on the ultrasound image at a time. The ultrasound unit must allow the sonographer to display another TI value as needed. The TI gives an indication of the possibility of an increase in temperature of the tissue in the ultrasound beam. A TI of 1.5 does not mean that the tissue will increase in temperature by 1.5° C, but tells the sonographer that this represents a higher rise in temperature when compared to a TI of 0.7.

MI evaluates for possible mechanical bioeffects, also referred to as "nonthermal effects," which are caused as the ultrasound waves pass through or near tissue that contains gas. It is affected by the pressure and frequency of the sound beam. The potential for a mechanical bioeffect increases as the pressure increases, and decreases as the frequency increases. The MI has a maximum setting of 1.9 for all uses except ophthalmic, which has a maximum limit of 0.23. One type of mechanical bioeffect is called "cavitation," which is the interaction of the sound waves with tiny gas bubbles in the tissue. These bubbles oscillate or can collapse in a violent implosion which can damage or destroy nearby cells. This occurs in a very small space around the bubble and affects only a few cells. Tissues that contain gas, such as the lungs and the digestive tract, are at a higher potential risk of an ultrasound-induced mechanical bioeffect. There are no mechanical bioeffects in the fetus since there are no gas bubbles; however, mechanical bioeffects are possible in the neonate, especially in the lung and intestine.

The sonographer should always use the lowest possible TI and MI values while still obtaining good quality diagnostic images.

EMERGING TECHNOLOGIES

The field of ultrasound continues to evolve with new technologies and techniques. Recently, liver elastography (Fig. 31-19) and liver contrast enhanced ultrasound (CEUS) have been approved by the FDA. In pediatric patients, elastography is currently approved for liver applications. CEUS have been approved for liver lesions and urinary reflux by the FDA. It is acceptable to use either technique for other organs and is called "off label use." Off label means using the technology for exams not approved by the FDA. In these instances, the patient must be informed that the exam has not yet been approved by the FDA. Having the

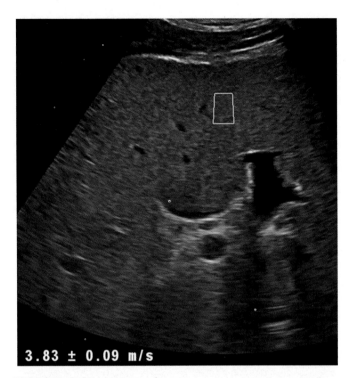

FIGURE 31-19. Liver elastography.

patient sign a consent form is optional and should be based on the policies for off label use of contrast agents used in magnetic resonance imaging (MRI) and computed tomography (CT).

The purpose of elastography is for staging liver fibrosis to potentially avoid the patient from having a liver biopsy. Elastography is helpful in patients being followed for nonalcoholic fatty liver disease (NAFLD), patients with chronic viral hepatitis, and other diseases that lead to liver fibrosis. Elastography evaluates the speed of sound through an area of defined liver tissue and is used primarily to evaluate and stage the liver for fatty liver infiltration and the degree of fibrosis. Ten measurements are obtained and can be reported in either meters per second (m/s) or kilo Pascals (kPa), which is a unit for stiffness. The speed or pressure will increase with diseased liver tissue from parenchymal disease such as fatty liver and cirrhosis. The more advanced the disease, the higher the numbers.

To perform the exam, the patient must be fasting. Fasting guidelines should be followed based upon age of the pediatric patient. Non-fasting patients will have artificially high numerical values. If the non-fasting patient has normal values, then they do not need to be rescheduled as the fasting value will be normal also. The patient should be in a supine or slight left lateral decubitus position of not more than 30°. For point shear wave elastography (pSWE), a spot in the liver is chosen that meets the following criteria:

1. Measurement should be taken in the right lobe of the liver between the ribs (intercostal scan window).

2. Find the best window to obtain using the most optimal B-mode image.

3. The region of interest (ROI) box should be placed approximately 2 centimeters below the liver capsule, not the skin surface.

4. The ROI box should be placed so that it is in a line perpendicular to the liver capsule.

5. Do not place the ROI box so that it touches or includes any of the following: large vessels, bile ducts, ligaments, Glisson's capsule, air, acoustic shadow, bone, and/or the gallbladder.

6. Five to ten measurements are obtained from the same spot which means that the ROI should not be moved to a different location with the patient in neutral breathing. The patient should not hold their breath as this increases the pressure inside the liver.

7. The protocol for 2D SWE is the same as for pSWE, except that only five measurements are needed, and reverberation artifacts must be avoided.

The mean value is used for reporting and will be seen in the reporting chart. To ensure that the five to ten numbers represent a good data set, the sonographer should check the IQR/M (interquartile ratio divided by the mean) found on the reporting page. For kPa, this value should be < 30% or 0.3 and for m/s < 15% or 0.15. If the IQR/M is greater than these numbers then the obtained value should be evaluated and any outliers deleted, Additional images need to be taken to replace the deleted values.

The purpose of this exam is to diagnose the patient with a likely normal liver and those that have compensated advanced chronic liver disease. NAFLD is not as common in the pediatric population, and other diseases that can require a liver elastography exam include cystic fibrosis, autoimmune hepatitis, biliary atresia, after a Kasai procedure, or congenital heart disease with Fontan surgery or viral hepatitis. Charts are still being developed and evaluated for pediatric patients. For NAFLD, it is possible to use the adult chart as this issue continues to evolve.

According to the Society of Radiologists in Ultrasound: it is expert opinion that each patient becomes his or her own control, using the stiffness delta changes over time to evaluate the efficacy of the treatment or the progression of disease—remembering that the measurement reflects stiffness and not fibrosis.

CEUS requires special software in the ultrasound unit. The contrast agent used in CEUS is a gas enclosed in shell. Some materials the outer shell may be comprised of include lipids, albumin, polymers, or galactose. The gas core may contain air, nitrogen, or perfluorocarbon. When activating contrast mode, the unit will automatically lower the MI. This is because a high MI would destroy the microbubbles. CEUS is helpful to evaluate liver masses to determine probability of malignancy (Fig. 31-20). The contrast is usually given to the patient via IV in the antecubital vein followed by a saline flush to push the contrast into the vein. Two people are required, usually the sonographer who is scanning and the radiologist, as timing of the contrast is critical for the diagnosis. A contrast timer must be started at the time of the injection.

It is in the sonographer's scope of practice, found on the Society of Diagnostic Medical Sonography (SDMS) website at www.sdms.org to be able to insert the IV, as other radiology imaging technologists are taught to insert an IV as part of their training.

There are three phases of liver CEUS. The first is the arterial phase which begins about 10 seconds after injection and ends after approximately 30 to 45 seconds. This is followed by the portal venous phase, which starts at 30 to 45 seconds and ends at approximately 120 seconds. Finally, there is the late phase, which can also be called "washout," which starts after 120 seconds. The contrast will remain in the body for 4 to 8 minutes. The injected gas bubbles leave the body as the patient exhales. Unlike CT and MRI contrast agents, ultrasound contrast is not nephrotoxic and is intravascular meaning it does not leak into surrounding tissue.

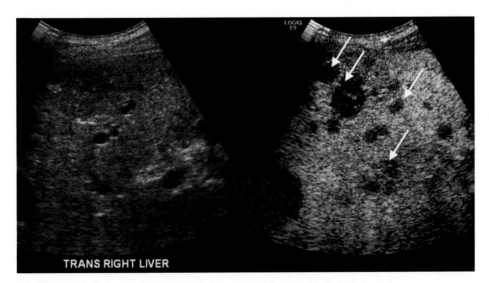

FIGURE 31-20. Contrast enhanced ultrasound in a patient with liver metastasis.

The usual feature of a malignant lesion is hyper-enhancing, with the tumor brighter than the normal liver tissue, in the arterial phase. In the portal venous phase and the late phase, the lesion can be hypo-enhancing, iso-enhancing, or non-enhancing (no contrast in the mass). Benign lesions typically are hypo- or iso-enhanced in the portal venous and late phase.

CEUS can also be used to evaluate the pediatric patient for urinary reflux, saving the patient from radiation acquired during radiographic, fluoroscopic, and CT imaging exams, and is called a "contrast-enhanced voiding urosonography." A urinary catheter is placed in the bladder and a bolus of contrast is injected into the bladder, called an "intravesical injection."

If there is reflux, the contrast will be visualized retrograde filling the ureter. Unlike a voiding cystourethrogram, each kidney must be evaluated separately.

Another new technology is called microflow imaging (MFI) which can visualize smaller vessels and slower flow then power Doppler. The image resembles a CEUS image. Different manufacturers will have their own term for this technology.

There are technologies still being developed and yet to be discovered. The sonographer should keep abreast of these developments and how they can benefit their patient by reading journals and attending conferences, especially the annual AIUM or SDMS conferences where new technologies are unveiled.

Lab Value Correlation

32

During review of this section, it is important to note that lab values can differ among facilities. Values provided in this text should serve as a general guideline (see Table 32-1.), as electronic records will provide the range of normal values per institution. For registry-review purposes, it is more important to note which lab values elevate or decrease with various pathologies, versus knowledge of the exact normal value range.

BLOOD UREA NITROGEN (BUN)

BUN level rises as kidney function decreases. However, with vascular transplant rejection, BUN increases. A normal BUN level is between 7 and 20 mg/dL, or in a more generalized blood panel between 5 and 25 mg/dL.

CREATININE

The level of creatinine within the blood rises as kidney disease progresses. Creatinine increases with vascular transplant rejection, interstitial transplant rejection, and transplant acute tubular necrosis. A creatinine level of >1.2 in women and >1.4 in men may be an early indication the kidneys are not functioning properly. In adults, a generalized normal creatinine range varies between 0.6 and 1.2 mg/dL. In pediatric patients 3 to 18 years of age, the normal creatinine range is lower at 0.5 to 1.0 mg/dL, with the mean serum creatinine concentration being slightly higher in boys.

LIVER FUNCTION TESTS

Various liver enzyme tests observed via blood drawn demonstrate the liver function.

Alkaline Phosphatase (ALP)

ALP values help in detecting liver disease, bone disorders or any condition involving bone growth or increased bone cell activity, and blocked bile ducts. ALP increases with biliary duct obstruction. A gamma-glutamyl transferase panel is drawn in addition to ALP to distinguish between liver and bone diseases. ALP panels may also increase during pregnancy. Normal ALP levels are between 14 and 127 units per litre (U/L).

TABLE 32-1 • Normal Lab Values*	
Laboratory Tests	**Lab Values**
BUN	5-25 MG/DL
Creatinine	0.5-1.0 MG/DL
ALP	14-127 U/L
ALT	4-51 U/L
AST	5-46 U/L
Lipase	10-60 U/L
Amylase	23-85 U/L
Bilirubin	0.1-1.5 MG/DL
Serum Alpha-Fetoprotein	<10 ng/mL
LDH	290-2000 U/L < 10 days 180-430 U/L 10 days to 2 years 110-295 U/L 2 years to 12 years 100-190 U/L >12 years
Prothrombin Time	11-13.5 seconds

*May vary slightly by institution.

Alanine Aminotransferase (ALT)

ALT panels are drawn to detect liver injury and disease. High ALT may indicate acute hepatitis, especially if ALT levels are higher than aspartate aminotransferase (AST). Normal ALT range is between 4 and 51 U/L.

Aspartate Aminotransferase (AST)

AST panels are drawn to detect liver damage. The normal AST range lies between 5 and 46 U/L.

Lipase

Lipase increases with acute pancreatitis. Normal lipase levels fall between 10 and 60 U/L.

Amylase

Amylase increases with acute pancreatitis, although is not as specific as lipase. Normal amylase levels fall between 23 and 85 U/L.

Bilirubin

Bilirubin increases with liver disease, blood disorders, and blockage of bile ducts. When bilirubin is increased jaundice may be visualized. Normal bilirubin panels measure between 0.1 to 1.5 mg/dL. Direct (conjugated) bilirubin is created by liver hepatocytes. Indirect (unconjugated) bilirubin is created by breakdown of red blood cells. Total bilirubin is a lab value incorporating direct and indirect bilirubin. Increased total and indirect bilirubin are commonly seen in newborns between age 1 and 3 days because of liver immaturity. Alternately, biliary atresia, a congenital disorder can also increase total and indirect bilirubin.

Serum Alpha-Fetoprotein (AFP)

Serum AFP is a glycoprotein that increases with hepatoblastoma, hepatocellular carcinoma, infantile hemangioendothelioma, scrotal yolk sac tumor, and scrotal endodermal sinus tumors. The normal range for serum AFP is less than 10 ng/mL; when measurement is greater than 500 ng/mL, tumor should be suspected.

Lactate Dehydrogenase (LDH)

LDH is a liver function test that increases when cell injury and cell death occur. LDH may be moderately increased with mononucleosis. LDH may be mildly increased with hepatitis, cirrhosis, and obstructive jaundice. LDH panels are most commonly drawn to detect myocardial infarction, but can also detect hemolytic anemia, blood flow deficiency, muscular dystrophy, tissue death, liver disease, pancreatitis, and other conditions. Normal LDH levels range between 290 and 2,000 U/L in a newborn, 180 and 430 U/L in a pediatric patient 10 days to 2 years of age, 110 and 295 U/L in a 2- to 12-year-old, and 100 and 190 U/L in patients greater than 12 years of age.

Prothrombin Time

Prothrombin time increases with liver disease and cell damage and is drawn to measure length of time taken for blood to clot. The normal prothrombin time is 11 to 13.5 seconds.

White Blood Cells (WBCs)

WBCs may be increased with inflammatory processes.

Glucose

Glucose correlates with presence of sugar within the blood. Glucose elevation is associated with chronic liver disease, overactive endocrine glands, and diabetes.

33

Hemodynamics

Hemodynamics refers to the circulation of blood, including the mechanisms and forces by which circulation occurs. Arterial and venous hemodynamics vary as the vessels have different components and driving forces. All circulation begins with the heart. As a basic review, oxygenated blood exits the left ventricle during ventricular systole. It travels through the aorta and is disseminated through various arteries in the body. The aorta and bodily arteries react by pulsating to continue the circulation of blood. Arteries contain three wall layers, including the inner intima, middle media, and outer adventitia. Arterioles, which are very small distal arteries, contain only two layers—the tunica intima and media. Capillaries are the distal-most branches of the small arterioles. Capillary walls are one cell thick, containing only endothelium.

Blood flow within the body is classified as laminar or turbulent. Laminar flow is normal physiologic flow. Plug and parabolic flow are forms of laminar flow. With parabolic flow the blood moves in concentric circles with the fastest blood flow in the center of the vessel and the slowest blood flow along the walls of the vessel, causing the blood to have a parabolic or "D" shaped profile. (Fig. 33-1). Parabolic blood flow is seen in long vessels like the aorta. With plug flow, all the blood layers travel at relatively the same speed and the curve of the "D" becomes flattened (Fig. 33-2). Plug flow is seen in short vessels. As blood squeezes through an area of narrowing within a vessel, called stenosis, the velocities will increase followed by chaotic, turbulent waveforms post-stenosis.

Arterial waveforms are displayed on spectral Doppler as triphasic, biphasic, or monophasic. Triphasic waveforms

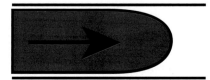

FIGURE 33-1. Parabolic flow with "D," or bullet-shaped profile.

FIGURE 33-2. Plug flow with flattened profile, all layers of blood travel at roughly the same speed.

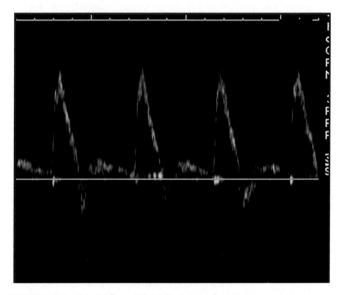

FIGURE 33-3. Arterial flow with triphasic waveform.

demonstrate a sharp upstroke, rapid downstroke, and reversed flow in diastole followed by another peak above the baseline (Fig. 33-3). A biphasic waveform displays a sharp upstroke, rapid downstroke, and has reversed flow in diastole (Fig. 33-4). A monophasic waveform has an upstroke followed by a downstroke and will not have any flow in diastole (Fig. 33-5).

Total energy within the circulatory system is the sum of kinetic, pressure, and gravitational energy. Pressure energy is a form of potential energy, meaning it has the potential to perform work and is noted in units of millimeters of Mercury,

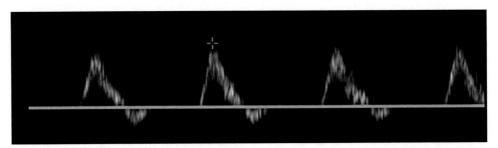

FIGURE 33-4. Arterial flow with biphasic waveform.

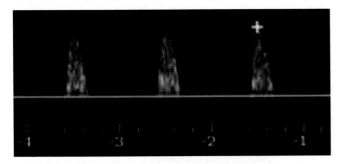

FIGURE 33-5. Arterial flow with monophasic waveform.

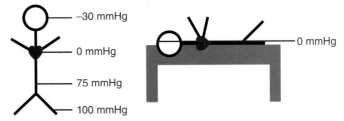

FIGURE 33-6. Hydrostatic pressures upright and supine.

mmHg. Gravitational and hydrostatic pressures are forms of potential energy.

> **Note:** To better understand potential energy one can think of the difference between a skydiver and a marathon runner. The skydiver does not need to exert any muscular effort to skydive—gravity does the work! Therefore, there is potential energy to move effortlessly simply by being elevated off of the ground. However, the marathon runner must rely on his/her own exertion and muscular energy to move.

Bernoulli's principle states that in a normal, closed vascular system, energy in two locations should be equal, with the difference between locations being the gradient. Pressure gradient involves blood flowing from high to low pressure areas. After blood disperses oxygen throughout the body, it travels through the capillaries into the veins.

Veins generally have thinner walls and are much more pliable than arteries. Veins also have three layers—the inner intima, middle media, and outer adventitia. The middle tunica media in veins is much thinner than it is in the arteries. Veins can stretch to accommodate a higher volume of blood and collapse during times of reduced volume. Venous pressure is lower than its arterial counterpart, and circulatory pressure can be obtained at heart level where hydrostatic pressure is 0 mmHg. Measured pressure is obtained by adding circulatory and hydrostatic pressures. In an upright individual, hydrostatic

pressure increases below heart level and decreases above heart level. When the patient lies supine, hydrostatic pressure is 0 mmHg throughout the venous system (Fig. 33-6).

Veins contain one-way valves which will open with the force of blood moving through them and then shut to prevent a back flow or reversal of blood flow. Veins are reactionary and do not circulate blood on their own as they react to arterial pulses. When the muscular walls of the arteries contract to force blood to move, that flow eventually pushes the blood into the veins at the capillary level. Venous blood continues to flow toward the heart and the veins expand and collapse because of the amount of blood the arteries are circulating. Body movement and muscle contraction also press on the veins, helping to move blood toward the heart.

Blood with lower levels of oxygen then returns to the right atrium of the heart, flows into the right ventricle, through the pulmonary arteries, and into the lungs where gas exchange between oxygen and carbon dioxide takes place. Blood then flows through the pulmonary veins, into the left atrium, and back through the left ventricle to begin the recirculation process.

Along with the cardiac cycles, respiration affects venous flow due to a change of intra-thoracic and abdominal pressures, which causes slight changes in the height of the spectral Doppler signal. Spectral venous waveforms are phasic and continuous or pulsatile. Continuous flow is flow in one direction that has variations with respiration (Fig. 33-7) and pulsatile venous waveforms have blood flow above and below the baseline (Fig. 33-8) and are seen in veins near the heart as well as caused by fluid overload due to conditions such as congestive heart failure.

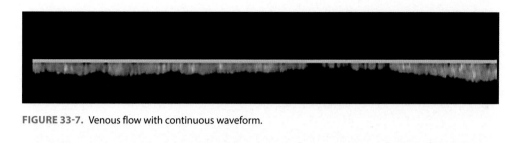

FIGURE 33-7. Venous flow with continuous waveform.

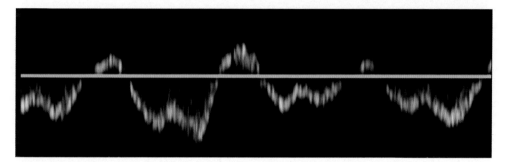

FIGURE 33-8. Venous flow with pulsatile venous waveform.

34

Artifacts

An artifact in ultrasound is an imaging error where the echo does not represent actual body tissue. Artifacts may be caused by machine malfunction, machine assumptions like using 1540 m/s for echo placement and that a sound wave travels in a straight line, operator error, or the interaction of sound waves with tissue. Several artifacts can be present in a single image. There are more artifacts than those that will be discussed and only the most common artifacts a sonographer may encounter are included in this section. Some artifacts are helpful indicators of structural characteristics while others degrade the image as they either obscure anatomy or make it difficult to discern between what is real and what is an artifact.

GRAYSCALE ARTIFACTS

Acoustic Shadow Artifact

One artifact that can be both helpful and problematic is a posterior acoustic shadow. This is a common artifact that results when the sound beam passes through a highly attenuative structure, such as calcium, causing no echoes to be produced underneath this structure (Fig. 34-1). The shadow is caused as the structure absorbs the sound beam, which is the most common cause, or totally reflects the sound beam back to the transducer. The helpful aspect of this artifact is that it suggests that the reflecting object contains calcium, as is seen with gallstones and bone. The acoustic shadow is best demonstrated when using harmonics. The problematic aspect of an acoustic shadow is that any normal or abnormal tissue in the area of the acoustic shadow, deep to the highly attenuating structure, will not be seen.

Edge Shadowing Artifact

A similar appearing artifact but with a different cause is edge shadowing. This artifact occurs when the sound beam strikes a

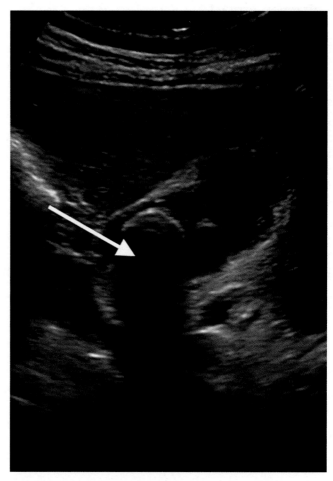

FIGURE 34-1. Shadowing artifact posterior to highly attenuating gallstones within the gallbladder.

smooth, rounded structure causing the sound waves to refract, or bend, along the side edges of the structure producing an acoustic shadow. Examples of structures which can produce an edge shadow include a cyst, oval or round solid homogenous mass, and the fetal head (Fig. 34-2).

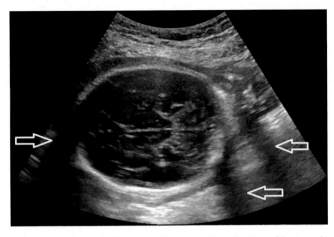

FIGURE 34-2. Edge shadowing artifact caused by refraction of the sound beam.

Refraction Artifact

A refraction artifact results when there is a change in direction of the sound waves as they travel from one medium into another (Figs. 34-3 and 34-4). A refraction artifact can only occur with oblique incidence and when the two mediums have different propagation speeds. A refraction artifact will not occur if the propagation speed of both mediums is the same or with normal incidence, which is when the sound beam hits the reflecting structure at a right angle. This artifact is very difficult to appreciate on an image.

Mirror Image Artifact

A mirror image artifact is created when sound rebounds from a strong reflector and is redirected toward a second structure and then back to the transducer, causing a replica of the structure to be incorrectly placed on the image (Fig. 34-5). The artifactual

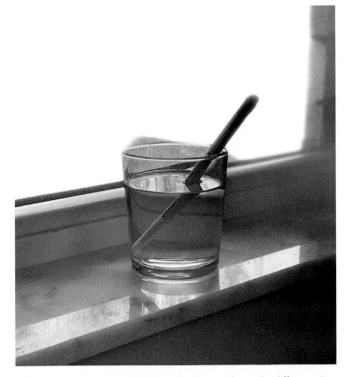

FIGURE 34-4. Visual representation of refraction due to the difference in propagation speed between air and water.

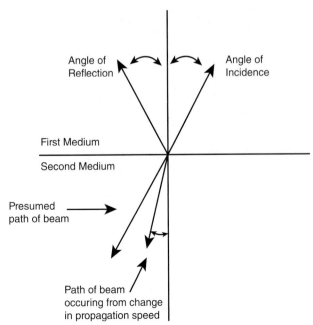

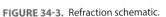

FIGURE 34-3. Refraction schematic.

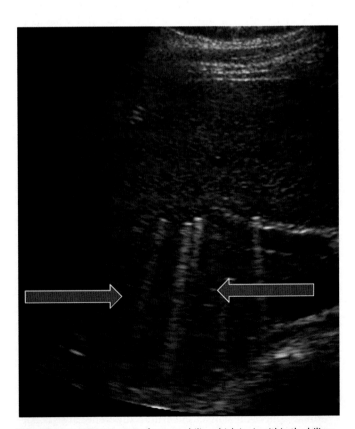

FIGURE 34-5. Mirror image of pneumobilia, which is air within the biliary system. Recall that air is a strong acoustic reflector.

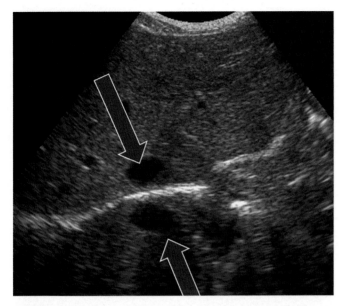

FIGURE 34-6. Mirror image of the inferior vena cava (IVC) across the diaphragm.

copy of the structure will be displayed deeper than the true reflector. The most common place to see an acoustic mirror artifact is across the diaphragm, where it can cause liver tissue to appear in the thoracic region (Fig. 34-6).

Acoustic Enhancement

Enhancement is another helpful artifact and can be thought of as the opposite of an acoustic shadow. It is also called "posterior enhancement" and "through-transmission." It occurs when the sound beam passes through a lowly attenuative structure, such as fluid, causing the echoes directly posterior to the structure to be brighter than the echoes on either side (Fig. 34-7). This helps to differentiate fluid-filled lesions from solid lesions. Some solid masses can be very homogenous and appear like a cyst but will

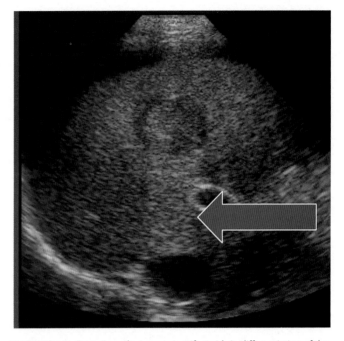

FIGURE 34-8. Posterior enhancement artifact aids in differentiation of the demonstrated abscess from a solid lesion.

lack acoustic enhancement, while some solid looking masses, such as an abscess or hematoma, will display acoustic enhancement allowing the mass to be characterized as containing fluid (Fig. 34-8).

Reverberation Artifact

A reverberation artifact (Figs. 34-9 and 34-10) demonstrates multiple equally spaced echoes at increasing depths. These reverberation echoes will decrease in intensity with depth. A reverberation artifact results when the sound wave is trapped between two strong reflectors causing it to be bounced between

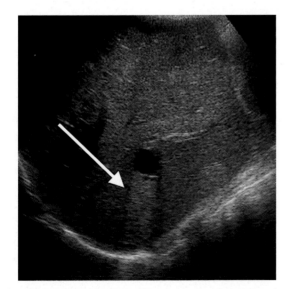

FIGURE 34-7. Posterior enhancement artifact seen as an area of increased echogenicity posterior to a liver cyst.

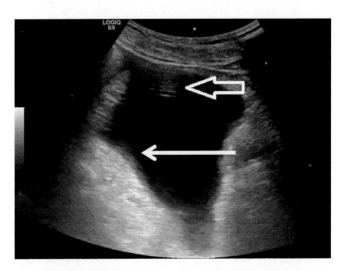

FIGURE 34-9. Reverberation artifact, wide arrow, at the top of the bladder. The echoes at the bottom of the bladder and are caused by a slice thickness artifact, thin solid arrow.

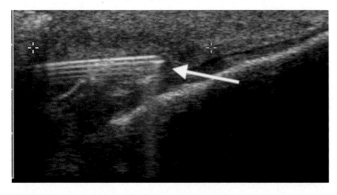

FIGURE 34-10. Reverberation from a biopsy needle.

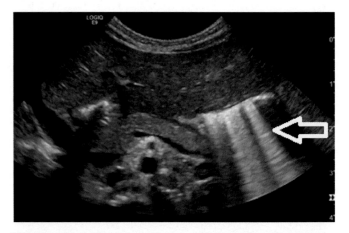

FIGURE 34-12. A ring-down artifact caused by gas in the stomach.

these reflectors, which are positioned parallel to the ultrasound beam. Reverberation artifacts are often seen posterior to the anterior wall of a structure that contains fluid, such as the urinary bladder or a cyst.

Ring-Down and Comet Tail Artifacts

Both ring-down and comet tail artifacts are types of compressed reverberation artifacts that appear as solid hyperechoic lines directed downward. They can be similar in sonographic appearance but will have different mechanisms as to their cause. A ring-down artifact is caused by air or gas (Fig. 34-11). Usually, a ring-down artifact is not as bright as a comet tail artifact and they can be longer in length. If there is a lot of gas or air together, it can create multiple ring-down artifacts (Fig. 34-12) and results in what is called "dirty" shadowing, which is an acoustic shadow that is not black but full of noise, causing the shadow area to appear filled-in. A comet tail artifact is created by solid objects such as crystals and metal. Examples include adenomyomatosis in the gallbladder (Fig. 34-13) and mechanical heart valves.

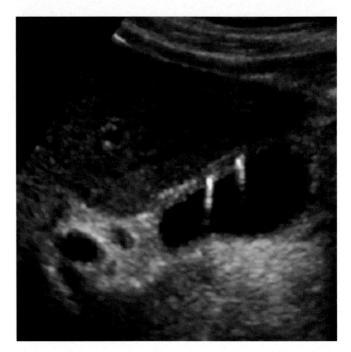

FIGURE 34-13. A comet tail artifact caused by solid crystals in the wall of the gallbladder.

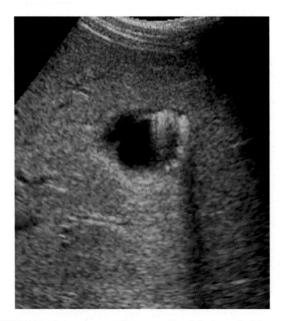

FIGURE 34-11. A ring-down artifact caused by air in the wall of the gallbladder from emphysematous cholecystitis.

Slice Thickness Artifact

Slice-thickness artifact (Fig. 34-14) is also called "section-thickness" or "partial-volume artifact." This artifact is related to the dimension of the sound beam perpendicular to the imaging plane and occurs due to the beam dimension being wider than the reflector. This artifact appears as echoes toward the bottom of curved cystic structures. By placing the focal zone near the area of the artifact, it may be noticeably diminished. It is important to differentiate this artifact from echoes produced by thick fluid, blood, or other pathology. Sometimes changing the transducer type will help to clear up the artifact. Activating the harmonic and/or compound imaging controls may help to clean up the artifact. Another option is to turn the patient on their side while scanning. If the echoes are real, the sonographer will see them floating downward to the dependent portion of the

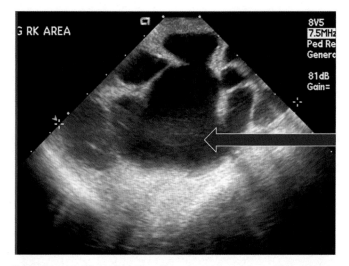

FIGURE 34-14. Slice thickness artifact appearing as echoes within a cystic structure.

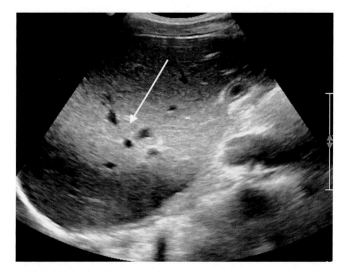

FIGURE 34-15. Focal banding artifact.

fluid-filled structure, whereas with a slice thickness artifact the echoes will either disappear or be there automatically.

Side Lobe Artifact

Side lobes are ultrasound beams that originate radially (off-axis) from the main beam. They are caused by the radial expansion of piezoelectric elements and are seen primarily in linear-array transducers. Strong reflectors that are in the path of the side lobes may create echoes that appear to have originated from within the main beam. New manufacturing transducer methods are helping to decrease side lobe artifacts.

Grating Lobes

Grating lobes are also ultrasound beams that originate radially (off-axis) from the main acoustic beam and are caused by the spacing between the individual elements in a transducer. Like side lobes, a strong echo in a grating lobe can be displayed on the image as if it originated from the main beam. Grating lobes have been reduced with new methods and transducer technologies such as subdicing the piezoelectric elements.

Focal Banding

Focal banding is when there is a horizontal band of echoes with increased intensity due to either the position of a focal zone or an improperly positioned time gain compensation, TGC, control (Fig. 34-15). The TGC controls can be used to correct focal enhancement.

Anisotropy Artifact

An anisotropy artifact is dependent on the angle of the insonating beam and occurs when the sound beam does not interact perpendicularly with a structure, causing echoes to be diminished in strength or not seen. This artifact is best seen with musculoskeletal, MSK, images and can cause tendons to appear as if they have tendinosis or a tear. This artifact may be corrected by

adjusting the transducer so that the sound beam interacts with the tendon at a 90-degree angle.

COLOR DOPPLER ARTIFACTS

Color Doppler Noise Artifact

Color Doppler noise artifact results from small amplitude echoes generated by electrical interference, signal processing, and spurious reflections. Color Doppler noise artifact is more likely to affect hypoechoic regions compared to areas of increased echogenicity. Sometimes decreasing color gain can reduce this artifact. This is sometimes referred to as "color flash" or "color confetti" artifact.

Color Aliasing Artifact

Color aliasing artifact (Figs. 34-16 and 34-17) occurs when the Doppler sampling rate, i.e., pulse repetition frequency

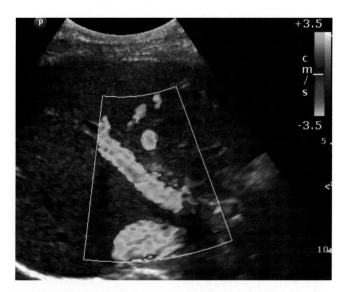

FIGURE 34-16. Color Doppler aliasing within the portal vein.

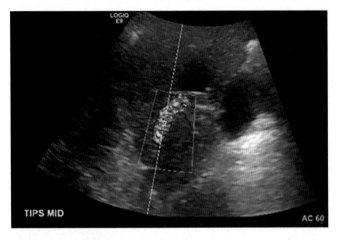

FIGURE 34-17. Color Doppler aliasing within a transjugular intrahepatic portosystemic shunt, TIPS.

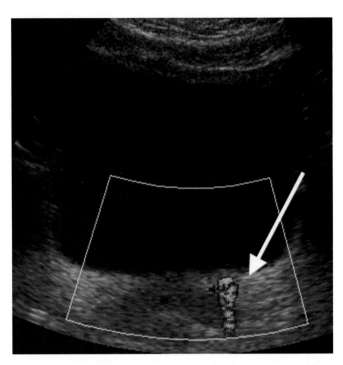

FIGURE 34-19. Color Doppler twinkle artifact from a small stone at the uterovesical junction, UVJ.

(PRF), is not fast enough to display the Doppler frequency shift. This artifact is unrelated to direction of flow and may be visualized when Doppler frequency shift surmounts ½ the PRF. It is seen as a mosaic pattern of colors inside the vessel, making it difficult to evaluate direction of flow. It is eliminated by increasing the color velocity scale, also known as the "PRF."

Color Twinkling Artifact

Color Doppler twinkle artifact (Figs. 34-18 and 34-19) appears as a focal or downward projection of numerous alternating colors at or posterior to a highly reflective structure. This is commonly visualized during imaging of renal calculi. Color twinkle artifact has a greater sensitivity compared to posterior shadowing artifact in the demonstration of small calculi. Calculi which have a rough surface more readily produce twinkling artifact. To enhance demonstration of twinkle artifact, the operator can decrease scale (PRF) setting and adjust the focal zone to directly below the suspected calculi.

SPECTRAL DOPPLER ARTIFACTS

Spectral Doppler Aliasing Artifact

Spectral Doppler aliasing artifact is a common artifact associated with the spectral Doppler tracing. The maximum height of the spectral Doppler display is determined by the Nyquist limit which is ½ PRF. When spectral Doppler aliasing artifact occurs, the peak of the Doppler spectrum appears below the baseline, under the main part of the signal (Fig. 34-20). Aliasing of the spectral Doppler waveform can be corrected by increasing scale (PRF), adjusting baseline shift, using a lower frequency transducer, choosing an alternative sonographic

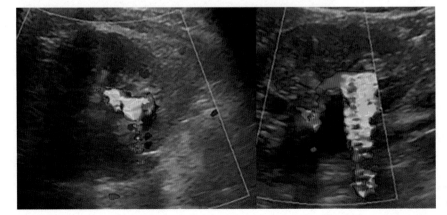

FIGURE 34-18. Color Doppler twinkle artifact posterior to renal calculi (stones).

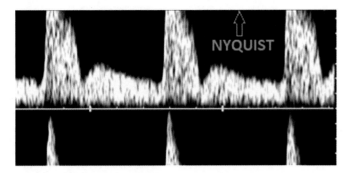

FIGURE 34-20. Spectral Doppler aliasing, the peak of the spectral waveform surpasses the Nyquist limit.

window with a shallower sample volume depth, or utilizing a continuous-wave Doppler transducer as they are not subject to aliasing but do not create an anatomic image.

Spectral Doppler Mirror Image Artifact (Crosstalk)

Spectral Doppler mirror image artifact is also called "crosstalk." It appears as a mirrored waveform below the baseline of the signal above the baseline (Fig. 34-21). It can be caused by a Doppler angle that is close to 90° or when the Doppler gain is too high. Improving the Doppler angle so that it is <60° or decreasing the Doppler gain can eliminate this artifact. The sonographer should differentiate spectral Doppler mirror image artifact from true bidirectional flow by changing the Doppler angle, decreasing Doppler gain, and/or evaluating flow with color Doppler.

Spectral Doppler Spectral Broadening Artifact

Spectral Doppler is electronically obtained via fast Fourier transform (FFT), with the spectral broadening index based upon FFT analysis. Spectral broadening artifact is associated with turbulent flow of varying direction and speed. Spectral broadening demonstrates a filled in spectral window (Fig. 34-22) due to a wider range of velocities and Doppler shifts present within a sample volume.

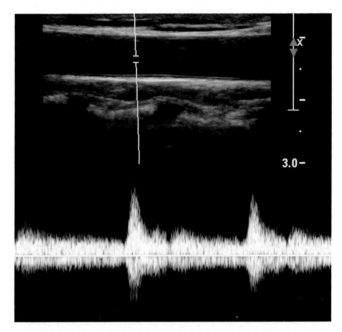

FIGURE 34-21. Mirror imaging of the spectral Doppler waveform.

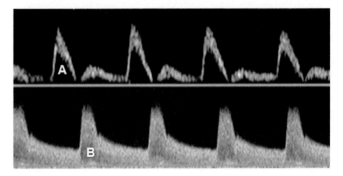

FIGURE 34-22. Letter A represents the spectral window and letter B represents filling in of the spectral window (spectral broadening).

35

Patient Care

PATIENT HISTORY

A thorough medical history is important in performing a diagnostic medical sonography exam.

It is the responsibility of the sonographer to verify that the imaging order is appropriate for the diagnosis. Before starting the exam, the sonographer must check two patient identifiers to verify that they are scanning the correct patient. The sonographer should review previous imaging reports, lab test results, and prior surgical procedures, especially when pathology is being followed. The primary caregiver will usually be the source of the pediatric patients' history which will include their birth and postnatal history. Children above the age of 4 may be able to point to any areas of pain or discomfort.

The sonographer should provide professional patient and family-centered care, using interpersonal skills, like verbal and nonverbal communication skills. The sonographer should introduce themselves and answer any questions or concerns that the caregiver may have that falls within the sonographer's scope of practice. The sonographer should also address any concerns or fears the patient may have to aid in their cooperation. AIDET is an acronym for acknowledge, introduce, duration (of exam), explanation, and thanking the patient and the patient's family or caregiver for allowing the sonographer to provide their care. AIDET is a good starting point for providing adequate care during each exam. The sonographer's mannerisms should be caring and sincere. The exam should be explained using terminology the patient and caregiver will understand. The patient's caregiver, or healthcare personnel caring for a pediatric inpatient,

should accompany the patient when their exam is in the ultrasound department. The sonographer should talk to the pediatric patient at eye level and follow the communication techniques which are discussed in the following section for the patient's age.

AGE SPECIFIC COMMUNICATION

The sonographer should be aware of age specific care and communication. This is a requirement of the Joint Commission on Accreditation of Healthcare Organizations (JCAHO), as each age group will respond differently to the medical care provided.

Neonates

Neonates are prone to rapid heat loss due to a lack of brown adipose tissue. This makes it important to keep the neonate in their isolation unit using the portholes for scanning. When scanning the neonate's head, the sonographer should make sure to wipe the gel off immediately after scanning as it is a significant source of heat loss.

Infants (birth to 1 year)

Use a soothing voice and smile when talking. Allow the caregiver to help comfort the infant. Having the caregiver hold the infant in their lap or on their shoulder like they are burping the infant may be helpful in keeping the child calm. For exams requiring images of the bladder, always scan the bladder first, especially in young infants, as they may void once clothing is removed or while pressing on the abdomen or pelvic area with the transducer while scanning.

Toddlers (1-3 years)

Make eye contact and smile before approaching the child, using a friendly voice. Provide the child with recommended safe toys, allowing opportunities to play. A caregiver's cell phone or tablet may be used to entertain the child.

Age (3-5 years)

Explain the exam in words that the child will understand. You can demonstrate what the exam entails by scanning on yourself or the patient's caregiver. Lower yourself to the child's eye level as much as possible. A caregiver's cell phone or tablet may be used to entertain the child.

School Age (5-10)

These patients may be inquisitive and ask questions about the procedure and if it will hurt. Always be honest and when permissible, allow the child to make some decisions about their care while with you. You can demonstrate what the exam entails by scanning on yourself or the patient's caregiver.

Adolescents (10-15 years)

This age group will start to want some privacy. Make sure that they are properly covered and use a professional approach. It is important to treat the patient more as an adult than a child.

PATIENT POSITIONING

Some commonly used patient positions are discussed below:

- Supine: recumbent, face up (Fig. 35-1). Most often used position for sonographic examinations.
- Prone: recumbent, face down (Fig. 35-2).
- Oblique: lying supine and rotated toward the right (right posterior oblique [RPO]) or left (left posterior oblique [LPO]) side (Fig. 35-3), usually between 45 and 60°. RPO position can aid in visualization of the left-sided abdominal organs, such as the left kidney and spleen. LPO may help visualize the common bile duct and gallbladder. Right

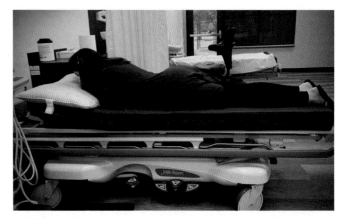

FIGURE 35-2. Prone position.

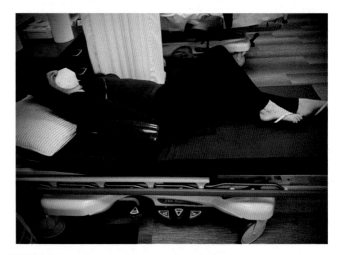

FIGURE 35-3. LPO position.

anterior oblique (RAO) and left anterior oblique (LAO) positions are infrequently used in sonographic imaging.

- Lateral/Decubitus: lying on the right (right lateral decubitus) (Fig. 35-4) or left (left lateral decubitus) side. Sometimes referred to as right side up, RSU, or left side up, LSU.
- Upright/Erect: seated or standing; in a semi-upright position the patient is seated at a 45 to 60° angle.

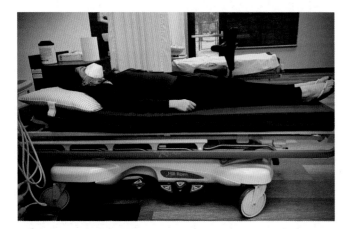

FIGURE 35-1. Supine position.

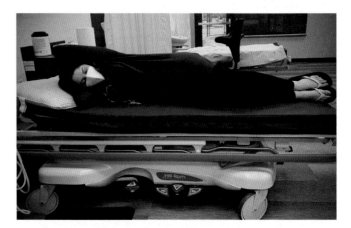

FIGURE 35-4. Right lateral decubitus position.

- Trendelenburg: the patient's head is positioned lower than the feet (Fig. 35-5).
- Reverse Trendelenburg: the patient's head is positioned higher than the feet (Fig. 35-6).
- Sims: recumbent LAO with right leg forward, in front of the left leg (Fig. 35-7). Not used in routine imaging; may be encountered for ultrasound-guided block of the sciatic nerve using subgluteal approach in an operating room setting.

It may be necessary to modify patient positioning to complete a protocol depending on patient cooperation. Pediatric patients may be scanned while sitting on a parent or caregiver's lap or lying on a parent or caregiver in a semi-upright position. If the infant is in an isolette or incubator and must be moved, the nurse should be notified and assist with moving the patient. Precautions should be taken while scanning as to not disrupt the placement of intravenous lines, oxygen tubing (tanks, flowmeters, cannulas, etc.), or catheters.

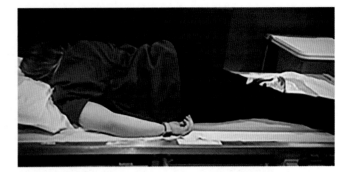

FIGURE 35-7. Sims position.

ANATOMICAL AND SCAN PLANES

Anatomical planes are imaginary lines which divide the body into anatomical segments (Fig 35-8). Sonographic scan planes may vary slightly from the true anatomical plane, as not all organs in the body lie in a true longitudinal or transverse fashion. Transducer placement and angle of insonation will determine the sonographic scan plane.

The sagittal anatomical plane divides the body into right and left halves. It is also called the "longitudinal plane." The

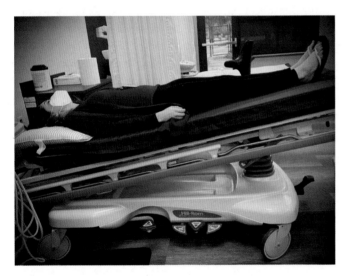

FIGURE 35-5. Trendelenburg position.

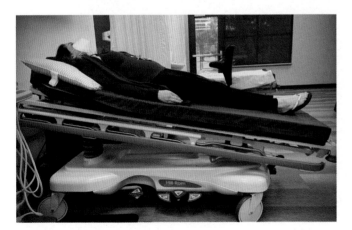

FIGURE 35-6. Reverse Trendelenburg position.

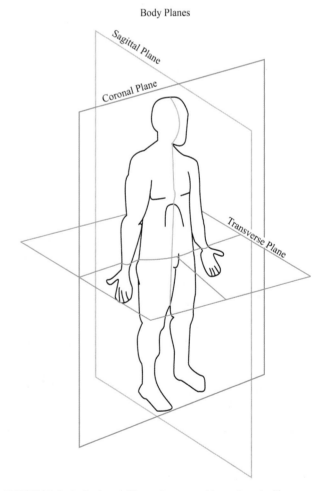

FIGURE 35-8. Body planes. (Illustration created by and used with permission from Isaiah Forestier.)

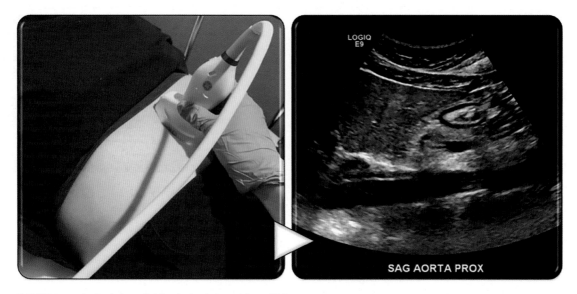

FIGURE 35-9. Sagittal plane divides the body into right and left.

sagittal scan plane (Fig 35-9) correlates to the long-axis view of an organ. When scanning an organ like the abdominal aorta, the true anatomical plane and scan planes usually correlate. However, some organs, such as the kidneys, lie at a slight oblique angle within the body. To produce a true long-axis view of organs which lie obliquely in the body, the transducer must be manipulated slightly from the true anatomical plane.

The transverse anatomical plane divides the body into superior and inferior halves. The transverse scan plane displays the short-axis view of an organ and divides the organ of interest into superior and inferior halves (Fig 35-10).

The coronal anatomical plane divides the body into anterior and posterior halves (Fig 35-11). The coronal scan plane divides the organ or area of interest into anterior and posterior halves. For abdominal scanning, the coronal scan plane is obtained by placing the transducer on the far right or left side of the body. A coronal scan plane is also used with intracranial, transvaginal (endovaginal), and translabial scanning.

SONOGRAPHIC WINDOWS

Sonographic windows are regions where the sound beam leaving the transducer can enter the body. Each sonographic window provides optimal images or views of specific organs. For example, the transtemporal acoustic window provides optimal views of the circle of Willis and the abdominal scan window allows for imaging of the pancreas. Each sonographic window correlates to the area of transducer placement (Fig 35-12). There are many sonographic windows located throughout the body. Some sonographic windows encountered in pediatric scanning include:

- Transabdominal: Through the anterior abdomen or pelvis
- Intercostal: Between the rib spaces
- Coronal: Through the right or left side of the body
- Prone: From the back
- Transfontanelle: Through the anterior, posterior, mastoid, or sphenoid fontanelles

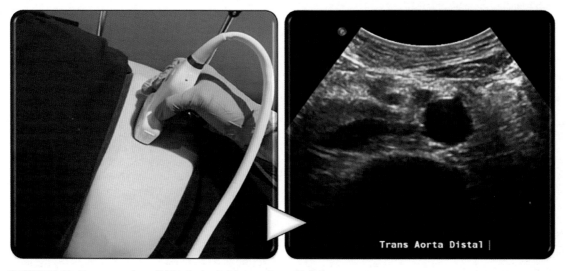

FIGURE 35-10. Transverse plane divides the body into superior and inferior.

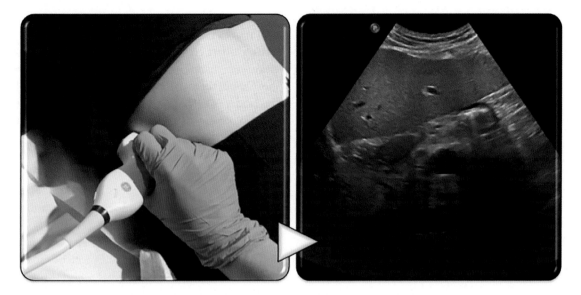

FIGURE 35-11. Coronal plane divides the body into front and back.

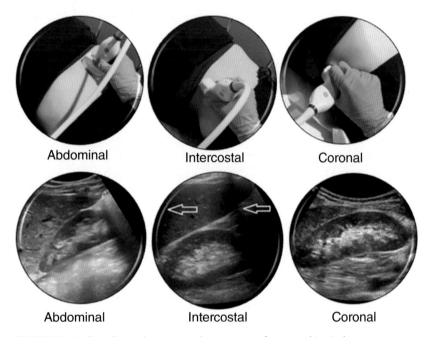

FIGURE 35-12. Transducer placement and appearance of sonographic windows.

- Transtemporal: Through the right or left temple
- Suboccipital: Below the occipital bone
- Transorbital: Across the orbit
- Posterior paraspinal: Adjacent to the spinal column
- Transthoracic: Through the chest wall
- Subcostal (subxiphoid): Beneath the costal margin
- Supraclavicular: Above the clavicle
- Infraclavicular: Below the clavicle
- Suprasternal: Above the sternum
- Parasternal: Beside the sternum
- Transsternal: Across the sternum

- Subdiaphragmatic: Below the diaphragm
- Translabial: Across the labia
- Transvaginal: Through the vaginal canal

ETHICS AND LEGAL CONSIDERATION

Ethical Considerations

The sonographer's responsibility includes performing diagnostic sonographic examinations, optimizing the sonographic image, and providing accurate information within the sonographer's scope of practice.

The sonographer should accurately represent their level of expertise to employers and receive additional training as necessary. Sonographers should abide by the profession's Code of Ethics set forth by the Society of Diagnostic Medical Sonography.

Legal Considerations

It is the sonographer's responsibility to protect the privacy of their patients as defined by the Health Insurance Portability and Accountability Act (HIPAA).

All patients have the right to make decisions for themselves including the right to refuse an exam. In the case of a pediatric patient, this may include the patient's primary caregiver. The sonographer should ensure that informed consent, usually verbal, has been obtained prior to beginning an exam or that written consent has been obtained before an interventional procedure. The types of consent needed are determined by hospital policy.

INFECTION CONTROL AND PRECAUTIONS

Hospital-acquired infections (HAIs) are infections that a patient develops while in the hospital, that is, they did not have the infection prior to being admitted. These infections could be prevented with proper hygiene techniques. HAIs add a financial burden to the health care system, costing billions of dollars. According to the Centers for Disease Control and Prevention (CDC), about 1 in 31 hospital patients develop an HAI, affecting an estimated 687,000 patients annually. Approximately 72,000 patients will die from an HAI each year. HAIs are a serious problem in health care worldwide.

Recent evidence has shown that the ultrasound department is a potential source where the patient may obtain an infection. As a sonographer, it is important to do our part in reducing the risk of HAIs. Many pathogens, such as vancomycin-resistant enterococci (VRE), methicillin-resistant *Staphylococcus aureus* (MRSA), *Clostridium difficile (C. diff)*, and COVID-19, can last on surfaces for days or even weeks. As sonographers we need to protect not only our patients, but be mindful of protecting ourselves and our families as well.

Proper hand washing is essential to help prevent the spread of infection, especially when scanning the neonate or immune-compromised pediatric patient. Personal protective equipment (PPE) includes gloves, a mask, a gown, and eye protection. Infants born before 37 weeks gestational age or with a birth weight of less than 2,500 grams are at an increased risk for developing an HAI. Hands should be washed before and after changing gloves, between each patient, before eating, and after using the restroom. Many of these pathogens will be found on our hands and can enter our body through our mouths, thereby infecting us. Because we are infected does not mean that we will develop the disease, but we will be a carrier who can infect others. While alcohol-based hand sanitizers can be used, some pathogens, such as *C. diff* can only be removed from our hands by using soap and water. The CDC website offers great advice on which method to use to properly clean your hands as well as current techniques. As we learn more about these pathogens these guidelines are changing, and the reader is encouraged to visit their website at www.cdc.gov to keep abreast of current recommendations. Many inpatient and intensive care units also require the wearing of a gown and mask. It is important to be aware of latex allergies and to wear appropriate non-latex gloves. Infants with spina bifida are at a risk to develop latex allergies as they get older, so using non-latex gloves should always be used as a precaution. Many facilities no longer have latex gloves.

The sonographer must ensure that the ultrasound unit and transducers are properly disinfected, especially between patients. The disinfection process will destroy the pathogens on the transducer and ultrasound unit. Unfortunately, not all disinfection agents can be used for the transducers and the ultrasound unit. The sonographer should consult the manufacturer's website, which will have a section devoted to cleaning and disinfection products that can be safely used to disinfect the ultrasound unit and the transducers. It is important to only use the products that the manufacturer has deemed safe to use on their equipment, as using the wrong product can void any warranties. When possible, a product that can be used on all transducers and the unit is preferred, so that the wrong product is not accidentally used.

A disinfection method must be used to destroy any potential pathogens on the transducer before it is used on the next patient. Transducers can undergo high level disinfection, HLD, or low level disinfection, LLD. How the transducer was used will determine which type of disinfection is required, which is based on Spaulding's classification. If the transducer has come in contact with mucous membranes, such as during a transvaginal or transrectal ultrasound, that transducer must be disinfected using a HLD method. Studies have shown that there are pathogens on the handles of both endovaginal (EV) and transrectal transducers, therefore, using a device or method that can perform a HLD on the handle is preferred. All other transducers can possibly be treated with LLD. At the time of publication, there is some controversy on which disinfection level method should be used on a transducer that was covered with a sterile cover and used for an interventional procedure. According to Spaulding's classification system a HLD method should be used, however, some physicians state that there is no evidence that any patient has been infected when a LLD method is used. As research continues, the sonographer should continue to check both the AIUM and SDMS for any updates or decisions. Some studies have shown that pathogens are left on a transducer after LLD, and HLD is encouraged to stop the spread of these pathogens.

Besides disinfecting the transducer, other aspects of infection prevention need to be understood, such as transducer storage, gel concerns, disinfecting the ultrasound unit, scanning table, and the examination room. Some recent guidelines that the sonographer should be aware of to reduce the risk of a HAI include how to store transducers. For example, transducers marked as clean should be stored in a cabinet, drawer, or transducer storage cabinet. The sonographer should only have the necessary transducers on the ultrasound unit for the exam to be performed, and should not refill gel bottles from a large container unless the bottles have been sterilized. Single use gel packets are currently being encouraged. It is beyond the scope of this chapter to go into the detail needed to truly understand disinfection practices, and the reader is encouraged to learn more about this important subject by attending disinfection lectures, listening to webinars on infection prevention, and reading appropriate articles.

HLD of all transducers is easier to perform if the transducer can be disinfected in the scanning room. The use of 35% hydrogen peroxide for HLD is popular in health care, including outside of the ultrasound department. Current research has shown that not all HLD methods kill human papillomaviruses (HPV), which have been found on EV transducers after HLD. If the department performs a lot of EV examinations, a method that kills HPV should be used so as not to possibly infect patients.

The reader is encouraged to read the American Institute of Ultrasound in Medicine (AIUM) official statement: Guidelines for Cleaning and Preparing External- and Internal- Use Ultrasound Transducers Between Patients, Safe Handling, and Use of Ultrasound Coupling Gel to help understand the importance of proper disinfection and the correct method to use. This guideline can be found on their website at www.aium.org. The Society of Diagnostic Medical Sonography (SDMS) also has published guidelines called: SDMS Guidelines for Infection Prevention and Control in Sonography: Reprocessing the Ultrasound Transducer. There is also an appendix with updated information and other helpful information. These can be found at www.sdms.org.

Sterile Field

For a space to be considered sterile, there must be no microorganisms present. A sterile field is necessary for surgical and interventional procedures, biopsies, drainages, and aspirations. Areas above the waist in gowned healthcare staff and above the tabletop are considered sterile. When preparing the patient for a sterile procedure, the area of interest is cleaned using an antibacterial solution (betadine, etc.). This solution is applied to the skin using a sterile sponge, starting at the area of interest, and moving outwards in a circular fashion. When assisting with a sterile procedure, the sonographer should wear sterile gloves and gown and use a sterile cover that covers both the transducer and the cord. Additionally, the sonographer should use sterile gel and keep their hands above waist-level during a procedure. Usually one hand will become "dirty" as it

is needed to adjust ultrasound system controls and document images. It is important to remember to not touch the sterile field with this hand.

Interventional Procedures

Interventional procedures include paracentesis, thoracentesis, abscess drainage, and various biopsies (renal, etc.) which will require using a sterile field. A biopsy may be performed using a core-biopsy-automated hollow core needle, called a "biopsy gun," which obtains a piece of tissue, or by using a fine needle aspiration (FNA) technique which obtains a sample of cells. The purpose of a biopsy is to determine characteristics of a tissue, and the biopsied tissue is sent to pathology. Drainages, including para- and thoracentesis consists of the removal of bodily fluids (Fig. 35-13(a) to (c)) for diagnostic or therapeutic purposes. Interventional procedures may be contraindicated when patients are taking anticoagulation medications or have chronic coagulopathy conditions. Before a procedure, the patient will have their blood work checked to assess their bleeding times.

EMERGENT PROCEDURES

From time to time the pediatric sonographer may encounter a time-sensitive positive finding in which prompt treatment is required for optimal patient outcome. When a sonographer visualizes a positive emergent finding, standard operating procedure for each institution should be followed. Typically, this includes contacting the radiologist for an expedited report. Particular pathologies, such as testicular torsion, have an allotted time for potential organ salvage of 6 hours following symptomatic onset. For this reason, prompt examination, an expedited report, and treatment of the patient is crucial. In pediatric imaging, the most common emergent procedures include evaluation for intussusception, appendicitis, and hypertrophic pyloric stenosis. The most common surgical emergency in the pediatric setting is appendicitis. Additional findings which are considered critical and time-sensitive are outlined in Table 35-1. It is important to note that not all etiologies listed are truly emergent, however they could be commonly encountered in the emergency department and critical care setting. Refer to Section II for specific information pertaining to pathologic conditions.

PATIENT SAFETY

A sonographers' responsibilities include but are not limited to:

- Ensuring that the bed or stretcher siderails are up, wheelchairs and stretchers are locked, careful monitoring of the patient, especially young children, keeping the patient comfortable, and instructing the patient and/or the patient's caregiver of their roles. No child should be left on an ultrasound scanning stretcher or bed without an adult by their side.

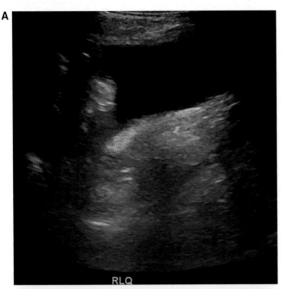

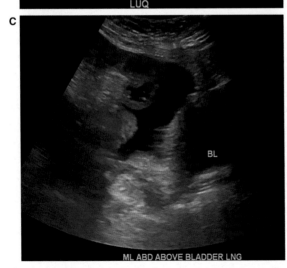

FIGURE 35-13. Ascites check prior to marking for paracentesis.

ERGONOMICS

In addition to patient safety, sonographers should be mindful of proper body mechanics in the work setting to reduce potential musculoskeletal work-related injuries.

In a study by Pike et al., 20% of sonographers who were symptomatic suffered career-ending injuries:

1. The onset of work-related musculoskeletal disorder (WRMSD) symptoms occurs as early as six months from the start of employment with a 15% incidence, increasing to 45% after three years, and as high as 72% after ten years of employment.

2. For this reason sonographers have a responsibility to maintain a safe work environment and to work on risk-reducing modifications during scanning and other work-related activities.

There are established methods for proper ergonomics that every sonographer should strive for that can include but are not limited to:

- Varying the types of exams performed and scanning positions including sitting and standing which allows for different muscles to be used.
- Take frequent mini-breaks throughout the workday between patients, microbreaks when possible during the exam and all breaks including meal breaks.
- Make use of all the adjustments of the ultrasound unit, exam table, and scanning chair used during the exam to reduce abduction and reach.
- Have the patient move closer to the edge of the exam table, toward the sonographer.
- Incorporate exercises and stretches daily, including between patients. Talk to a physical therapist about exercises and needed equipment, such as stretch bands and pulleys, to perform at home.
- Consider using accessories such as a transducer cable support device and positioning sponges.
- Wear properly fitting gloves.

TABLE 35-1 • Etiologies Frequently Encountered in the Acute-Care Setting

Abdominal	Pelvic	Scrotal	Cranial	MSK	Miscellaneous
Intussusception, Malrotation, Volvulus	Ovarian Torsion	Testicular Torsion	Parenchymal Etiologies	Acute Hip Effusion (i.e., Transient Synovitis, Septic Arthritis)	Focused Assessment with Sonography for Trauma (FAST)
Appendicitis	Hydrocolpos, Hydrometrocolpos, Hematametrocolpos	Testicular Appendage Torsion	Subdural and Extra-Axial Collections (i.e., hematoma)		Foreign Body Localization and US-Guided Percutaneous Drainage
Pyloric Stenosis	Abscess	Testicular Rupture			
Acute Pyelonephritis, UPJ Obstruction, Obstructive Nephrolithiasis	Ectopic Pregnancy in Adolescents	Hematocele			
Pancreatitis, Pancreatic Abscess, Pseudocyst, Hemorrhage, Necrosis		Intrascrotal Inguinal Hernia with Absent Peristalsis (Incarceration)			
Cholecystitis, Choledochal Cysts		Epididymitis			
		Orchitis			
		Abscess			

Sources: Cogley JR, O'Connor SC, Houshyar R, Dulaimy KA. Emergent pediatric us: What every radiologist should know. *RadioGraphics*. 2012;32(3):651–665; Saigal G, Therrien JR, Kuo F. Ultrasound in pediatric emergencies. *Appl Radiol*. 2014;43(8):6–16. Available at link.gale.com/apps/doc/A381588161/AONE?u=anon~2892c6ba&sid=googleScholar&xid=2e9d5d02 (accessed March 5, 2022).

36

Most Common Anomalies and Disease Processes

NEUROSONOGRAPHY

- The most common aperta (non-skin-covered) spinal dysraphism is myelocele and myelomeningocele.
- The most common intracranial hemorrhage site in preterm infants is the subependymal germinal matrix of the lateral ventricle.
- The second most common benign nerve sheath tumor is schwannoma.
- Astrocytoma is the most common brain tumor and glioblastoma is the most common type of astrocytoma.
- The most common benign nerve sheath tumor is neurofibroma.

THORAX AND ABDOMINAL SONOGRAPHY

- The most common neonatal abdominal mass is multicystic dysplastic kidney.
- The most common cause of intestinal obstruction in children between 3 months and 3 years is intussusception.
- The most common malignant liver mass in infants and children is hepatoblastoma.
- The most common benign hepatic tumor in infants less than 6 months of age is infantile hemangioendothelioma.
- The second most common benign liver mass is mesenchymal hamartoma.

- The most common primary hepatic neoplasm is hepatocellular carcinoma, or hepatoma.
- The most common form of malignant disease in the liver is metastasis.
- The most common cause of portal hypertension in the United States is cirrhosis.
- The most common viral hepatitis in the United States is hepatitis A.
- The most common carbohydrate metabolism inborn error is glycogen storage disease.
- The most common lysosomal storage disorder is Gaucher disease.
- The most common tumor to metastasize to the gallbladder is malignant melanoma.
- The most common benign splenic neoplasm is cavernous hemangioma.
- The most common malignant splenic neoplasm in Hodgkin and non-Hodgkin patients is lymphoma.
- The most common endocrine islet-cell tumor of the pancreas is insulinoma.
- The second most common endocrine islet-cell tumor of the pancreas is gastrinoma.
- The most common malignant pancreatic tumor is adenocarcinoma.
- The most common complication of acute pancreatitis is pseudocyst formation.

- The most common cystic mass of the pancreas is a pseudocyst.
- The most common benign stomach tumor is leiomyoma.
- The most common malignant gastrointestinal neoplasm in childhood is gastric lymphoma.
- The most common malignant gastrointestinal tumor is adenocarcinoma.
- The most common primary retroperitoneal tumor that metastasizes from fat is liposarcoma.

REPRODUCTIVE SONOGRAPHY

- The most common primary germ cell tumors of the scrotum are mature teratoma (infants) and yolk sac carcinoma (adolescent).
- The neoplasm most associated with crytorchidism is seminoma.
- The most common malignant paratesticular tumor is rhabdomyosarcoma.
- Seminomas are malignant germ cell tumors that are rare in children, however are the most common testicular tumor in adults, followed by embryonal cell carcinoma.
- The most common benign ovarian tumor is cystic mature teratoma, or dermoid cyst.

SUPERFICIAL SONOGRAPHY

- The most common and least aggressive thyroid carcinoma is papillary carcinoma.
- The second most common thyroid carcinoma is follicular carcinoma.
- The most common malignant neurogenic tumors of the neck are neuroblastoma and neurofibroma.
- The third most common malignant tumor with cervical involvement in children is cervical lymphoma.
- The most common soft tissue sarcoma of childhood is rhabdomyosarcoma.
- The most common benign breast mass in young women is fibroadenoma.

VASCULAR SONOGRAPHY

- The most common vascular soft tissue tumor of infancy is soft tissue hemangioma.

URINARY SYSTEM AND ADRENAL SONOGRAPHY

- The most common benign solid renal tumor of infancy is mesoblastic nephroma, or fetal renal hamartoma.

- The most common renal malignancy and second most common malignant solid tumor in children is Wilms tumor, or nephroblastoma.
- The most common benign bladder tumors are leiomyoma and papilloma.
- The most common malignant bladder tumor in childhood is bladder rhabdomyosarcoma.
- The most common neonatal renal mass is multicystic dysplastic kidney.
- The most common renal anomaly is horseshoe kidney.
- The most common congenital anomaly of the urinary tract is partial or complete renal collecting system duplication.
- The most common disorder of the urinary tract in children is urinary tract infection.
- The most common cause of renal artery stenosis in children is fibromuscular dysplasia.
- The most common cause of acute renal failure is acute tubular necrosis.
- The most common cause of renal transplant allograft failure is acute rejection.
- The most common perinephric fluid collection is lymphocele.
- The most common cortical renal mass with painless hematuria is renal adenoma.
- The second most common childhood tumor and most common solid malignant extracranial tumor in children is neuroblastoma, an adrenal medullary neoplasm arising in the adrenal gland.
- The most common inherited cause of adrenal insufficiency is congenital adrenal hyperplasia.
- The most common of the rare stromal adrenal tumors is adrenal hemangioendothelioma.
- The most common neonatal adrenal mass arises secondary to adrenal hemorrhage.
- The fourth most common metastatic site in the body is the adrenal glands.

MISCELLANEOUS

- The most common general malignancy of childhood is leukemia.
- The most common cause of inflammatory tenosynovitis in children is juvenile rheumatoid arthritis and overuse syndrome.
- The most common cause of painful hip and joint effusion in children is toxic synovitis, or transient synovitis.

37

Autosomal Dominant and Autosomal Recessive Disorders of the Body

AUTOSOMAL DOMINANT

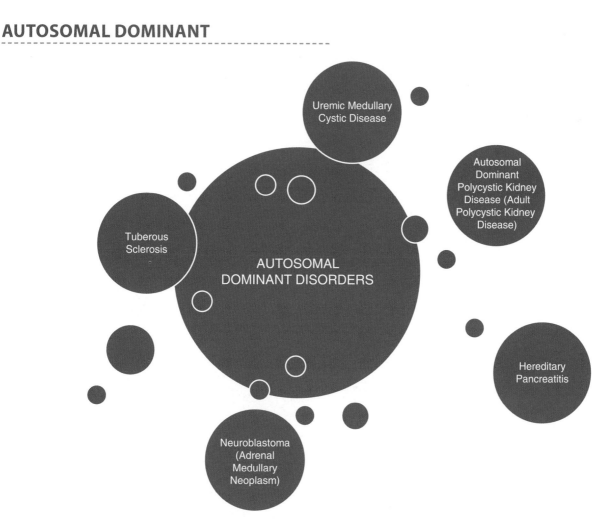

FIGURE 37-1. Autosomal Dominant Disorders

AUTOSOMAL RECESSIVE

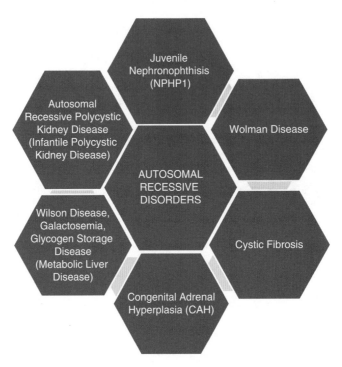
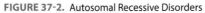

FIGURE 37-2. Autosomal Recessive Disorders

38

Same-Name Pathology

This section discusses pathologies which can affect numerous areas of the body and describes the sonographic appearance in each anatomical region.

TERATOMA

A teratoma is a germ cell tumor. A mature teratoma is generally benign with low malignant potential and immature teratoma is more often malignant. Increased levels of alpha-fetoprotein are seen with immature teratoma. A mature teratoma is also called a "dermoid cyst," or "cystic teratoma." Immature teratoma contains immature fetal tissue, primitive neuroectoderm, and mature tissue elements. Tissue types such as hair, teeth, muscle, and bone may occur within a teratoma, creating sonographic signs such as "dermoid mesh" and "tip of the iceberg" sign. The "dermoid mesh" sign, also called the "dot-dash pattern," is created by the presence of hair within the lesion, creating echogenic lines of varying lengths. "Tip of the iceberg" sign is created in the presence of teeth, calcification, or Rokitansky nodule fat, in the anterior aspect of an otherwise cystic mass, which creates a posterior shadowing artifact. A teratoma can occur in numerous locations throughout the body.

Pancreatic Cystic Teratoma	Cystic tumor with fat, bone, soft tissue, and calcification. "Tip-of-the-iceburg" or "dermal mesh" signs may be demonstrated.
Gastric Teratoma	Benign, complex, cystic, and echogenic mass containing fluid, fat, and calcification. Calcification within the tumor may represent bone.
Scrotal Teratoma	Well-defined, heterogeneous mass containing hypoechoic areas of serous fluid and hyperechoic components of calcification with shadowing.
Ovarian Mature Teratoma	Complex mass of variable echogenicity. This mass may contain calcification, "tip-of-the-iceburg" sign, and fluid-fluid level. Appearance depends upon components including sebum, serous fluid, calcium, hair, or fat. If hair is present within the mass, "dermoid mesh" sign may be visualized.
Ovarian Immature Teratoma	Malignant germ cell tumor appearing as a solid echogenic mass with fine scattered calcifications.
Cervical Teratoma	Heterogeneous cystic mass with calcifications. This mass is located within the anterior neck. May be visualized in utero and palpable upon physical neonatal screening. Can cause severe airway problems and other issues related to delivery.
Intracranial Teratoma	Large echogenic mass with calcification and cystic areas of necrosis and degeneration. With intracranial teratoma, midline brain structures become displaced and hydrocephalus may be present.

LEUKEMIA

Leukemia is an excess of immature differentiated white blood cells. This hematopoietic neoplasm begins in the bone marrow. Types of leukemia include acute myeloid leukemia, chronic myeloid leukemia, acute lymphoblastic leukemia, and chronic lymphocytic leukemia. Sonographic appearance of leukemia usually involves enlargement of affected organs.

Renal Leukemia Spread	Nephromegaly with maintained reniform shape, decreased renal echogenicity, loss of corticomedullary differentiation, multiple masses, and hydronephrosis due to ureteral obstruction.
Hepatic Leukemia Spread	Hepatomegaly, ascites, lesions of varying echogenicity within the liver, and para-aortic lymph node enlargement.
Splenic Leukemia Spread	Splenomegaly, discrete red-pulp nodules during active stages and leukemia remission.

LYMPHOMA

Blasts refer to immature cells that arise from bone marrow. Lymphoma is a malignancy of the lymphoblasts or lymphocytes. Lymphoma can affect many regions of the body, including the central nervous system, head, neck, thorax, hepatobiliary organs, spleen, gastrointestinal tract, genitourinary organs, skin, and musculoskeletal system. Imaging appearance varies with location and stage of lymphoma.

Pancreatic Lymphoma Spread	Diffusely enlarged homogeneous, hypoechoic pancreas with anechoic masses mimicking pancreatic cysts. Widespread lymph node enlargement is present with pancreatic lymphoma.
Gastric Lymphoma Spread	Gastrointestinal wall thickening, hypoechoic polypoid mass with intramural and extramural extension within the abdomen, and widespread lymph node enlargement.
Renal Lymphoma Spread	Multiple homogeneous lymphomatous cortical renal masses of varying echogenicity with absent distal acoustic enhancement, hydronephrosis, and ureteral dilatation as enlarged retroperitoneal nodes compress the ureters.
Cervical Lymphoma Spread	Bilaterally enlarged painless, homogeneous, hypoechoic lymph nodes with central and peripheral Doppler flow.
Hepatic Lymphoma Spread	Well-defined homogeneous, hypoechoic to anechoic septated nodules within an enlarged liver.
Splenic Lymphoma Spread	Splenomegaly, multiple avascular hypoechoic to anechoic masses without acoustic enhancement, and surrounding widespread retroperitoneal lymph nodes.

LYMPHANGIOMA

Lymphangioma is an abnormal lymph node channel development that leads to formation of cystic masses. This mass often causes swelling in areas which are affected.

Pancreatic Lymphangioma	Congenital obstructive, hypoechoic, septated, multicystic, serous fluid-filled mass surrounded by a thin capsule.
Cervical Lymphangioma	Thin-walled loculated mass with acoustic enhancement, resulting from congenital blockage of lymphatic draining canals.
Hepatic Mesenchymal Hamartoma (Lymphangioma)	Benign, congenital, multilocular, encapsulated, mucoid mass with echogenic septations.
Splenic Lymphangioma	Benign, congenital, avascular, multilocular cyst with echogenic septations and calcified components.

HAMARTOMA

Hamartoma is a benign malformation comprised of many abnormal, disorganized cells in their region of origin. Hamartoma can occur in various regions of the body and it is not uncommon for hamartoma to mimic malignancy.

Renal Cystic Hamartoma	Cystic noncommunicating mass with echogenic septations.
Renal Hamartoma, (Angiomyolipoma)	Small bilateral hyperechoic lesions in the renal cortex. Potential to cause renal failure if complete renal parenchyma invasion occurs.
Liver Hamartoma (Mesenchymal Hamartoma)	Multilocular encapsulated mucoid mass with echogenic septations.
Splenic Hamartoma	Well-defined, benign, hypoechoic lymphoid tissue mass with complex and cystic changes.

HEMANGIOMA

A hemangioma is a benign, vascular tumor. This etiology is categorized as congenital or infantile. Congenital hemangioma is fully-formed at birth while infantile hemangioma may proliferate throughout infancy and into early childhood. Hemangioma readily demonstrates flow with Doppler imaging.

Soft Tissue Skin Hemangioma	Physically appears as a bluish skin discoloration. This well-defined, vascular, superficial soft-tissue mass has varying echogenicity. Along with sacral dimple, soft tissue skin hemangioma is predisposing to occult dysraphism of the spine.
Cervical Hemangioma	Congenital, hypoechoic, hypervascular, endothelial cell mass.
Hepatic Cavernous Hemangioma	Well-defined, hyperechoic, homogeneous mass with slow blood flow.
Splenic Hemangioma	Well-defined homogeneous, hyperechoic, hypervascular mass.

RHABDOMYOSARCOMA

Rhabdomyosarcoma is a malignancy which has a variable appearance and is not sonographically distinguishable from other types of sarcoma. Biopsy is required for a definitive diagnosis.

Bladder	Malignant, echogenic, pedunculated soft-tissue mass projecting into the bladder with a "bunch of grapes" complex cystic appearance.
Cervical	Malignant hypoechoic mass with calcifications, central or peripheral Doppler flow, and enlarged surrounding lymph nodes.
Liver	Malignant, large, and solid nonspecific tumor.
Paratesticular	Most common malignant paratesticular tumor. Appearance is variable, but often inhomogeneous.
Soft Tissue	Rhabdomyosarcoma is the most common malignant soft tissue tumor of childhood. Appearance is variable, but often inhomogeneous.
Vaginal	Malignant, large, heterogeneous tumor that usually occurs in female infants and in early childhood.

PYOGENIC ABSCESS

Pyogenic abscess is a confined region of inflammation and tissue necrosis resulting from parasites, bacteria, or fungus. With these collections it is not uncommon for small gas bubbles and associated artifact to be visualized.

Hepatic Pyogenic Abscess	Spreads via the portal venous system. Appearance includes hepatomegaly, round hypoechoic masses within the right lobe with thick irregular walls, internal debris and septation. Hypoechoic gas pockets with shadowing and ring-down artifact may be visualized, along with clinical symptom of fever.
Splenic Pyogenic Abscess	Results from hematogenous seeding of infection. Splenic pyogenic abscess appearance includes a hypoechoic complex mass with internal echoes, fluid-fluid levels, echogenic foci with shadowing and ring-down artifact, and surrounding lymphadenopathy.

Medical Root Terms

LET'S BREAK IT DOWN!

Knowledge of prefix, suffix, and word roots is beneficial for determining the meaning of pathological terms and/or other etiologies on the registry examination a sonographer may be unfamiliar with. For example, a question pertains to inflammation of the fallopian tubes. A sonographer's understanding of the prefix "salping-" (fallopian tubes) and suffix "-itis" (inflammation) is helpful in determining the correct answer choice while weeding out the alternative distractor choices.

Prefixes

Some of the prefixes and their meaning are listed below.

PREFIXES	MEANING	EXAMPLES(S)
A-, an-	Without	Anechoic, anencephaly
Ab-	Away from	Abduct
Abdomino-, abdomin-	Pertaining to the abdomen	Abdominal
Acous-	Related to hearing, sound	Acoustic
Acro-	Extremity	Acroataxia
Ad-	Toward	Adduct
Adeno-	Gland, related to a gland	Adenonoma, adenopathy
Adip-, Adipo-	Fat, fatty	Adipose tissue
Adren-, adreno-	Related to the adrenal glands	Adrenal
Amni-	Amnion	Amniocentesis
Andr-	Male	Androgen
Angio-	Blood vessel	Angiography, angioedema, angioma
Anis-, aniso-	Unequal, uneven	Anisotropy
Ante-	Before, forward	Antepartum
Anti-	Against	Antibacterial, antibody

Antr-	Antrum	Antrum of the stomach
Aort-	Aorta	Aortic stenosis
Appendic-	Appendix	Appendicolith
Ateri-, aterio-	Related to the artery	Arteriosclerosis
Arthro-	Joint, limb	Arthropathy, arthrolithiasis
Atel-	Incomplete, partial	Atelectasis
Axill-	Armpit	Axilla
Bi-	Two, twice	Bistable
Blast-, blasto-	Developing cell, bud	Blastocyst, myeloblast
Brachi-	Arm	Brachial
Brady-, brachy-	Slow, less, small	Bradycardia, brachycephalic
Burs-	Sac, cavity	Bursitis
Calc-	Calcium	Calculus
Carcin-, carcino-	Cancer	Carcinoma
Cardi-, cardio-	Heart	Tachycardia
Carp-, carpo-	Related to the wrist	Carpal tunnel
Caud-	Below, lower part of body	Caudal
Ceph-, cephal-, cephalo-	Head, toward the head	Cephalic
Cere-, cerebr-, cerebro-	Brain	Cerebellum, cerebral spinal fluid
Cerv-	Neck	Cervical spine
Chol-, chole-, cholagi-	Bile, bile duct	Cholangitis
Cholecyst-	Gallbladder	Cholecystitis
Choledocho-	Common bile duct	Choledocholithiasis
Chondr-	Cartilage	Chondromalacia
Chori-	Chorion	Human chorionic gonadotropin (HCG)
Colp-	Vagina	Hydrocolpos, hematometrocolpos
Contra-	Opposite	Contralateral
Cost-	Rib	Intercostal
Cutan-, cutane-	Skin	Cutaneous
Cyan-. cyano-	Blue	Cyanosis
Cyst-, cysto-	Bladder, cyst, sac	Cystitis
Cyt-, cyte-, cyto-	Cell	Cytology, Cytolysis
Derm-, derma-, dermat-	Skin, dermis	Subdermal, dermatitis

Di-, dif, dis-	Separate, two	Diamniotic, dizygotic
Dia-	Through, across	Dialysis
Dors-	Toward the back	Dorsal
Duodeno-	Duodenum, top of stomach	Duodenum
Dys-	Difficult, painful	Dysphagia, dysmenorrhea
Ecto-, ectop-	Outside	Ectopic, ectoderm
Em-, en-	In, within, before	Enteric
Encephal-	Pertaining to the brain	Encephalocele
Endo-	Inside	Endovaginal, endoderm
Enter-, entero-	Intestine, intestinal	Enteric
Epi-	Around, above, upon	Epithelium, epididymis
Esophago-	Esophagus	Esophagitis
Eryth-, erythr-	Red	Erythema
Ex-, exo-, extra-	Away from, out of, outside	Exocrine
Fibr-	Fibrous tissue	Fibroid
Galact- galacto-	Milk	Galactocele
Gastr-, gastro-	Stomach	Gastritis
Gloss-, glott-	Tongue	Glossitis
Glyco-, gluco-, gluca-	Sugar, related to sugar	Glucagon
Gravid-	Pregnancy, related to pregnancy	Gravida
Gyn-. Gyno-, gyne-	Woman, related to women	Gynecology, gynecomastia
Hema-, hemato-, hemo-	Blood	Hematemesis
Hemi-	Half	Heminephrectomy
Hepat-	Liver	Hepatomegaly
Hetero-	Different	Heterogeneous
Hist-, histo-, histio-	Tissue	Histology
Homo-	Same	Homogeneous
Homeo-	Body	Homeostasis
Hydro-, hydr-	Water, Fluid	Hydrocele, hydronephrodis
Hyper-	Increased, extreme	Hyperechoic, hypertension
Hypo-	Below, less	Hypoechoic
Hyster-	Uterus	Hysterectomy
Infra-	Below	Infrasound

Inter-	Between	Interface
Intra-	Within	Intraperitoneal
Ipsi-	Same	Ipsilateral
Iso-	Same, similar	Isoechoic
Leuk-, leuc-	White	Leukocyte
Lipo-	Fat	Lipoma, angiomyolipoma
Lith-	Stone, calculi	Lithotripsy, appendicolith
Macro-	Large, enlarged	Macrosomia, macrocephaly
Mamm-, mammo-, masto-	Breast, related to the breast	Mammography
Mega-	Large, enlarged	Splenomegaly, hepatomegaly
Mening-, meningo-	Meninges	Meningocele
Mes-, meso-	Middle	Mesoderm
Metr-, metro-	Related to the uterus	Metrorrhagia
Micro-	Small	Microcephaly
Mono-	Single, singular	Monoamniotic, monozygotic
Multi-	Many	Multigravida
Musculo-	Muscle	Musculoskeletal
Myo-, my-	Muscle	Myomectomy
Myco-	Fungus	Mycophage
Myel-	Spinal cord	Lipomyelocele, myelocystocele
Necr-	Death	Necrosis
Neo-	New	Neoplasm
Nephr-, nephro-	Kidney	Nephritis, nephron
Neuro-	Nerve	Neuropathy, neurosonography
Oligo-	Less, Few	Oligohydramnios, oliguria
Omphal-, omphalo-	Related to the umbilicus	Omphalocele
Oophor- oophoro-, ovario-	Related to the ovary	Oophorectomy
Osteo-	Bone	Osteomyelitis
Para-	Abdominal, alongside, nearby	Paracentesis
Patho-	Diseased, diseased state	Pathology
Pelvo-, pelvi-	Pelvic	Pelvis, pelviectasis
Peri-	Around	Periumbilical
Periton-	Peritoneum	Peritoneal

Phleb-	Vessel, blood vessel	Phlebitis, phlebotomy
Poly-	Increased, more, many	Polyhydramnios
Post-	After	Postpartum
Pseudo-	False	Pseudoaneurysm
Pyel-	Renal pelvic	Pyelonephritis
Pyo-	Pus	Pyonephritis, pyosalpinx
Re-	Again	Recur
Ren-, reno-	Related to the kidney	Renal
Retro-	Behind	Retroperitoneum
Salpin-, salpingo-	Related to fallopian tubes	Salpingitis, salpingectomy
Sclero-	Hard	Ateriosclerosis
Splen-, spleno-	Related to the spleen	Splenomegaly
Spondy-	Spine	Spondylitis
Sten-, steno-	Narrow	Stenosis
Sub-	Below	Subcutaneous
Supra-	Above	Suprasternal
Tachy-	Fast	Tachycardia
Therm-	Temperature	Hypothermic
Thora-, thorac-, thoraco	Chest	Thoracentesis
Thrombo-	Clot	Thrombosis
Thymo-	Thymus	Thymopharyngeal, thymosin
Thyro-	Thyroid	Thyromegaly
Tracheo-	Trachea	Tracheotomy
Trans-	Through, across	Transmission, transfusion
Tri-	Three, triple	Triplet
Ultra-	Above, excessive	Ultrasound
Umbili-, umbilic-	Belly button, umbilicus	Umbilical
Varic-, varico-	Swollen, twisted vein	Varicocele
Vaso-, vasculo-	Blood vessel	Vasodilate
Veno-, vena-	Venous	Arteriovenous fistula, inferior vena cava
Ventricul-	Related to the ventricles	Ventriculitis
Xantho-	Yellow	Xanthogranulomatous

Suffixes

Some of the suffixes and their meaning are listed below.

SUFFIXES	MEANING	EXAMPLE(S)
-algia	Pain	Myalgia
-angio	Vessel	Hemangioma
-apheresis	Removal, removal of	Thrombocytapheresis
-capnea	Carbon dioxide	Hypocapnea
-cele	Herniation, pouching	Meningocele, hydrocele
-centesis	Puncture	Paracentesis, thoracentesis
-cidal	To kill	Germicidal
-crine	To secrete	Endocrine, exocrine
-dynia	Pain	Mastodynia
-echo, -echoic	Related to echoes	Hypoechoic, hyperechoic
-ectasis	Dilate, Stretch	Ductal ectasia
-ectomy	Removal, excision	Hysterectomy, cholecystectomy
-ema	Swelling	Edema
-emesis	Vomit	Hematemesis
-emia	Related to blood, blood condition	Anemia
-gen	From, of a specific kind, born in	Heterogeneous
-genesis, -genic	Origin, produced from	Organogenesis
-gram, -graphy	Recording	Sonogram, sonography
-ia, -iasis	Condition	Lithiasis, giardiasis
-iatry	Field of medicine, component	Podiatry
-itis	Inflammation	Cholecystitis, appendicitis
-lith	Stone	Appendicolith, lithiasis
-lysis	To dissolve	Hemolysis
-malacia	Softening	Osteomalacia
-megaly	Enlarged, large	Hepatomegaly, splenomegaly
-oid	Similar, like	Carcinoid
-ologous	In relation to, relating to	Analogous, homologous
-oma	Tumor, swelling	Gastrinoma
-opathy	Disease	Lymphadenopathy
-oscopy	To view, view	Cystoscopy, Endoscopy
-osis	A process, pathologic condition	Diverticulosis

-ostomy	Opening, mouth	Duodenostomy
-otomy	To cut	Laparotomy, episiotomy
-penia	Decrease	Thrombocytopenia
-phage	To eat	Macrophage
-plasia	Formation, to form	Hyperplasia
-pnea	Breath, air	Apnea, dyspnea
-ptosis	Downward, to fall	Nephroptosis
-rrhage, -rrhagia, -rhage	Discharge	Hemorrhage
-rrhea, -rhea	Excessive flow	Dysmenorrhea
-sarcoma	Malignant tumor of the connective tissues	Angiosarcoma
-stasis	Standing still	Homeostasis, hemostasis
-stomy	Opening	Ostomy
-tension, -tensive	Related to blood pressure	Hypertension, hypotension
-trophy, -trophic	Growth, nourish	Dystrophy, hypotrophic
-uresis	Micturition	Enuresis
-uria	Urine	Proteinuria
-xia	Oxygen	Hypoxia, hypoxic

Sections III, IV, V Review: Sonographic Instrumentation, Patient Care, and Helpful Correlations

1. What is the propagation speed of sound in soft tissue?
    a. 330 m/s
    b. 1540 m/s
    c. 1580 m/s
    d. 4080 m/s

2. What artifact is frequently demonstrated posterior to a highly attenuating structure?
    a. Posterior enhancement
    b. Edge shadow
    c. Shadowing
    d. Reverberation

3. What can the sonographer adjust to decrease aliasing of a spectral Doppler waveform?
    a. Increase the gain
    b. Increase the PRF
    c. Increase the filter
    d. Decrease the frame rate

4. Which is the narrowest part of the ultrasound beam?
    a. Fresnel zone
    b. Focal zone
    c. Fraunhofer zone
    d. Huygens zone

5. Which of the following would increase temporal resolution?
    a. Increase number of focal zones
    b. Increase depth
    c. Decrease sector width
    d. Decrease frequency

6. Which type of transducer produces a rectangle image shape?
    a. Linear array
    b. Vector array
    c. Annular array
    d. Curved linear array

7. Total energy is the sum of kinetic, gravitational, and _____ energies.
    a. Inertial
    b. Pressure
    c. Electric
    d. Acoustic

8. Which type of flow is seen when the capillaries are open during systole?
    a. Triphasic
    b. Monophasic
    c. High resistance
    d. Low resistance

9. Which type of waveform is demonstrated?

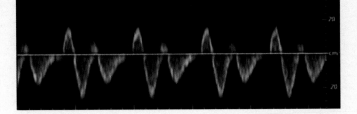

    a. Phasic venous flow
    b. Forward flow
    c. Turbulent flow
    d. Pulsatile venous flow

10. While supine, hydrostatic pressure at the ankle is
    a. 100
    b. 60
    c. 30
    d. 0

11. Relative motion between the transducer and blood flow creates a change in frequency known as
    a. Time of flight
    b. Doppler shift
    c. Fundamental frequency
    d. Bandwidth

12. **Which type of transducer does not create an anatomic image?**

    a. Phased array

    b. Linear sequential

    c. Continuous wave

    d. Convex

13. **What is the most common error associated with Doppler ultrasound?**

    a. Aliasing

    b. Ghosting

    c. Crosstalk

    d. Clutter

14. **The top of a spectral Doppler display is known as the**

    a. Baseline

    b. Spectral gain

    c. Nyquist limit

    d. Sample volume size

15. **Which of the following is related to spectral broadening?**

    a. Plug flow

    b. Laminar flow

    c. Parabolic flow

    d. Turbulent flow

16. **How should the patient be positioned for a paracentesis?**

    a. Supine or lateral decubitus

    b. Prone or lateral decubitus

    c. Lateral decubitus or left posterior oblique

    d. Lateral decubitus or right posterior oblique

17. **For which procedure is a radiologist required to be present?**

    a. Pyloric ultrasound

    b. Ultrasound of the appendix

    c. Paracentesis

    d. Ascites check

18. **For which sonographic procedure should sterile gel be used?**

    a. Pyloric ultrasound

    b. Renal biopsy

    c. Ultrasound of the appendix

    d. Pre-transplant evaluation

19. **Devices that convert energy from one form to another are called**

    a. Currents

    b. Elements

    c. Transducers

    d. Phantoms

20. **What transducer component shortens the pulse to decrease ringing?**

    a. Backing layer

    b. Matching layer

    c. Acoustic insulator

    d. Electrical shield

21. **The range of frequencies emitted above and below the resonant frequency is called**

    a. Scale

    b. Bandwidth

    c. Harmonics

    d. Baseline

22. **As frame rate increases, which resolution is improved?**

    a. Spatial

    b. Elevational

    c. Axial

    d. Temporal

23. **Which of the following is an ultrasound frequency?**

    a. 15 Hz

    b. 10 kHz

    c. 18,000 Hz

    d. 22 kHz

24. **Which transducer would most optimally demonstrate the infant spinal cord?**

    a. 3-8 MHz linear transducer

    b. 5-17 MHz linear transducer

    c. 3-5 MHz curved transducer

    d. 4-12 MHz curved transducer

25. **Which of the following lab values increase with decreasing renal function?**

    a. Lactate dehydrogenase

    b. Amylase

    c. Bilirubin

    d. Blood urea nitrogen

26. Which of the following is a grayscale artifact?

    a. Aliasing

    b. Spectral broadening

    c. Anisotropy

    d. Crosstalk

27. Which of the following frequencies will have the best axial resolution?

    a. 1 MHz

    b. 5 MHz

    c. 10 MHz

    d. 15 MHz

28. With which age group could the sonographer begin providing opportunity for medical play such as allowing the patient to touch the ultrasound gel or transducer?

    a. Infant

    b. Toddler

    c. School Age

    d. Adolescent

29. Which age group lacks brown adipose tissue?

    a. Neonates

    b. Infants

    c. Toddlers

    d. Adolescents

30. Which body plane separates the body into front and back halves?

    a. Sagittal

    b. Transverse

    c. Coronal

    d. Longitudinal

31. The bending of a sound wave during transmission is

    a. Reflection

    b. Refraction

    c. Resolution

    d. Rarefaction

32. How should an endocavitary transducer be cleaned?

    a. Low-level disinfection

    b. Medium-level disinfection

    c. High-level disinfection

    d. Sterilization

33. When performing an abdominal exam on a 14-year-old patient, which transducer should the sonographer select?

    a. C1-5 MHz

    b. C10-14 MHz

    c. L4-10 MHz

    d. L6-15 MHz

34. Which portion of the transducer emits the sound beam?

    a. Piezoelectric element

    b. Backing material

    c. Focusing lens

    d. Matching layers

35. Which of the following is defined as the progressive weakening of the amplitude of the sound beam?

    a. Absorption

    b. Attenuation

    c. Scattering

    d. Reflection

36. The best Doppler signal is achieved with which Doppler angle?

    a. 0°

    b. 45°

    c. 60°

    d. 90°

37. Which of the following is a benefit of power Doppler?

    a. Decreased flow sensitivity

    b. Increased flow sensitivity

    c. Doppler angle dependency

    d. Decreased spatial resolution

38. A 12-year-old patient is referred for abdominal distention. During the abdominal sonogram, the sonographer notes a hyperechoic, multifocal mass in the liver, consistent with hepatocellular carcinoma. Which laboratory value would the sonographer expect to be elevated with this patient?

    a. Serum alpha-fetoprotein

    b. Lipase

    c. Amylase

    d. Alkaline phosphatase

39. Which laboratory values are increased in acute pancreatitis?

    a. BUN and creatinine

    b. ALP and bilirubin

    c. Lipase and amylase

    d. Bilirubin and AFP

40. Which artifact is seen posterior to a simple cyst?

    a. Acoustic shadowing

    b. Enhancement

    c. Refraction

    d. Reflection

41. Edge shadowing is a common artifact in sonographic imaging that is the result of which of the following processes on the sound beam?

    a. Increased impedance

    b. Refraction

    c. Decreased impedance

    d. Compressed reverberation

42. The color twinkle artifact is commonly seen posterior to which structure?

    a. Simple cyst

    b. Complex cyst

    c. Calcification (calculi)

    d. Multifocal mass

43. Which artifact is seen with when the sound beam is perpendicular to blood flow, or the spectral gain is too high?

    a. Spectral broadening

    b. Mirror image

    c. Color twinkle

    d. Spectral aliasing

44. The lack of which tissue causes rapid heat loss in neonates?

    a. Black adipose

    b. Brown adipose

    c. Black fibrous

    d. Brown fibrous

45. The position in which the patient's feet are higher than the head is

    a. Trendelenburg

    b. Decubitus

    c. Supine

    d. Upright

46. Hospital acquired infections affect how many patients annually?

    a. 1 in 21

    b. 1 in 31

    c. 2 in 21

    d. 2 in 31

47. Which pathogen can only be removed or killed with hand washing?

    a. VRE

    b. MRSA

    c. C. Diff

    d. HPV

48. What percentage of hydrogen peroxide is commonly used for high-level disinfection in healthcare?

    a. 25%

    b. 35%

    c. 45%

    d. 55%

49. What is the most common malignant liver mass in infants and children?

    a. Hemangioendothelioma

    b. Hemangioma

    c. Focal nodular hyperplasia

    d. Hepatoblastoma

50. What is the most common islet-cell tumor of the pancreas?

    a. Insulinoma

    b. Gastrinoma

    c. Adenocarcinoma

    d. Pseudocyst

51. What is the most common testicular tumor in a pediatric patient?

    a. Rhabdomyosarcoma

    b. Yolk sac carcinoma

    c. Choriocarcinoma

    d. Seminoma

52. What is the most common soft tissue sarcoma in childhood?

    a. Lymphoma

    b. Fibroadenoma

    c. Rhabdomyosarcoma

    d. Neuroblastoma

53. **What is the most common malignant bladder tumor?**

    a. Leiomyoma

    b. Papilloma

    c. Rhabdomyosarcoma

    d. Nephroblastoma

54. **Which disorder is autosomal dominant?**

    a. Cystic fibrosis

    b. Tuberous sclerosis

    c. Wolman disease

    d. Wilson disease

55. **Which type of teratoma appears as an echogenic mass with calcifications and cystic areas of necrosis and degeneration?**

    a. Ovarian

    b. Cervical

    c. Intracranial

    d. Scrotal

56. **The sonographic appearance of lymphoma is described as**

    a. Single hypoechoic lesion

    b. Multiple hypoechoic areas

    c. Single hyperechoic area

    d. Multiple hyperechoic areas

57. **Rhabdomyosarcoma in which location will appear as a "bunch of grapes" with a complex, cystic appearance?**

    a. Bladder

    b. Liver

    c. Cervical

    d. Testicular

Appendices

1. C
   - Sonography of the neonatal brain is performed through the fontanelles (anterior, posterior, mastoid, and sphenoid) of the pediatric skull. The fontanelles allow for an acoustic window throughout the first year of life and begin to close near 9 months of age. The anterior fontanelle is the most common acoustic window used for sonography of the neonatal brain.

2. A
   - By three weeks gestation the neural tube is completely formed with the cephalic end of the tube closing before the caudal end. The caudal end of the neural tube forms the spinal cord while the cranial end forms the brain.

3. C
   - In healthy infants the position of the conus medullaris should be located above the L2-L3 disc space, with the cord ending between T12-L2. A conus tip below the level of the L2-L3 disc space is suggestive of a tethered cord.

4. D
   - The pancreas is an organ composed of exocrine and endocrine tissues, as well as fibrous stroma parenchyma, vessels, nerves, and lymphatics. The endocrine tissues are made of islet cells, which make up 2% of the pancreas.

5. B
   - Hepatic ligaments and fissures include the falciform ligament, ligamentum teres, ligamentum venosum, and main lobar fissure. The ligamentum teres is a remnant of the fetal umbilical vein which is also known as the round ligament of the liver. This ligament runs along the free edge of the falciform ligament from the umbilicus into the left lobe.

6. D
   - Riedel's lobe is a congenital variant more common in females projecting (tongue-like projection) from the anterior right lobe of the liver to the iliac crest.

7. A
   - The spleen is a homogeneous organ, more echogenic than the kidney and equal to or more echogenic than the liver. The spleen is held in place by the gastrosplenic and splenorenal ligaments and may be enlarged if it's seen extending below the inferior margin of the left kidney.

8. C
   - The location of the appendix is at the lower end of the cecum, a portion of the large intestine, in the right lower abdominal quadrant.

9. C
   - The small bowel is located centrally and large bowel peripherally within the abdomen. The average thickness of the small bowel wall is between 2-3 mm. Wall thickening greater than 3 mm may indicate bowel disease along with increased color Doppler suggesting intestinal inflammation.

10. A
    - The largest salivary gland is the parotid gland. This gland is located inferior to the earlobe and is comprised of two lobes. The larger superficial lobe makes up 80% of the parotid, while the smaller deep lobe makes up only 20%. Normally the parotid gland is homogeneous and hyperechoic to the adjacent masseter muscle, surrounded by small lymph nodes.

11. B
    - The thyroid is a mid-level homogenous structure surrounded by the strap, sternocleidomastoid and longus colli muscles. The strap muscles are made up of sternohyoid, sternothyroid, thyrohyoid, and omohyoid.

12. B
    - The thymus changes appearance as the patient ages, being largest in neonatal patients and young infants. The thymus begins developing between 6-8 weeks gestational age and is located anterior to the great vessels and posterior to the sternum. The view that allows best visualization of the thymus is transsternal, over the sternum. The thymus may be more difficult to visualize with increasing age, as the thymus begins to atrophy and undergoes fatty replacement as patients reach puberty.

13. D
    - Cartilaginous structures have well-defined echogenic margins with hypoechoic echotexture in relation to muscle and bone. Major joint spaces in the body that can be visualized with ultrasound include the hip, knee, ankle, foot, shoulder, elbow, wrist, and hand.

14. A
- In both the upper and lower extremities, central arteries should normally demonstrate a triphasic flow pattern with forward flow acceleration in systole, reversal of flow in early diastole, and low amplitude antegrade flow during late diastole. With exercise and warmth antegrade diastolic flow will increase and will decrease with vasoconstriction. Arterial occlusion is noted when there is absence of Doppler signal or color flow.

15. C
- Arteries can easily be differentiated from veins because the lumen of a normal artery is anechoic and the walls are thicker than those of the adjacent veins, and arteries will not collapse when pressure is applied to them with the transducer. Arterial layers include the tunica intima, tunica media, and tunica adventitia.

16. D
- The three aortic branches that arise from the celiac axis are common hepatic, left gastric, and splenic arteries. Of these branches, the left gastric is the smallest branch and the splenic is the largest. The common hepatic artery further bifurcates into the proper hepatic and gastroduodenal artery.

17. B
- Normal intracranial arterial blood flow patterns are assessed with RI and flow velocity. RI and flow velocity are dependent on prematurity and vary by age in full-term neonates. In premature infants under thirty weeks of gestational age, diastolic flow in the intracranial arteries may be absent (important to note, other factors can affect this in infants, i.e., patent ductus arteriosus [PDA]). In full-term infants antegrade flow is present throughout systole and diastole. Normal intracranial arterial blood flow patterns will show systolic and diastolic velocities increasing and resistive indices decreasing as gestational age increases.

18. A
- The main renal arteries can be seen branching off the abdominal aorta and course posterior to the main renal veins. Branches of the main renal artery include the parenchymal, intrarenal, segmental, interlobar, and outermost arcuate arteries. The main renal arteries should readily demonstrate a low-impedance waveform, indicating appropriate perfusion to the kidneys.

19. B
- The normal PSV in adults is 100–180 cm/sec, and the normal EDV is 25–50 cm/sec. The normal ratio of renal artery PSV to aortic PSV (RAR) is less than 3.5. The main renal artery peak systolic velocity (PSV) ranges from 30-52 cm/sec in neonatal patients and 100-110 cm/sec in older children. The PSV decreases the further the artery branches into the renal parenchyma. Systolic acceleration time (AT) is usually equal to or less than 0.07 seconds throughout the start of systolic upstroke to early systolic peak (ESP).

20. D
- The left gonadal vein enters the left renal vein then into the inferior vena cava, whereas the right gonadal vein enters directly into the inferior vena cava.

21. C
- The anterior fontanelle is the main acoustic window, although the brain can be visualized through the posterior and mastoid fontanelles for axial views. The mastoid fontanelle is most used to evaluate the posterior fossa, which includes the cerebellum and area of the fourth ventricle, although it can enable evaluation of other structures (i.e., circle of Willis, posterior ventricles).

22. B
- The aorta becomes the abdominal aorta after it passes through the diaphragm. The aorta has multiple abdominal branches including the celiac axis, superior mesenteric artery, renal arteries, gonadal arteries, inferior mesenteric artery, and eventually bifurcates to form the iliac vessels.

23. C
- The celiac axis is the first branch off the abdominal aorta. The three aortic branches that arise from the celiac axis are common hepatic, left gastric, and splenic arteries.

24. A
- Branches of the main renal arteries include the parenchymal, intrarenal, segmental, interlobar, and outermost arcuate arteries in the bilateral kidneys.

25. A
- Hepatic ligaments and fissures include the falciform ligament, ligamentum teres, ligamentum venosum, and main lobar fissure. The ligamentum venosum separates the left lobe from the caudate lobe. The ligamentum venosum is the obliterated ductus venosus which in fetal life shunts blood between the umbilical vein and IVC to bypass the liver.

26. C
- The inferior and superior vena cava return blood to the right atrium of the heart. Flow in the proximal inferior vena cava is influenced by activity of the right atrium of the heart and shows back-pressure changes with spectral Doppler imaging.

27. B
- The thyroid gland contains right and left lobes connected by an isthmus and is covered by a fibrous tissue capsule. The trachea is located directly posterior to the thyroid isthmus.

28. D
- Sonography of the neonatal brain is performed through the fontanelles (anterior, posterior, mastoid, and sphenoid) of the pediatric skull. The fontanelles allow for an acoustic window throughout the first year of life and begin to close near 9 months of age. However, the acoustic windows via these fontanelles may become limited even within the first 3 to 6 months of life.

29. A
- The anterior fontanelle is the main acoustic window, although the brain can be visualized through the posterior and mastoid fontanelles for axial views. The anterior (bregma, frontal) fontanelle closes around two years of age.

30. B
- The cerebellum is located in the posterior fossa. This structure is separated from the cerebrum by the tentorium cerebelli and is connected to the brainstem. The cerebellum, like the supratentorial brain (i.e., cerebrum), consists of gray and white matter. The cerebellum is the largest component of the hindbrain and is made up of two hemispheres, connected by the vermis. The cerebellum controls posture, balance, and voluntary movements.

31. C
- A 7.5 MHz phased array or vector transducer is used for premature infants, and a 5 MHz transducer is needed for larger older infants. Imaging includes coronal anterior to posterior views, followed by sagittal midline to right and midline to left. Superficial sagittal sinus and mastoid views may also be obtained. In the anterior-most coronal view of the neonatal brain the interhemispheric (longitudinal) fissure is seen dividing the cerebrum into right and left hemispheres, in addition to the ethmoid sinus, orbital roofs, and frontal lobe.

32. B
- Length of fasting time is based upon the patient's age. General guidelines for patient preparation and fasting include the following: a newborn less than one year of age should fast 2 hours (particularly important in cases of suspected biliary atresia). Patients less than 5 years of age should be NPO 4 hours prior to an abdominal ultrasound. Patients greater than 5 years of age should remain NPO for 6 hours. Adolescents approaching adulthood should be fasting a full 8 hours prior to abdominal ultrasound exam to reduce bowel gas artifact and fully distend the gallbladder.

33. C
- The main pancreatic duct is known as the duct of Wirsung, which joins the CBD. The normal duct of Wirsung measures less than 3 mm in the head of the pancreas. The head of the pancreas sits in the C-loop of the duodenum which is commonly termed the "romance of the abdomen".

34. C
- The appendix is a compressible, blind-ending structure which normally measures less than 6mm in maximum diameter.

35. C
- Zone IIA of the neck correlates to the upper internal jugular region, or more specifically anteromedial to the internal jugular vein at the level of the parotid gland.

36. A
- The diaphragm is a muscle that separates the thoracic and abdominal cavities. The diaphragm is dome-shaped, with the right dome slightly more superior due to the large underlying right hepatic lobe. Sonographically the diaphragm appears as a smooth, slightly curved, echogenic line adjacent to the spleen and liver.

37. B
- To best view structures of the pediatric chest, imaging approaches may include supraclavicular, suprasternal, parasternal, trans-sternal, intercostal, sub-xiphoid, sub-diaphragmatic, and posterior paraspinal acoustic windows, depending on the region of interest to be imaged. Ultrasound of the chest is often performed to rule out pleural effusion. It is preferred that the patient is sitting for this procedure, however it may be performed supine when necessary.

38. C
- The femoral head is the superior-most portion of the femur. At birth, the femoral head is cartilaginous and hypoechoic to bone. The femoral head ossification center develops between the second and eighth months of life.

39. D
- In this image, the hip joint is being imaged in coronal view. Examination of the hip is most successfully performed in patients under six months of age.

40. C
- The greater saphenous veins of the lower extremity are superficial and are the body's longest veins.

41. A
- The common iliac artery (CIA) arises from the bifurcation of the distal abdominal aorta, further dividing into the internal and external iliac arteries. The external iliac arteries continue to form the common femoral arteries of the lower extremities.

42. B
- An artery is a hollow muscular tube enclosed in a sheath, whose purpose is to carry blood away from the heart. Arteries have three layers, including the tunica intima, tunica media, and tunica adventitia. The endothelial tunica intima is the innermost layer. The muscular tunica media is in the middle and can handle high pressure. The adventitial layer is the outermost layer and comprised of connective tissue.

43. B
- In healthy infants the position of the conus medullaris should be located above the L2-L3 disc space, with the cord ending between T12-L2. A conus tip below the level of the L2-L3 disc space is suggestive of a tethered cord.

44. B
   - The appendix is a compressible, blind-ending structure which normally measures less than 6 mm in maximum diameter. If the structure the sonographer is evaluating appears continuous and a blind end cannot be detected, the sonographer may have identified the terminal ileum, which can mimic the appearance of the appendix when compressed.

45. A
   - This anterior coronal image demonstrates the orbital roofs, area of the ethmoid sinus, and interhemispheric fissure dividing the right and left frontal lobes of the brain.

46. C
   - The epididymis sits posterolateral to each testicle and functions to store and move sperm from each teste into the spermatic cord (vas deferens). The epididymal heads are hypoechoic, hypovascular, ovoid to triangular structures that have a continuous body and tail.

47. A
   - The major intracranial arteries include the anterior cerebral, middle cerebral, posterior cerebral, and internal carotid arteries. The circle of Willis is made up from the branches of the internal carotid arteries and basilar artery. This creates the network of vessels that perfuse brain tissue. Anteriorly, the circle of Willis is formed by the right and left anterior cerebral arteries which communicate via the anterior communicating artery. Likewise, posteriorly the connection is via the posterior cerebral arteries and posterior communicating arteries, where the basilar artery joins them.

Section II Answer Key:

1. C
   - Renal cell carcinoma is associated with von Hippel Lindau syndrome, urogenital malformations, tuberous sclerosis, and Beckwith-Wiedemann syndrome. Renal cell carcinoma presents in 2-4% of patients with tuberous sclerosis.

2. A
   - Sturge-Weber syndrome is a neurocutaneous syndrome associated with vascular malformation lesions. Sturge-Weber patients may have nevus flammeus, which is a slow flow vascular lesion with abnormal venous spaces and normal arterial components

3. B
   - Simple meningoceles are posterior herniations through a bony vertebral defect. These herniations are simple, only filled with cerebrospinal fluid. This causes the appearance of a cyst-like mass within the posterior subcutaneous tissues.

4. C
   - Hematologic elements secondary to extracorporeal oxygenation (ECMO) related to splenic pooling of damaged red blood cells during ECMO can cause splenic enlargement.

5. A
   - Complications of splenic torsion and infarct include abscess formation, bowel obstruction, pancreatitis, or necrosis of the pancreatic tail, and if venous congestion is present gastric varices may develop.

6. C
   - With cystic fibrosis there is abnormally thick luminal secretions which lead to pancreatic duct obstruction, glandular atrophy, fibrosis, fatty replacement, and exocrine dysfunction. This can lead to symptoms of abdominal pain, fat intolerance, steatorrhea, and failure to thrive in 90% of cystic fibrosis or affected patients. The sonographic appearance of cystic fibrosis within the pancreas can include a hyperechoic fatty pancreas, possible cyst formation, calcifications, and atrophy.

7. D
   - Solid pseudopapillary tumors are low-grade malignant and arise from the pancreatic tail. These exocrine lesions are large generally measuring around 9 centimeters. They have a well-defined, complex sonographic appearance with areas of hemorrhage and cystic degeneration.

8. B
   - Approximately 50% of children with severe acute pancreatitis have extra-pancreatic fluid collections that lack a well-defined capsule. Other extra-pancreatic abnormalities associated with severe acute pancreatitis are bowel wall thickening, gallbladder wall thickening, pericholecystic fluid, and splenic involvement including infarct, hemorrhage, or abscess. Pseudocyst formation is the most common complication of acute pancreatitis.

9. C
   - Idiopathic fibrosing pancreatitis is characterized as chronic pancreatitis of unknown cause, where pancreatic parenchyma begins to replace with fibrous tissue. This replacement can cause obstructive jaundice as fibrotic tissues narrows the common bile duct. Idiopathic fibrosing pancreatitis is associated with inflammatory bowel disease and is not associated with pseudocyst formation.

10. D
   - Hypertrophic pyloric stenosis (HPS) is considered an acquired gastric outlet obstruction of the pylorus' circular muscle, resulting in narrowing of the pyloric channel. Positive findings include inability to view gastric emptying, wall thickness equal or greater than 3 millimeters, and an elongated pyloric channel greater than 17 millimeters. Symptoms typically present between 2 to 6 weeks of age and may continue up to 5 months. Clinical findings include projectile nonbilious vomiting, an olive-shaped mass palpated in the epigastrium region, and gastric hyperperistalsis. Hypertrophic pyloric stenosis is 4 to 5 times more likely to occur in males.

11. A
- Pyloric stenosis appears as a hypervascular target or bullseye sign in transverse orientation. This bullseye represents thick hypoechoic muscle surrounding the echogenic mucosa. In sagittal orientation, pyloric stenosis resembles a hypervascular thickened pyloric muscle which surrounds an elongated pyloric channel.

12. B
- Intussusception is telescoping of a proximal segment of intestine, the intussusceptum, into a caudal segment of bowel, the intussuscipiens. Intussusception is the most common acute abdominal disorder of early childhood. This disorder is most common between 3 months to 3 years of age, with peak occurrence between 5 to 9 months.

13. D
- A duplication cyst is a spherical or tubular structure that is lined with GI epithelium and contains smooth muscle in its wall. Enteric duplication cysts may occur anywhere along gastrointestinal tract and are usually attached directly to bowel, sharing the bowels blood supply.

14. A
- Gastric lymphoma is the most common malignant gastrointestinal neoplasm in childhood. Most gastric lymphomas are a non-Hodgkin subtype and include a palpable mass with abdominal pain. Sonographic findings include gastrointestinal wall thickening, hypoechoic polypoid mass with intra- or extra-mural extension, splenomegaly, and surrounding lymph node enlargement.

15. C
- Horseshoe kidney is the most common renal anomaly occurring in approximately 1/400 births. Horseshoe kidney has a 2:1 male predominance with the most common fusion site being at the kidney's lower poles connected by a midline isthmus. The isthmus of the horseshoe kidney may have fibrous tissue or functioning renal parenchyma, with the ureters crossing in front of the isthmus.

16. B
- Autosomal Recessive Polycystic Disease (ARPKD) is also known as infantile polycystic kidney disease. Autosomal recessive polycystic disease is inherited as a recessive characteristic. With this disease innumerable bilateral 1–2-millimeter cysts are seen throughout the medulla representing dilated collecting tubules that extend into the cortex of the kidneys. Sonographic findings in neonatal patients include bilateral renal enlargement, overall increase in parenchymal echogenicity with a hypoechoic peripheral rim, poor corticomedullary differentiation, and dilated bile ducts.

17. C
- Medullary sponge kidney disease, also known as medullary tubular ectasia, is a sporadic, non-inherited disorder involving cystic dilation of renal pyramid collecting tubules.

18. B
- Angiomyolipoma is often associated with tuberous sclerosis (80%) or other phakomatoses (20%). Angiomyolipoma is also associated with lymphangioleiomyomatosis and may occur in patients with neurofibromatosis type 1 (NF1) or von Hippel-Lindau syndrome (vHL).

19. D
- Multicystic dysplastic kidney disease is a non-hereditary developmental anomaly due to early in-utero urinary tract obstruction that occurs within the first ten weeks of gestation. Multiple non-communicating renal cysts of various sizes separated by fibrous tissue contain primitive dysplastic elements in the kidneys. Most cases of multicystic dysplastic kidney disease are diagnosed during prenatal ultrasound.

20. A
- Renal duplication artifact occurs more frequently in the left kidney than in the right. Refractive duplication artifact can be easily confused with duplication of the renal collecting system. With refractive duplication artifact, refraction of sound at the interface between the kidney and spleen or liver and adjacent fat creates an image appearing similar to duplication of the superior aspect on the kidney or simulates a suprarenal mass.

21. D
- Clinical signs and symptoms of intussusception may include stool changes such as diarrhea or a "currant jelly" stool appearance, resulting from a combination of blood and mucous in the stool. Additionally, clinical presentation of intussusception can have variation based on age. Infants tend to be lethargic, have stool changes, and swelling of the abdomen. Young children more often experience vomiting and will draw the knees upward and cry during intermittent spells of abdominal pain. Sonographic findings include a transverse donut or target sign. This target sign represents a complex mass with concentric hypoechoic and hyperechoic rings. The echogenic portion of these rings consists of mucosa and submucosa, with the hypoechoic portion being the muscularis. Some other sonographic findings associated with intussusception include inversion of mesenteric vessels, peritoneal fluid, and dilation of small bowel proximal to the site of intussusception.

22. D
- Pyonephrosis is an accumulation of purulent exudate within the hydronephrotic kidney. This accumulation of exudate occurs due to an obstructive uropathy, ureteral calculi, or ureteral stricture. The most

common cause is Escherichia coli retrograde entering the kidney. Sonographic findings include dilated collecting system with mobile debris and debris in urine, bright echoes with dirty shadowing due to gas, and a fluid-debris level.

23. C
   - Duplication of the renal collecting system can be partial or complete and is the most common congenital anomaly of the urinary tract. S difference of greater than 1 cm in renal length in pediatrics raises suspicion for renal duplication, which can be partial or complete.

24. A
   - A renal to aortic ratio, or renal artery ratio (RAR) is calculated by dividing the highest renal artery peak systolic velocity (PSV) by the aortic PSV at a level distal to the superior mesenteric artery and proximal to renal artery origin. A normal RAR is less than or equal to 3.5.

25. B
   - Predominantly a newborn disease, renal vein thrombosis usually occurs because of severe dehydration, hemoconcentration secondary to blood loss, sepsis, or diarrhea. Sonographic findings of renal vein thrombosis include edema, hemorrhage, adrenal hemorrhage if the left renal vein is involved, acute enlarged kidney with increased echogenicity, absent corticomedullary differentiation, and absent venous signal around the thrombus in the main renal vein to inferior vena cava junction. These findings are followed by chronic decreased echogenicity and atrophied heterogeneous kidney if left untreated.

26. C
   - Mesoblastic nephroma, also known as fetal renal hamartoma, is the most common renal tumor in the neonate. This benign process presents in the first six months of life.

27. A
   - Angiomyolipoma, also referred to as renal hamartoma, is a renal neoplasm with a varying amount of mature adipose tissue (i.e., fat-poor in pediatrics), smooth muscle, and blood vessels. Usually an incidental finding, angiomyolipoma is a small hyperechoic neoplasm in the renal cortex that causes hematuria, abdominal pain, and anemia secondary to hemorrhage.

28. D
   - Wilms tumor, or nephroblastoma, is the most common renal malignancy in children. This pathologic process accounts for 90% of all pediatric renal malignancies and presents before five years of age.

29. C
   - Acute lymphoblastic leukemia is the most common general malignancy of childhood, most prevalent in children 3-5 years of age.

30. B
   - Renal medullary carcinoma is an aggressive neoplasm of epithelial origin within the renal medulla. This malignant process is commonly found in patients with sickle cell trait and hemoglobin sickle cell disease. The right kidney is most susceptible to renal medullary carcinoma, usually occurring in the second to third decade of life.

31. A
   - Rhabdoid tumor is a rare aggressive malignant neoplasm of the renal medulla. This medullary tumor accounts for only 2% of malignancies and occurs around 18 months of age. Clinical findings include abdominal mass, fever, hypertension, and hypercalcemia. Sonographic findings include a large heterogeneous intrarenal mass with indistinct margins, infiltration of the renal hilum, and possible extension into the renal vein and inferior vena cava.

32. C
   - In young pediatric patients the transplant kidney is anastomosed to the distal aorta and IVC within the intraperitoneal cavity. In older pediatric patients the transplant kidney is anastomosed to the iliac vessels in the retroperitoneum. The normal sonographic appearance of a transplant kidney should be similar to a native kidney. The resistive index (RI) should fall between 0.4 to 0.8 with a mean RI of 0.6.

33. B
   - Transplant acute tubular necrosis occurs in first twenty-four hours after transplant resulting from prolonged ischemia. Sonographic findings include graft enlargement, increased cortical echogenicity, loss of corticomedullary differentiation, enlarged hypoechoic pyramids, reversed diastolic flow, and high resistive index.

34. A
   - During fetal development, the umbilicus and anterior bladder wall communicate via the urachus. This tubular channel normally closes during the fourth to fifth month of gestation. If the urachus does not completely close it can result in a patent urachus, urachal sinus, urachal diverticulum, or urachal cyst. Urachal cysts may occur when the channel is closed at the umbilicus and bladder but remain open in the center resembling a cyst.

35. C
   - Rhabdomyosarcoma of the bladder is the most common childhood bladder tumor involving the submucosal trigone region. This malignant mass generally occurs between 2 to 6 years of age and 14 to 18 years of age. Sonographic findings include an echogenic pedunculated soft tissue mass that projects into the bladder lumen. This mass occurs with a complex cystic appearance resembling bunches of grapes, focal wall thickening, and capacity for deep invasion of the bladder is diminished as the bladder

wall becomes deformed and rigid. Hydronephrosis and perivesical invasion, as well as metastases to pelvic lymph nodes can be seen.

36. D
- Wolman disease is an autosomal recessive inborn error of lipid metabolism due to lysosomal acid lipase deficiency and massive cholesterol accumulation throughout the body. Sonographic appearance includes bilaterally enlarged echogenic adrenal glands with prominent necrotic areas and shadowing calcifications in the adrenal cortex.

37. C
- Neuroblastoma is the most common solid extracranial malignant tumor in children, arising in the adrenal medulla or ganglion chain. This adrenal medullary neoplasm has an autosomal dominant inheritance pattern related to an abnormality in the short arm of chromosome 16. Neuroblastoma can present with findings of metastases and has multiple stages. The treatment for neuroblastoma depends on the stage of the tumor. Sonographic appearance includes a suprarenal or paraspinal hyperechoic mass with areas of calcification, necrosis, cystic change, and fluctuating vascularity. This mass may appear hypoechoic in neonatal patients.

38. D
- Spermatoceles are painless palpable masses resulting from cystic dilatation of the efferent tubules. Spermatoceles are seen in the epididymis head and only occur post-pubertal, whereas epididymal cysts can arise anywhere within the epididymis and may occur at any age. Spermatoceles also contain spermatozoa, where epididymal cysts contain no spermatozoa.

39. A
- Cryptorchidism is an incomplete descent of the testicle. Testicular descent is generally completed at birth but may continue postnatally and should be complete by 3 months of age. An undescended teste poses risk for infertility and malignancy. 80% of undescended testicles are located within the inguinal canal. Orchiopexy, or the surgical moving of the undescended teste into the scrotal sac, does not relieve the risk for malignancy or infertility due to underlying testicular dysplasia.

40. D
- Testicular tumors are more common before the age of 2 and at the start of puberty. A teratoma, which is usually benign, is the most common in infants and yolk sac tumor in older boys. Seminomas are malignant germ cell tumors that are rare in children, however are the most common testicular tumor in adults. This neoplasm is commonly associated with cryptorchidism and is usually found later in adolescence if discovered during a pediatric age. The second most common testicular germ cell tumor in an adult is an embryonal cell carcinoma.

41. D
- Mature teratoma, a benign ovarian tumor, is also referred to as cystic teratoma or dermoid cyst. This typically unilateral neoplasm is the most common benign ovarian tumor, accounting for approximately 90% of all benign ovarian tumors. Mature teratomas contain all three germ-cell layers: ectoderm, mesoderm, and endoderm. These masses range anywhere between five millimeters to thirty centimeters in size. Sonographic appearance is complex with multiple appearances, including hypoechoic with echogenic and anechoic components to solid with calcification. This calcification is referred to as tip of the iceberg sign. Mature teratomas may have a fluid-fluid level if sebum, serous fluid, calcium, hair, or fat is involved. When hair is an internal component, it is referred to as a dermoid mesh sign.

42. B
- Yolk sac tumor is otherwise known as endodermal sinus tumor. This lesion presents in prepubescent boys around two years of age. Approximately 80% of these tumors are located in the scrotum and are associated with elevated serum alpha-fetoprotein levels.

43. B
- Cystic Hygroma, also known as cervical lymphangioma, is a benign mass that is endothelial lined, dilated lymphatic space due to a congenital blockage of the lymphatic drainage canals. Sonographically, a cystic hygroma appears as a thin-walled loculated mass, with increased echogenicity, acoustic enhancement, and low velocity Doppler signals may be seen within the septations.

44. D
- Neck neuroblastoma is the most common neurogenic tumor of the neck, along with neurofibroma. Sonographically both a neuroblastoma and neurofibroma appear similar as a paraspinal round or oval echogenic mass, hyperechoic to the adjacent muscle. Echotexture can be homogeneous or heterogeneous, with mild to moderate Doppler flow and scattered calcifications. Age is the only indication to differentiate neuroblastoma from neurofibroma, tissue-sampling must be performed for definitive diagnosis

45. B
- Extralobar, or congenital sequestration, is a congenital thoracic malformation of segmental lung tissue that has no connection to the bronchial tree or pulmonary arteries. ELS is also known as an accessory lung with abnormal vasculature and occurs less commonly than intralobar sequestration (ILS). ELS has its own pleura, separate from any surrounding lung tissue. The primary difference between ELS and ILS, is that ELS is pleura-covered. ELS can be visualized as early at sixteen weeks gestation in-utero and occurs more commonly in neonatal males than females.

46. A
- In patients with congenital, or Bochdalek, diaphragmatic hernias, 80% are seen unilateral and on the left side. A congenital diaphragmatic hernia can be diagnosed in-utero as an asymmetric chest with scaphoid abdomen. Major complications can occur as a result of a diaphragmatic hernia including pulmonary hypoplasia and persistent fetal circulation.

47. C
- On coronal extension and flexion views, the proximal femoral epiphysis, or femoral head, should be covered in the acetabulum by at least 50% of the ilium. Developmental hip dysplasia is diagnosed by findings of a shallow acetabulum or abnormal position of femoral head at rest and with stress.

48. B
- Tenosynovitis is inflammation of the tendon and synovium. The most common cause of inflammatory tenosynovitis in pediatric patients is juvenile rheumatoid arthritis or overuse syndrome, which causes tendon and sheath microtrauma leading to secondary inflammation.

49. A
- Toxic synovitis, otherwise known as transient synovitis, is the most common cause of painful hip and joint effusion in children between five to ten years of age. Clinically, patients present with hip or knee pain and a limp, low grade fever and mild leukocytosis. Sonographically there is fluid in the hip joint capsule, increased capsule to bone distance, and convex capsule margin.

50. C
- Ventriculitis is an intracranial infection where inflammatory exudate organisms gain ventricular access via route of the choroid plexus. Sonographic findings include ventricular dilatation, thickened ependymal lining, intraventricular septations and debris, and increased echogenicity of the choroid plexus.

51. B
- Hydrocephalus is dilatation of the ventricular system associated with increased intraventricular pressure. Hydrocephalus can be communicating (non-obstructive) or non-communicating (obstructive). Non-communicating intra-ventricular hydrocephalus is usually acquired or congenital, such as with Dandy-Walker syndrome. The most common cause of congenital hydrocephalus is aqueductal stenosis.

52. D
- Transcranial Doppler (TCD) is based on time-averaged mean of maximum velocity (TAMMX) where velocities less than 170 cm/sec are considered normal, 170-199 cm/sec are conditional, and greater than 200 cm/sec are read as abnormal. Transcranial Doppler sensitivity for diagnosing stenosis and occlusion is 86-94% accurate.

53. C
- Liver transplant is the only treatment for end-stage liver disease and is done via whole cadaveric allograft, split cadaveric allograft, or living related donor allograft. Hepatic artery thrombosis occurs in 40% of allografts in the first two post-operative months. Portal vein thrombosis occurs in 3-10% of pediatric liver transplants. Inferior vena cava thrombosis occurs in less than 1% of cases.

54. A
- Glycogen storage disease is a family of metabolic storage diseases. This autosomal recessive disorder is the most common carbohydrate metabolism inborn error characterized by excessive glycogen deposition in hepatocytes and proximal renal tubules. Type I glycogen storage disease known as Von Gierke disease is the most common form of glycogen storage disease in pediatrics. Van Gierke disease manifests in the neonatal period with marked hepatomegaly and hypoglycemia.

55. B
- Usually of viral origin, clinical findings of hepatitis include jaundice, liver failure, and abdominal pain. Sonography cannot diagnose hepatitis but can determine whether cause of jaundice is cholestatic or obstructive in nature. Sonographic findings include normal liver parenchyma with mild hepatitis. In more severe cases of acute hepatitis, hepatomegaly, increased portal venule wall echogenicity known as "starry sky" or "starry night" liver, enlarged porta hepatic nodes, gallbladder wall thickening with intraluminal sludge, and hypoechoic liver parenchyma may be prevalent.

56. B
- Fungal abscess is found in immunocompromised children due to Candida albicans or Aspergillus fungi. Sonographic appearance includes multiple small homogeneous hypoechoic lesions with hyperechoic wheel within a wheel or bullseye patterns throughout the liver, spleen, and kidneys. Fungal infection may mimic metastases, lymphoma, and other diseases.

57. C
- Infantile hepatic hemangioma, earlier known as hepatic infantile hemangioendothelioma, is the most common benign hepatic tumor in infants less than 6 months of age. Sonographic appearance is variable; however, color Doppler readily demonstrates increased flow due to prominent vascular channels throughout the mass.

58. D
- Hepatic adenoma is associated with oral contraceptive use, obesity, type I and III glycogen storage disease, metabolic syndrome, diabetes mellitus, and use of anabolic steroids – particularly in young males. This mass is made up of abnormal hepatocytes but does not contain Kupffer cells. Sonographic appearance includes a solitary heterogeneous, well-defined, hypoechoic, or hyperechoic encapsulated tumor comprised of hepatocytes.

59. A
- Hepatocellular carcinoma, or hepatoma, is the second most common malignant pediatric liver tumor. This malignancy most commonly occurs between five to fifteen years of age. Clinical findings include elevated serum alpha-fetoprotein, right upper quadrant mass, and abdominal distention. Sonographic appearance includes a hyperechoic multifocal or diffuse infiltrating mass with hypoechoic rim commonly in the right lobe with vascular invasion, areas of calcification or necrosis, and metastases.

60. C
- Soft tissue hemangioma is the most common vascular soft tissue tumor of infancy. Soft tissue hemangioma presents as a bluish skin discoloration. Sonographic appearance includes well-defined vascular superficial soft tissue mass of varying echogenicity.

61. A
- In reference to superficial etiologies, rhabdomyosarcoma is the most common malignant soft tissue tumor in children. Children less than six years of age are most affected by rhabdomyosarcoma. The most common presenting symptom of rhabdomyosarcoma is a growing mass or swelling wherever the tumor forms. Sonographic appearance is a heterogeneous well-defined irregular mass of low to medium echogenicity with increased flow on color Doppler.

62. B
- Hypertrophic pyloric stenosis (HPS) is considered an acquired gastric outlet obstruction of the pylorus' circular muscle, resulting in narrowing of the pyloric channel. Symptoms typically present between 2 to 6 weeks of age and may continue up to 5 months. Clinical findings include projectile nonbilious vomiting, an olive-shaped mass palpated in the epigastrium region, and gastric hyperperistalsis.

63. A
- Hematometrocolpos is defined as distention of the uterus and vagina with blood product due to obstruction from transverse membranes or septa.

64. A
- In healthy infants the position of the conus medullaris should be located above the L2-L3 disc space, with the cord ending between T12-L2. A conus tip below the level of the L2-L3 disc space is suggestive of a tethered cord.

65. A
- Normal gallbladder variants include Phrygian cap, junctional fold, septations, and Hartman's pouch. Junctional fold is the most common variant of the gallbladder, where the gallbladder folds at the neck region.

66. C
- Pleural effusion is a collection of fluid within the pleural space. Simple pleural effusions are without septations, debris, and internal echoes. A complicated pleural effusion may contain internal echoes, debris, or septations. Sonography is considered superior to CT and radiography in determining whether pleural effusion is containing loculated fluid pockets.

67. B
- In utero the spleen's importance is to aid in production of red blood cells, but this organ is haematopoietically inactive in child and adulthood. Postnatally hematopoiesis of the spleen can resume with disorders such as osteopetrosis and thalassemia major.

68. A
- Meckel's diverticulum is an insidious cause of right lower quadrant pain. It is the most common congenital anomaly of the GI tract. Meckel's diverticulum may be seen as a fluid filled structure with gut signature in the mid to lower abdomen which does not communicate with small bowel. Surrounding bowel loops will be seen peristalsing around this fluid filled structure.

69. C
- Simple pleural effusion is a completely anechoic collection of fluid within the pleural space. Simple pleural effusions are without septations, debris, and internal echoes. A complicated pleural effusion may contain internal echoes, debris, or septations. Sonography is considered superior to CT and radiography in determining whether pleural effusion is containing loculated fluid pockets.

70. D
- Tuberous sclerosis is a phakomatosis or neurocutaneous disorder is transmitted as an autosomal dominant trait. With tuberous sclerosis 90% of patients will have skin lesions, 90% will have seizures, and 50% will have mental retardation. Tuberous sclerosis is clinically characterized as a triad of adenoma sebaceum, mental retardation, and seizures. Only one-third of patients with tuberous sclerosis have this triad of symptoms.

71. B
- Occult spinal dysraphism is a skin-covered (i.e., closed) spinal malformation that can occur with or without an accompanying mass.

72. C
- Filar cysts are of no clinical significance and are an anatomic variant of the spinal cord.

73. A
- Gastrinomas are a pancreatic endocrine and functioning islet-cell tumor. Gastrinoma is the second most common islet-cell tumor seen in approximately 30% of pancreatic endocrine tumor patients.

74. B
- Hydrops is gallbladder distension without inflammation. Hydrops of the gallbladder measures greater than 3 centimeters in length in infants less than 1 year of age and greater than 7 centimeters in length in adolescents.

75. D
- Horseshoe kidney is the most common renal anomaly occurring in approximately 1/400 births. Horseshoe kidney has a 2:1 male predominance with the most common fusion site being at the kidney's lower poles connected by a midline isthmus.

76. C
- With thoracic outlet compression syndrome abnormal Doppler waveforms are encountered in the subclavian artery of the arm affected. For confirmation, multiple tests can be performed including Wright's test (extremity hyperabduction), the Eden test (military brace, shoulders pulled down), or Adson's test (head rotation toward side affected), etc. With these maneuvers, a waveform decrease would be visualized.

77. A
- Wilms tumor, or nephroblastoma, is the most common renal malignancy in children. This pathologic process accounts for 90% of all pediatric renal malignancies and presents before five years of age.

78. A
- Wilms tumor is categorized in stages I-V. With stage I the tumor is limited to the kidney alone and can be resected. In stage II the tumor extends beyond the kidney but may still be resected. In the third stage the Wilms tumor is confined to the abdomen without hematogenous spread. In stage IV hematogenous metastasis may be seen in the lung, liver, bone, and brain tissues. Lastly, stage V consists of bilateral renal involvement at the time of diagnosis.

79. B
- Nephroblastomatosis is the multifocal or diffuse renal involvement with nephrogenic rests. Nephroblastomatosis is a malignant nephrogenesis abnormality and potentially a precursor to Wilms tumor. In 30-40% of cases, nephrogenic rests induce Wilms tumors, and are found in 99% of bilateral Wilms tumors.

80. C
- Rejection is the most common cause of allograft failure. Acute rejection occurs within the first three months. Chronic rejection occurs 3 months to years after the transplant.

81. B
- Perinephric lymphocele is the most common perinephric fluid collection. This collections results from seepage of lymph from severed lymphatic vessels following transplant. Lymphocele typically develops two to eight weeks following surgery

82. D
- Cushing syndrome accounts for effects of various etiologies involving excess glucocorticoid. These may be endogenous or exogenous. Excess cortisol production from endogenous sources involves overproduction of cortisol and ACTH by ACTH-secreting tumors (i.e., pituitary adenoma) in 80% of cases. Adrenal adenomas make up the remaining 20%. Rare endogenous sources include primary pigmented nodular adrenal dysplasia (PPNAD), corticotropin-releasing hormone-secreting tumor, and adrenocorticotropic (ACTH)-independent macronodular adrenocortical hyperplasia (AIMAH). Comparatively, Cushing disease exclusively refers to excess glucocorticoid related to an adrenocorticotropic pituitary adenoma, which secretes hormones including cortisol.

83. A
- It can be helpful to understand medical terminology prefix, suffix, and root words to understand medical and pathological terms, particularly when ruling out answer choices on the registry. The prefix for blood can be expressed as hema-, hemat-, hemo-, or hemato-; These can be helpful in deciphering words such as hematemesis. The suffix -emesis means vomit, or vomiting, therefore the word hematemesis can be broken down into the meaning of vomiting blood.

84. D
- Cryptorchidism is an incomplete descent of the testicle. Testicular descent is generally completed at birth but may continue postnatally and should be complete by 3 months of age. An undescended teste poses risk for infertility and malignancy. 80% of undescended testicles are located within the inguinal canal.

85. C
- The appendix epididymis, or appendix testes, is comprised of embryologic remnants of blind-ending mesonephric tubules and Mullerian duct system. Torsion of the appendix teste is the one of the three most common causes of acute scrotal pain in prepubertal males, along with testicular torsion and epididymitis. Of the answer choices, appendix teste torsion would be the most appropriate.

86. B
- Precocious puberty is the onset of physical pubertal characteristics and hormone levels prior to 8 years of age. This may be caused by dysfunction of the ovaries or adrenal glands and can cause a premature onset of menses. Sonographically, the uterus and ovaries may appear like that of a pubertal patient.

87. B
- When the Mullerian ducts completely fail to fuse, didelphys uterus results. Sonographically, a duplicated vaginal canal, cervix, and uterus is seen.

88. D
- Salpingitis is inflammation of the fallopian tubes. Sonographic findings include fluid-filled, thickened fallopian tubes.

89. A
- A branchial cleft cyst is a congenital epithelial cyst that presents as a non-tender neck mass and has no internal

or external communication. In pediatric patients, branchial cleft cysts are the most common non-inflammatory masses located in the lateral neck region. The branchial apparatus contains 6 arches and 5 clefts. The branchial cleft is a groove between the arches in the cervical region's branchial network where branchial apparatus abnormalities may occur. Benign branchial cleft cysts most commonly occur within this groove, with 90-95% originating in the second branchial cleft.

90. C
- Hashimoto thyroiditis is an autoimmune disorder of the thyroid where antibodies attack the thyroid tissues. Hashimoto's is the most common cause of acquired hypothyroidism and most common thyroid dysfunction in pediatrics.

91. B
- Developmental dysplasia of the hip is caused by abnormal ligamentous laxity accentuated by excessive circulating maternal estrogen levels. Risk factors for DDH increase with family history, breech birth, oligohydramnios during pregnancy, torticollis, foot deformities, and neuromuscular problems. Clinical signs showing possibility of DDH include asymmetric skin folds on thigh, limited hip abduction, and abnormal Barlow and Ortolani maneuvers.

92. C
- The subependymal germinal matrix of the lateral ventricle is the most common bleeding site in premature infants. Subependymal germinal matrix hemorrhage is rarely seen in term infants and typically only visualized when term infants are small for gestational age.

93. C
- Sickle cell disease is a common cause of acute cerebral ischemic infarction in older infants and children. Sickle cell anemia can cause large vessel occlusion at the base of the brain leading to cerebral infarction and stroke. Transcranial Doppler (TCD) studies can detect or monitor MCA vasospasm, aneurysm, basilar artery obstruction, evaluate for ICA stenosis, and monitor real-time blood flow to the brain during surgical procedures. Transcranial Doppler sensitivity for diagnosing stenosis and occlusion is 86-94% accurate.

94. B
- A diffuse parenchymal disease involving presence of increased iron storage in the liver is hemochromatosis. Hemochromatosis can be further described as primary, secondary, or as transfusional iron overload. With primary hemochromatosis is a human leukocyte antigen (HLA)-linked inherited disorder where a mucosal defect in the intestinal wall leads to increased absorption of ingested iron. Secondary hemochromatosis is associated with red blood cell breakdown related to hemolytic anemia. Transfusional iron overload hemochromatosis is a type of secondary hemochromatosis and diffuse parenchyma disease involving presence of increased iron storage in the liver due to multiple blood transfusions.

95. A
- Hydatid Disease, or Echinococcosis, is a parasitic infection. Sonographic appearance includes complex cyst with multiple internal daughter cysts known as water lily sign. Clinical findings include enlarged liver, abdominal pain, and jaundice if bile duct is obstructed.

96. C
- Angiomyolipoma, also called renal hamartoma, is a renal neoplasm with a varying amount of mature adipose tissue (i.e., fat-poor in pediatrics), smooth muscle, and blood vessels. As these masses contain adipose tissue, they tend to appear hyperechoic on ultrasound.

Section III, IV, V Answer Key:

1. B
- Propagation speed is also referred to as velocity. It is the speed at which a wave front travels through a medium and is expressed unit of distance per unit of time. A familiar term is miles per hour. With Ultrasound meters per second is used and is abbreviated as either m/sec or m/s. It is determined by the density and stiffness of the medium. The average propagation speed of soft tissue is 1540 m/s or 1.54 millimeters per microsecond abbreviated as mm/μs. Air is 330m/sec, muscle 1580m/sec and bone 4080m/sec.

2. C
- A highly attenuative structure absorbs the sound beam and therefore there is nothing left to image deeper. This causes a black area, as there are no echoes, posterior or under the structure. Dense tissue, such as calcium, cause the shadow. Examples include gallstones, kidney stones, and bone.

3. B
- Aliasing occurs when the blood is moving faster than the ultrasound machine can process causing the signal to "wrap around" the baseline. When aliasing occurs the peak of the signal will be below the baseline directly under the signal. Aliasing will occur when the signal is greater than the Nyquist limit which is ½ PRF, pulse repetition frequency. Aliasing can be corrected by increasing the scale (PRF), lowering the baseline, or repositioning the patient and/or transducer to get the vessel closer to the transducer. Sometimes it is not necessary to get the peak velocity. For example, if the diagnosis for a stenosis is 200cm/sec or greater and the signal starts to alias at 210cm/sec, the artery has a stenosis, and it doesn't matter what the true peak velocity is as the diagnosis is the same.

4. B
- The best lateral resolution is in the focal zone, which is the area surrounding the focus (narrowest part of the ultrasound beam). The focal zone corresponds to an icon on the right side of the image. Focusing of the

sound beam is accomplished by manipulating the delay lines to the crystal which allows the sonographer to vary the focal zone. Newer ultrasound machines have continual focusing and do use focal zone icons.

5. C
   - The higher the frame rate, the better the temporal resolution. Essentially, any function that requires additional information to be displayed on the image, such as color Doppler, will reduce the frame rate and therefore the temporal resolution. Increasing the imaging depth or the number of focal zones will decrease the frame rate. Decreasing the sector width will increase the frame rate and therefore improve temporal resolution. The frequency of the transducer has no effect on the frame rate.

6. A
   - The shape of the image is determined by the shape of the transducer with the linear array family or the timing of the delay lines in the sector array family. The linear array produces a rectangle image that is determined by the shape and length of the transducer. Curved linear arrays, also referred to as curvilinear transducers, are a linear array transducer with the crystals arranged in an arc producing a trapezoid type of image with a concave or blunted near field. A sector array produces an arc or pie shaped image, and a vector array produces what is described as a flat top sector.

7. B
   - Total energy within the circulatory system is the sum of kinetic, pressure, and gravitational energy. Pressure energy is a form of potential energy, meaning it has the potential to perform work and is noted in units of mmHg.

8. D
   - Arterial waveforms are described by spectral Doppler as high or low resistance or triphasic, biphasic and monophasic. The capillaries will determine what happens in diastolic flow. When they are open during diastole blood continually is a forward flow and this type of Doppler signal is termed low resistance. Examples of low resistance signals are renal, internal carotid and hepatic arteries.

9. D
   - This image demonstrates a pulsatile venous waveform, which changes with cardiac contractions. This type of signal is normal in the hepatic and subclavian veins. With heart failure all the veins will display a pulsatile waveform.

10. D
   - When the patient lies supine, the hydrostatic pressure is in the ankle vessels is 0 mmHg as the leg is at the same level as the right atrium. Hydrostatic pressure is defined as the pressure exerted by fluid at rest due to the force of gravity.

11. B
   - A Doppler shift occurs when there is motion between the reflecting objects, such as the red blood cells, and the sound beam.

12. C
   - A continuous wave transducer contains two piezoelectric elements, one which continuously transmits the sound wave and the other that continually receives the returning echoes. As this is not a pulse echo technique an anatomic image cannot be created. CW-transducers are typically used in vascular imaging and have a duty factor of 100%.

13. A
   - Spectral Doppler aliasing artifact is a common error that occurs when the velocity of the blood flow is faster than the machine can process. This causes the Doppler signal to wrap around the baseline and display the peak of the signal under the main part of the signal.

14. C
   - The Nyquist limit is determined by ½ PRF, pulse repetition frequency, and is the fastest velocity that can be displayed without aliasing.

15. D
   - Spectral broadening demonstrates a filled in spectral window due to a wide range of velocities present within the sample volume due to turbulent flow.

16. A
   - For a paracentesis, which is an interventional procedure involving draining of ascites fluid from the abdominal cavity, the patient should be in a supine or lateral decubitus position. Position can also be facility-dependent, and an obliqued position may also be used to aid in pooling of fluid.

17. C
   - Interventional procedures are performed by a radiologist. The sonographer may be present for interventional procedures that are performed under ultrasound guidance, such as a paracentesis, thoracentesis, abscess drainage, and various types of biopsies such as renal, thyroid, and masses.

18. B
   - A sterile field is necessary for surgical and interventional procedures, biopsies, drainages, and aspirations. When assisting with a sterile procedure, such as a renal biopsy, the sonographer should don sterile gloves and gown, and a sterile probe cover should be used over the transducer and cord. Additionally, the sonographer should utilize sterile gel and keep their hands above waist-level during a procedure.

19. C
   - Transducers are devices that convert one form of energy into another form of energy, such as light

bulbs into light and heat. In diagnostic ultrasound, transducers convert electricity into mechanical (sound) energy and vice versa.

20. A
- The backing or damping material is a material bonded to the back of the crystal. Its purpose is to stop the crystal from ringing to produce a short pulse. This helps to shorten the spatial pulse length and increase resolution. The backing material is an epoxy resin impregnated with tungsten.

21. B
- Transducers do not emit a single frequency but rather a range of frequencies called bandwidth. Most ultrasound transducers are wide bandwidth, that is they emit a wide range of frequencies. This allows the sonographer to optimize the image for resolution or penetration without having to change the transducer.

22. D
- Frame rate is the number of frames displayed per second. It is measured in frames per second. Temporal resolution is the ability to resolve two events related by time. The higher the frame rate, the better the temporal resolution. Essentially, any function that requires additional information to be displayed on the image reduces frame rate such as increasing imaging depth, increasing sector size or number focal zones and using color Doppler.

23. D
- The human range of hearing is from a low of 20 Hz to a high of 20,000 Hz or 20 kHz. (The k is the abbreviation for kilo and is equal to 1,000). Hertz, abbreviated Hz, refers to the number of cycles per second. Ultrasound is any sound frequency above 20 kHz. Infrasound is any sound frequency below 20 Hz. Diagnostic ultrasound uses frequencies above 1 megahertz, MHz, which is equal to 1,000,000 cycles per second.

24. B
- To image the infant spinal, cord a high frequency linear array transducer between 5 – 17 MHz should be used. The transducer should be placed over the spinous processes.

25. D
- Blood urea nitrogen (BUN) levels rise as kidney function decreases. The creatinine will increase as well, and the eGFR or estimated glomerular filtration rate will decrease.

26. C
- A grayscale anisotropy artifact occurs when strong specular reflectors have variable echogenicities depending on the angle of insonation. Grayscale anisotropy artifact is most seen in tendon imaging and can cause the tendon to look like there is pathology present. This artifact is corrected by

adjusting the transducer to image the tendon at a 90° angle.

27. D
- Axial resolution is determined by the frequency of the transducer. The higher the frequency the better the resolution but unfortunately the amount of penetration is decreased as lower frequencies have better penetration.

28. B
- Age specific care and communication is a requirement by JCAHO as each age group responds differently to medical intervention. It is important for the sonographer to be aware of appropriate care based upon the patient's age. In the toddler stage (age 1-3 years) the sonographer should ensure friendly facial expressions and provide safe toys or opportunity for medical play prior to performing the procedure. This may include allowing the patient to touch the ultrasound gel prior to exam, use of transducer to "scan" a stuffed animal or doll, or exam distraction with use of bubbles, age-appropriate show, or game on a tablet, and so forth.

29. A
- Neonates are prone to rapid heat loss due to a lack of brown adipose tissue (BAT). This makes it important to keep the neonate in its isolate and use the portholes for scanning.

30. C
- The coronal imaging plane divides the body into front, anterior, and back, or posterior, halves. Transducer placement and orientation to achieve coronal views varies based on the anatomical region being imaged such as the abdomen, neonatal brain, or infant hip.

31. B
- Refraction is a change in the sound wave's direction or bending of the sound wave while passing between tissues. Refraction can only occur when there is a difference in velocity between the media, across the interface, and with an oblique angle of incidence.

32. C
- A disinfection method must be used to destroy the potential pathogens on the transducer. How the transducer was used will determine what type of disinfection is required and is based on Spaulding's classification. If the transducer touches mucous membranes, such as with an endocavitary vaginal or rectal ultrasound, the appropriate level of disinfection should be high level, HLD, according to the manufacturer's guidelines. The disinfection product should be used according to the manufacturer's directions. The sonographer should keep current on disinfection techniques. Currently, the AIUM does not recommend HLD requirement with a covered biopsy transducer.

33. A
  - The pediatric abdomen is evaluated in its entirety as an abdominal complete or abdominal limited ultrasound evaluation. Transducer selection is based upon patient habitus, ranging from a higher frequency selection for neonates and infants, to a low to mid frequency transducer for adolescents. A curvilinear 3-5 MHz transducer would be most appropriate for an adolescent patient, unless they have a thin body habitus where a higher frequency might be more appropriate. The highest frequency transducer that has the appropriate penetration should be used.

34. A
  - The piezoelectric element, sometimes referred to as the crystal, emits the sound beam and receives the echoes. Ultrasound piezoelectric elements are man-made as they are less expensive, more rugged, and more efficient in converting mechanical energy to electrical energy. However, they are not naturally piezoelectric and must be made piezoelectric by heating the crystal to its Curie temperature while in the presence of a strong electrical field. Transducers must never be heated above their Curie temperature, as it will cause the transducer to lose its piezoelectric properties. The thickness of the crystal and the propagation speed of sound in the crystal determines the frequency. The thicker the crystal, the lower the frequency.

35. B
  - Attenuation is the progressive weakening of the amplitude of the sound beam. It is dependent on frequency, density of medium and number of interfaces. It is caused by absorption, reflection, and scattering. Attenuation is directly related to frequency and distance, the higher the frequency or the longer the distance, the higher the rate of attenuation.

36. A
  - The most accurate Doppler measurement will come from angles that are parallel to blood flow, i.e., 0°, where the cosine is 1. As it is difficult to achieve angles of 0°, Doppler angles of less than 60° are used.

37. B
  - Power Doppler is an extension of the autocorrelation process of color Doppler and evaluates the power or intensity of the Doppler signal as opposed to its mean velocity. Benefits of power Doppler include increased flow sensitivity, quick evaluation of flow, angle independency, organ perfusion, increased spatial resolution meaning that the color does not bleed outside the vessel's wall and detection of low flow. The main disadvantage is that it does not provide flow direction information on all systems.

38. A
  - Hepatocellular carcinoma, or hepatoma, is the second most common malignant pediatric liver tumor. This malignancy most commonly occurs between five to fifteen years of age. Clinical findings include elevated serum alpha-fetoprotein, right upper quadrant mass, and abdominal distention. Alkaline Phosphatase (ALP) values help in detecting liver disease, bone disorders or any condition involving bone growth or increased bone cell activity, and blocked bile ducts. Normal Alkaline Phosphatase (ALP) levels are between 14 and 127 U/L.

39. C
  - Both lipase and amylase increase in the presence of acute pancreatitis, and elevated levels may be an indication for an abdominal ultrasound. Amylase levels increase quicker than lipase levels. However, lipase levels remain elevated longer than amylase levels and the patient may have a normal amylase but an elevated lipase.

40. B
  - Enhancement, also referred to as increased through-transmission, is the opposite of shadowing. It occurs when the sound beam interacts with a low attenuation structure, which is fluid, and the echoes posterior to the structure appear as a brighter echogenicity than the echoes on either side.

41. B
  - Edge shadow artifact occurs when sound strikes a smooth rounded structure at an angle. The sound will refract, or bend, and cause shadowing from the side edges. This artifact helps the sonographer to determine whether a structure such as a cyst, has a smooth border and a rounded or oval shape. It is important not to mistake an edge artifact for an acoustic shadow from a stone, especially with the gallbladder.

42. C
  - Color Doppler twinkling artifact is visualized as various colors, that looks like aliasing, portrayed in a comet-tail artifact fashion directly posterior to a calcified structure. This artifact is commonly seen with renal calculi and other calcifications and can increase the sonographic confidence that the echogenic structure is a small stone or other calcification. This is especially helpful when the stone is too small to cast an acoustic shadow such as a small stone at the UVJ, utero-vesical junction. To best demonstrate an acoustic shadow and color twinkle artifacts, the sonographer should utilize the highest transducer frequency and activate harmonics. In cases of urolithiasis, the sonographer should provide a split-screen image of the gray scale image and the twinkle-artifact of the stone.

43. B
  - A mirror image artifact, also called crosstalk, is when the Doppler signal is duplicated across the baseline causing the appearance of flow above and below the baseline. This can occur if the spectral gain is too high. If the blood flow is perpendicular to the sound beam the machine may have a difficult time deciding if flow is towards or away from the transducer so it displays

both. Creating an angle of < 60° or decreasing the gain will remove the artifact.

44. B
   - Neonates are prone to rapid heat loss due to a lack of brown adipose tissue (BAT). This makes it important to keep the neonate in its isolate and use the portholes for scanning. When scanning the neonate's head make sure to wipe the gel off immediately after scanning as it is a source of significant heat loss.

45. A
   - In Trendelenburg position, the patient's head is lower than the feet. With reverse Trendelenburg, the patient's head is higher than the feet or abdomen.

46. B
   - Hospital-acquired infections (HAIs) are preventable infections that a patient develops while in the hospital, that is they did not have the infection prior to being admitted. HAIs add a financial burden to the health care system, costing billions of dollars. According to the Centers for Disease Control and Prevention (CDC), about 1 in 31 hospital patients contract a HAI, affecting an estimated 687,000 patients annually. Washing our hands and properly disinfecting the transducers will help decrease the possibility of the patient obtaining an HAI from an ultrasound examination.

47. C
   - Proper hand washing is essential to help prevent the spread of infections, especially when scanning the neonate or immune compromised pediatric patient. Infants born before 37 weeks gestational age or with a birth weight of less than 2,500 grams are at increased risk. Hands should be washed before and after glove changing and between each patient, before we eat, and after using the restroom. Clostridium difficile (C. diff) is a pathogen that can only be removed with proper hand washing versus use of an alcohol-based sanitizer.

48. B
   - 35% hydrogen peroxide is used for high-level disinfection (HLD) in health care, including the ultrasound department for endovaginal (EV) and other transducers as required.

49. D
   - The most common malignant liver mass in infants and children is a hepatoblastoma. Up to 90% of cases are seen in patients less than five years of age, with peak occurrence between infancy to two years of age. Elevated serum alpha-fetoprotein, AFP, is seen 80-90% of cases. Sonographic appearance includes a well marginated echogenic mass. Large hepatoblastomas may have variable echogenicity but remain well-defined.

50. A
   - The most common endocrine islet-cell tumor of the pancreas is an insulinoma. Insulinoma is a pancreatic endocrine and functioning islet-cell tumor. This tumor is small, typically measuring around 2 centimeters. The second most common endocrine islet-cell tumor of the pancreas is a gastrinoma.

51. B
   - Testicular tumors are more common before the age of 2 and at the start of puberty. A teratoma, which is usually benign, is the most common in infants and a yolk cell tumor in older boys. Seminomas are malignant germ cell tumors that are rare in children, however are the most common testicular tumor in adults. This neoplasm is commonly associated with cryptorchidism and is usually found later in adolescence if discovered during a pediatric age. The second most common testicular germ cell tumor in an adult is an embryonal cell carcinoma.

52. C
   - Rhabdomyosarcoma is the most common soft tissue sarcoma of childhood. Approximately 35-40% of rhabdomyosarcomas arise in the head and neck. The most common head and neck locations for rhabdomyosarcoma to form is the nasopharynx, orbits, sinus, ear, neck, and skull base.

53. C
   - Rhabdomyosarcoma of the bladder is the most common childhood bladder tumor involving the submucosal trigone region. This malignant mass generally occurs between 2 to 6 years of age and 14 to 18 years of age.

54. B
   - Notable autosomal dominant disorders include tuberous sclerosis, hereditary pancreatitis, neuroblastoma, von Hippel-Lindau syndrome, uremic medullary cystic disease, and ADPKD. Autosomal recessive disorders pertaining to pediatric imaging include cystic fibrosis, ARPKD, juvenile nephronophthisis, Wolman disease, congenital adrenal hyperplasia, and metabolic liver diseases like Wilson disease, galactosemia, and glycogen storage disease.

55. C
   - Intracranial teratoma appears as a large echogenic mass with calcification and cystic areas of necrosis and degeneration. With intracranial teratoma, midline brain structures become displaced, and hydrocephalus may be present.

56. B
   - The typical appearance of lymphoma when it invades an organ is multiple hypoechoic areas. If it is a bilateral organ such as the testicles, both organs are usually affected. Lymphoma also has a diffuse appearance, and each individual mass may be hard to appreciate. Lymphoma will rarely enlarge the organ.

57. A
   - Bladder rhabdomyosarcoma is a malignant, echogenic, pedunculated soft-tissue mass projecting into the bladder with a "bunch of grapes" complex cystic appearance.

Text Abbreviations

ACA	Anterior Cerebral Artery	HIV	Human Immunodeficiency Virus
AFP	Alpha Fetoprotein	ICA	Internal Carotid Artery
AI	Accelerated Index	ICP	Intracranial Pressure
AIDS	Acquired Immunodeficiency Syndrome	IIA	Internal Iliac Artery
ALP	Alkaline Phosphatase	IIV	Internal Iliac Vein
ALT	Alanine Aminotransferase	IJV	Internal Jugular Vein
AO	Aorta	IMA	Inferior Mesenteric Artery
AOI	Area of Interest	IMV	Inferior Mesenteric Vein
AP	Anteroposterior	IUD	Intrauterine Device
ADPKD	Autosomal Dominant Polycystic Kidney disease	IV	Intravenous
ARPKD	Autosomal Recessive Polycystic Kidney Disease	IVC	Inferior Vena Cava
AST	Aspartate Aminotransferase	IVH	Intraventricular Hemorrhage
AT	Acceleration Time	LDH	Lactic Dehydrogenase
ATA	Anterior Tibial Artery	LFT	Liver Function Test
ATV	Anterior Tibial Vein	LH	Luteinizing Hormone
AVF	Arteriovenous Fistula	LHV	Left Hepatic Vein
AVM	Arteriovenous Malformation	LLD	Left Lateral Decubitus
BUN	Blood Urea Nitrogen	LPO	Left Posterior Oblique
CBD	Common Bile Duct	LPV	Left Portal Vein
CCA	Common Carotid Artery	LSV	Lesser Saphenous Vein
CFA	Common Femoral Artery	LUQ	Left Upper Quadrant
CFV	Common Femoral Vein	MCA	Middle Cerebral Artery
CHF	Congestive Heart Failure	MCDK	Multicystic Dysplastic Kidney
CIA	Common Iliac Artery	MHV	Middle Hepatic Vein
CIV	Common Iliac Vein	MI	Mechanical Index
CNS	Central Nervous System	MPV	Main Portal Vein
CSF	Cerebrospinal Fluid	MRA	Magnetic Resonance Angiography
CSP	Cavum Septum Pellucidum	MRI	Magnetic Resonance Imaging
CT	Computed Tomography	MRV	Magnetic Resonance Venography
DDH	Developmental Dysplasia of the Hip	MSK	Musculoskeletal
DFV	Deep Femoral Vein	NAFLD	Non–Alcoholic Fatty Liver Disease
DICA	Distal Internal Carotid Artery	NASH	Non–Alcoholic Steatohepatitis
DVT	Deep Venous Thrombosis	NEC	Necrotizing Enterocolitis
ECA	External Carotid Artery	NICU	Neonatal Intensive Care Unit
ECMO	Extracorporeal Membranous Oxygenation	NPO	Nil Per Os (Nothing by Mouth)
EDV	End Diastolic Velocity	NS	Non-Stress
EIA	External Iliac Artery	PCA	Posterior Cerebral Artery
EIV	External Iliac Vein	PCOS	Polycystic Ovarian Syndrome
FNH	Focal Nodular Hyperplasia	PET	Positron Emission Tomography
FSH	Follicle–Stimulating Hormone	PI	Pulsatility Index
FV	Femoral Vein	PICC	Peripherally Inserted Central Catheter
GB	Gallbaldder	PID	Pelvic Inflammatory Disease
GI	Gastrointestinal	Pop A	Popliteal Artery
GSV	Greater Saphenous Vein	Pop V	Popliteal Vein
HA	Hepatic Artery	PPE	Personal Protective Equipment
HCC	Hepatocellular Carcinoma	PRF	Pulse Repetition Frequency
hCG	Human Chorionic Gonadotrophin	PSV	Peak Systolic Velocity

PT	Prothrombin Time		SMV	Superior Mesenteric Vein
PTA	Posterior Tibial Artery		SPL	Spatial Pulse Length
PTV	Posterior Tibial Veins		STR	Stress
PV	Portal Vein		SV	Splenic Vein
PW	Pulsed Wave		T3	Triiodothyronine
RAO	Right Anterior Oblique		T4	Thyroxine
RAR	Renal Aortic Ratio		TAMX	Time Average Mean of the Max
RBC	Red Blood Cell		TCD	Transcranial Doppler
RCCA	Right Common Carotid Artery		TGC	Time Gain Compensation
RCI	Right Common Iliac		TIA	Transient Ischemic Attack
RHV	Right Hepatic Vein		TIPS	Transjugular Intrahepatic Portosystemic shunt
RI	Resistive Index		TOS	Thoracic Outlet Compression Syndrome
RLD	Right Lateral Decubitus		TPN	Total Parenteral Nutrition
RLQ	Right Lower Quadrant		TSH	Thyroid Stimulating Hormone
ROI	Region of Interest		UPJ	Ureteropelvic Junction
RPO	Right Posterior Oblique		UTI	Urinary Tract Infection
RPV	Right Portal Vein		UVJ	Urerterovesical Junction
RUQ	Right Upper Quadrant		VA	Vertebral Artery
SD	Standard Deviation		VCUG	Voiding Cystourethrogram
SFA	Superficial Femoral Artery		VUR	Vesicoureteral Reflux
SVC	Superior Vena Cava		WBC	White Blood Cell
SMA	Superior Mesenteric Artery			

Please note that all text abbreviations may not be included, however these are some of the most common encountered throughout the text.

References

1. Abboud B, El Hachem J, Yazbeck T, Doumit C. Hepatic portal venous gas: physiopathology, etiology, prognosis and treatment. World J Gastroenterol. 2009 Aug 7;15(29):3585-90. doi: 10.3748/wjg.15.3585. PMID: 19653334; PMCID: PMC2721230.

2. Abu Hishmeh M, Srivastava P, Lougheide Q, Srinivasan M, Murthy S. Massive spontaneous hemothorax as a complication of apixaban treatment. *Case Rep Pulmonol.* 2018 Oct 16;2018:8735036.

3. Adaletli I, Kurugoglu S, Kantarci F, Tireli GA, Yilmaz MH, Gulsen F, et al. Testicular Volume Before and After Hydrocelectomy in Children J Ultrasound Med. 2006;25:1131-1136.

4. Adigun OO, Reddy V, Sevensma KE. Anatomy, head and neck, basilar artery. [Updated 2021 Aug 11]. In: StatPearls [Internet]. Treasure Island (FL): StatPearls Publishing; 2022 Jan. Available from: https://www.ncbi.nlm.nih.gov/books/NBK459137/.

5. *Abdominal Doppler Ultrasound.* (2019, August 12). University of Washington. https://depts.washington.edu/usrad/protocols/general/tipps-pre-liver-transplant/

6. Aggarwal A, et al. Choledochal cyst. Radiopaedia. https://radiopaedia.org/articles/choledochal-cyst?lang=us.

7. AIUM-ACR-SPR-SRU practice parameter for the performance of an ultrasound examination for detection and assessment of developmental dysplasia of the hip. (2018). *Journal of Ultrasound in Medicine, 37*(11). https://doi.org/10.1002/jum.14829

8. AIUM practice guideline for the performance of a transcranial Doppler ultrasound examination for adults and children. *J Ultrasound Med.* 2012;31(9):1489-1500.

9. AIUM practice guideline for the performance of an ultrasound examination of the abdomen and/or Retroperitoneum. (2012). *Journal of Ultrasound in Medicine, 31*(8), 1301-1312. https://doi.org/10.7863/jum.2012.31.8.1301

10. AIUM practice guideline for the performance of renal artery duplex sonography. (2009). *Journal of Ultrasound in Medicine, 28*(1), 120-124. https://doi.org/10.7863/jum.2009.28.1.120

11. Aldoah B, Ramaswamy R. Effects of Hydrocele on Morphology and Function of Testis. *Annals of Medical and Health Sciences Research.* 2020;10(1):764-770.

12. Al-Mubarak et al. (2018, April 10). Air enema versus barium enema in intussusception: an overview. Retrieved from https://www.ijcmph.com/index.php/ijcmph/article/viewFile/3020/1981

13. Albright A, Pollack I, Adelson P. *Principles and Practice of Pediatric Neurosonography.* 3rd ed. New York: Thieme; 2014.

14. Alexandrov AV, Sloan MA, Wong LK, Douville C, Razumovsky AY, Koroshetz WJ, Kaps M, Tegeler CH, American Society of Neuroimaging Practice Guidelines Committee. J Neuroimaging. 2007 Jan; 17(1):11-8.

15. Ali Z, Lang S, Bakar D, Storm P, Stein S. Pediatric intracranial arachnoid cysts: comparative effectiveness of surgical treatment options. *Childs Nerv Sys.* 2013;30(3):461-469. doi:10.1007/s00381-013-2306-2.

16. American College of Radiology. (2016). ACR–SPR practice parameter for the performance of pediatric fluoroscopic contrast enema examinations. Retrieved from https://www.acr.org/-/media/ACR/Files/Practice-Parameters/FluourConEnema-Ped.pdf?la=en

17. Amini B, Bell D. Cavum septum pellucidum. *Radiopaedia.org.* https://doi.org/10.53347/rID-1066.

18. Ansari P. Hernias of the Abdominal Wall. Merck Manuals Professional Edition. https://www.merckmanuals.com/professional/gastrointestinal-disorders/acute-abdomen-and-surgical-gastroenterology/hernias-of-the-abdominal-wall. Published April 2020.

19. Aponte, E., & O'Rourke, M. (2020). Paracentesis. *StatPearls Publishing, LLC.* https://www.ncbi.nlm.nih.gov/books/NBK435998/

20. Applied Radiology. (2016, November 28). Selecting contrast media for pediatric fluoroscopy: a primer. Retrieved from https://appliedradiology.com/articles/selecting-contrast-media-for-pediatric-fluoroscopy-a-primer

21. Astrocytoma. Cleveland Clinic. https://my.clevelandclinic.org/health/diseases/17863-astrocytoma. Published September 5, 2018.

22. Bahgat E, El-Halaby H, Abdelrahman A, Nasef N, Abdel-Hady H. Sonographic evaluation of diaphragmatic thickness and excursion as a predictor for successful extubation in mechanically ventilated preterm infants. *Eur J Pediatr.* 2021;180(3):899-908. doi: 10.1007/s00431-020-03805-2.

23. Baker M, Anjum F, dela Cruz J. Deep Venous Thrombosis Ultrasound Evaluation. [Updated 2022 Jun 19]. In: StatPearls [Internet]. Treasure Island (FL): StatPearls Publishing; 2022 Jan. Available from: https://www.ncbi.nlm.nih.gov/books/NBK470453/.

24. Ballabh P. Intraventricular hemorrhage in premature infants: mechanism of disease. *Pediatr Res.* 2010;67(1):1-8. doi:10.1203/pdr.0b013e3181c1b176.

25. Ban C. H. Tsui, Santhanam Suresh, David S. Warner; Ultrasound Imaging for Regional Anesthesia in Infants, Children, and Adolescents: A Review of Current Literature and Its Application in the Practice of Extremity and Trunk Blocks. *Anesthesiology* 2010; 112:473–492 doi: https://doi.org/10.1097/ALN.0b013e3181c5dfd7

26. Bandarkar AN, Blask AR. Testicular torsion with preserved flow: key sonographic features and value-added approach to diagnosis. *Pediatric Radiology*. 2018;48(5):735-744. doi:10.1007/s00247-018-4093-0

27. Bani-Hani K. Agenesis of the gallbladder: difficulties in management. *J Gastroenterol Hepatol*. 2005;20(5):671-675. doi:10.1111/j.1440-1746.2005.03740.x.

28. Barata Tavares J, Bandeira A. Caudal regression syndrome. *Appl Radiol*. 2017;46(1):47A-47B.

29. Bosemani T, Orman G, Boltshauser E, Tekes A, Huisman T, Poretti A. Congenital abnormalities of the posterior fossa. *RadioGraphics*. 2015;35(1):200-220. doi:10.1148/rg.351140038

30. Barger et al. (2011). Radiographic procedures. In *Radiologic Technology Review* (5th ed., pp. 20-22). United States of America: RTS Publishing Company, Inc.

31. Beachy J. Investigating jaundice in the newborn. *J Neonatal Nurs*. 2007;26(5):327-333. doi:10.1891/0730-0832.26.5.327.

32. Bashir, O., Fahrenhorst-Jones, T. Left gastric vein. Reference article, Radiopaedia.org. (accessed on 13 Apr 2022) https://doi.org/10.53347/rID-16762

33. Baun J, Lange MD. *OB/GYN Sonography: An Illustrated Review*. Pasadena, CA: Davies Publishing, Inc.; 2016.

34. Becker C, Kharbanda A. Acute appendicitis in pediatric patients: an evidence-based review. Pediatr Emerg Med Pract. 2019 Sep;16(9):1-20. Epub 2019 Sep 2. PMID: 31461613.

35. Beckwith JB. Nephrogenic rests and the pathogenesis of Wilms tumor: developmental and clinical considerations. *Am J Med Genet*. 1998 Oct 2;79(4):268-273.

36. Behari S, Garg K, Malik N, Jaiswal A. Chiari III malformation with hypertelorism and microcephaly in a neonate: case report and a review of the literature. *J Pediatr Neurosci*. 2008;3(2):169-171. doi:10.4103/1817-1745.43652.

37. Behr S, Courtier J, Qayyum A. Imaging of müllerian duct anomalies. *RadioGraphics*. 2012;32(6):E233-E250. doi:10.1148/rg.326125515.

38. Bell D, Gaillard F, et al. Splenosis. Radiopaedia. https://radiopaedia.org/articles/splenosis?lang=us.

39. Bell D, Agrawal R, et al. Congenital lobar overinflation. Radiopaedia. https://radiopaedia.org/articles/congenital-lobar-overinflation?lang=us.

40. Bell D, Iqbal S, et al. HIV-associated salivary gland disease. Radiopaedia. https://radiopaedia.org/articles/hiv-associated-salivary-gland-disease?lang=us.

41. Bell D, Radswiki, et al. Spinal dysraphism. Radiopaedia. https://radiopaedia.org/articles/spinal-dysraphism-3?lang=us.

42. Bennett JC, Maffly RH, Steinbach HL. The significance of bilateral basal ganglia calcification. Radiology. 1959;72(3):368-378.

43. Benson C, Bluth E. *Ultrasonography in Obstetrics and Gynecology: A Practical Approach*. 2nd ed. New York: Thieme; 2011.

44. Berte N, Filfilan A, Mainard L, Mansuy L, Lemelle JL. Co-existing infantile hepatic hemangioma and mesenchymal hamartoma in a neonate. *J Surg Case Rep*. 2018 Jan 23;2018(1):rjx260.

45. Botz B, Agrawal R, et al. Pulmonary sequestration. Radiopaedia. https://radiopaedia.org/articles/pulmonary-sequestration?lang=us.

46. Botz B, Reddy V U, et al. Diaphragmatic paralysis. Radiopaedia. https://radiopaedia.org/articles/diaphragmatic-paralysis-1?lang=us.

47. Caffey J, Kuhn J. *Caffey's Pediatric Diagnostic Imaging*. 1st ed. Philadelphia, Pa: Mosby; 2004.

48. Capillary Vascular Malformations: Port Wine Stains. https://www.chop.edu/conditions-diseases/capillary-vascular-malformations-port-wine-stains. Published August 4, 2014.

49. Caroli disease. Genetic and Rare Diseases Information Center. https://rarediseases.info.nih.gov/diseases/6002/caroli-disease/cases/30757. Published July 19, 2017. Accessed July 3, 2021.

50. Carpenter G, et al. External jugular vein. Radiopaedia. https://radiopaedia.org/articles/external-jugular-vein?lang=us.

51. Carsote M, Ghemigian A, Terzea D, Gheorghisan-Galateanu AA, Valea A. Cystic adrenal lesions: focus on pediatric population (a review). *Clujul Med*. 2017;90(1):5-12. doi:10.15386/cjmed-677

52. Casas-Melley AT, ed. Intussusception. KidsHealth. https://kidshealth.org/en/parents/intussusception.html. Published February 2020.

53. Cascio S, Siddiqui MM, Barrett AM. Is screening ultrasound of the urinary tract indicated in infants with hypertrophic pyloric stenosis? *Acta Paediatrica*. 2007;94(1):23-25. doi:10.1111/j.1651-2227.2005.tb01782.x

54. Centers for Disease Control and Prevention. (2019, December 9). *Aortic aneurysm*. CDC. https://www.cdc.gov/heartdisease/aortic_aneurysm.htm

55. Chaudhary, V., & Bano, S. (2013). Thyroid ultrasound. *Indian Journal of Endocrinology and Metabolism*, 17(2), 219. https://doi.org/10.4103/2230-8210.109667

56. Chavhan GB, Parra DA, Mann A, Navarro OM. Normal Doppler Spectral Waveforms of Major Pediatric Vessels: Specific Patterns. *RadioGraphics*. 2008;28(3):691-706. doi:10.1148/rg.283075095

57. Childhood Thyroid Cancer Treatment. National Cancer Institute. https://www.cancer.gov/types/thyroid/patient/child-thyroid-treatment-pdq. Published February 18, 2021.

58. Chitkara U, Cogswell C, Norton K, Wilkins I, Mehalek K, Berkowitz R. Choroid plexus cysts in the fetus: a benign anatomic variant or pathologic entity? report of 41 cases and review of the literature. *Obstet Gynecol*. 1988;72(2):185-189.

59. Chung CJ, Armfield KB, Mukherji SK, Fordham LA, Krause WL. Cervical neurofibromas in children with NF-1. *Pediatric Radiology*. 1999;29(5):353-356. doi:10.1007/s002470050605

60. Chung EM, Travis MD, Conran RM. Pancreatic tumors in children: radiologic-pathologic correlation. Radiographics. 2006;26:1211–1238

61. Cicin I, Saip P, Guney N et al. Yolk sac tumours of the ovary: evaluation of clinicopathological features and prognostic factors. *Eur J Obstet Gynecol*. 2009;146(2):210-214. doi:10.1016/j.ejogrb.2009.02.052.

62. Cincinnati Children's Hospital Medical Center. (n.d.). Air enema for intussusception. Retrieved from https://www.cincinnatichildrens.org/health/a/air-enema

63. Cogley JR, O'Connor SC, Houshyar R, Dulaimy KA. Emergent pediatric us: What every radiologist should know. *RadioGraphics*. 2012;32(3):651-665.

64. Congenital splenic cyst –case study. *J Med Life*. 2011;4(1):102-104. Available at: http://www.medandlife.ro/archive/151-vol-iv-iss-1-january-march-2011/case-presentation-vol-iv-iss-1/378-congenital-splenic-cyst.

65. Craig M. *Essentials of Sonography and Patient Care*. 3rd ed. St. Louis, MO: Elsevier; 2013.

66. Cuna, A.C., Reddy, N., Robinson, A.L. *et al*. Bowel ultrasound for predicting surgical management of necrotizing enterocolitis: a systematic review and meta-analysis. *Pediatr Radiol* 48, 658–666 (2018). https://doi.org/10.1007/s00247-017-4056-x

67. Curry R, Tempkin B. *Sonography: Introduction to Normal Structure and Function*. 3rd ed. St. Louis, MO: Elsevier; 2011.

68. D'Arcy C, Pertile M, Goodwin T, Bittinger S. Bilateral congenital adrenal agenesis: a rare disease entity and not a result of poor autopsy technique. *Pediatr Dev Pathol*. 2014;17(4):308-311. doi:10.2350/14-03-1455-cr.1.

69. D'Souza, D. (n.d.). *Renal artery stenosis | Radiology reference article | Radiopaedia.org*. Radiopaedia.org, the wiki-based collaborative Radiology resource. Retrieved July 3, 2020, from https://radiopaedia.org/articles/renal-artery-stenosis?lang=us

70. D'Souza, D., & Kabbani, A. (n.d.). *Abdominal aortic aneurysm*. Radiopaedia.org. Retrieved July 3, 2020, from https://radiopaedia.org/articles/abdominal-aortic-aneurysm?lang=us

71. D'Souza, D., & Morgan, M. (n.d.). *Portal hypertension*. Radiopaedia.org. Retrieved July 3, 2020, from https://radiopaedia.org/articles/portal-hypertension?lang=us

72. Das J, Dossani RH. Cavum septum pellucidum. [Updated 2022 Apr 9]. In: StatPearls [Internet]. Treasure Island (FL): StatPearls Publishing; 2022 Jan. Available from: https://www.ncbi.nlm.nih.gov/books/NBK537048/.

73. Davis Medical Electronics Inc. Transducers. https://www.davismedical.com/ReplacementUltrasoundTransducers.aspx

74. Davis SL, ed. Venous Malformations (for Parents) - Nemours KidsHealth. KidsHealth. https://kidshealth.org/en/parents/venous-malformations.html. Published January 2021.

75. DeBruyn R. *Pediatric Ultrasound: How, Why, and When*. 2nd ed. New York: Churchill Livingston. Elsevier; 2010.

76. Deeg K, Rupprecht T, Hofbeck M. *Doppler Sonography in Infancy and Childhood*. Cham: Springer International Publishing; 2015.

77. Degrate L, Misani M, Mauri G, et al. Mature Cystic Teratoma of the Pancreas. Case Report and Review of the Literature of a Rare Pancreatic Cystic Lesion. *Journal of the Pancreas*. 2011;13(1):66-72. http://www.serena.unina.it/index.php/jop.

78. del Rosario J, ed. Intestinal malrotation. KidsHealth. https://kidshealth.org/en/parents/malrotation.html. Published March 2017.

79. Deng F, et al. Multilocular cystic renal neoplasm of low malignant potential. Radiopaedia. https://radiopaedia.org/articles/multilocular-cystic-renal-neoplasm-of-low-malignant-potential?lang=us.

80. Dodd GD. An American's guide to Couinaud's numbering system. *American Journal of Roentgenology*. 1993;161(3):574-575. doi:10.2214/ajr.161.3.8352108

81. Dogra V, Gottlieb R, Oka M, Rubens D. Sonography of the scrotum. *Radiology*. 2003;227(1):18-36. doi:10.1148/radiol.2271001744.

82. Dremmen MHG, Bouhuis RH, Blanken LME, et al. Cavum Septum Pellucidum in the General Pediatric Population and Its Relation to Surrounding Brain Structure Volumes, Cognitive Function, and Emotional or Behavioral Problems. *American Journal of Neuroradiology*. 2019;40(2):340-346. doi:10.3174/ajnr.a5939

83. Ecury-Goossen GM, Camfferman FA, Leijser LM, Govaert P, Dudink J. State of the art cranial ultrasound imaging in neonates. J Vis Exp. 2015 Feb 2;(96):e52238.

84. Edelman S. *Understanding Ultrasound Physics*. 4th ed. Woodlands, Tex.: ESP; 2012.

85. El-Feky M, Gilcrease-Garcia B, et al. Pediatric cystic nephroma. Radiopaedia. https://radiopaedia.org/articles/pediatric-cystic-nephroma?lang=us

86. El-Feky M, Weerakkody Y, et al. Pulmonary sequestration (intralobar). Radiopaedia. https://radiopaedia.org/articles/pulmonary-sequestration-intralobar?lang=us.

87. Eidlitz-Markus T, Zeharia A, Haimi Cohen Y, Konen O. Characteristics and management of arachnoid cyst in the pediatric headache clinic setting. *Headache: J Head Face Pain*. 2014;54(10):1583-1590. doi:10.1111/head.12470.

88. Ellis H. Anatomy of the gallbladder and bile ducts. *Surgery*. 2011;29(12):593-596. doi:10.1016/j.mpsur.2011.09.011.

89. Epelman M, Dinan D, Gee MS, Servaes S, Lee EY, Darge K. Müllerian Duct and Related Anomalies in Children and Adolescents. *Magnetic Resonance Imaging Clinics of North America*. 2013;21(4):773-789. doi:10.1016/j.mric.2013.04.011

90. Esmaeili M, Keshaki M, Younesi L, Karimani A, Otoukesh H, Esmaeili M. Ultrasound measurement of kidney dimensions in premature neonates. Int J Pediatr. 2020;8(10): 12235-12242.

91. Esposito F, Mamone R, Di Serafino M, Mercogliano C, Vitale V, Vallone G, Oresta P. Diagnostic imaging features of necrotizing enterocolitis: a narrative review. Quant Imaging Med Surg. 2017 Jun;7(3):336-344. doi:10.21037/qims.2017.03.01. PMID: 28812000; PMCID: PMC5537125.

92. Fajardo R, DeAngelis G. Septate uterus. Appl Radiol. 2011; 40(9):26-27. Available at: http://www.appliedradiology.com/articles/septate-uterus.

93. Fallon S, Orth R, Guillerman R et al. Development and validation of an ultrasound scoring system for children with suspected acute appendicitis. *Pediatr Radiol*. 2015;45(13):1945- 1952. doi:10.1007/s00247-015-3443-4.4

94. Farooq S, Whitehead H. Mayer-Rokitansky-Küster-Hauser syndrome. Radiopaedia.org. https://doi.org/10.53347/rID-10786.

95. Fasouliotis S, Achiron R, Kivilevitch Z, Yagel S. The human fetal venous system. *J Ultrasound Med.* 2002;21(10):1145-1158. doi:10.7863/jum.2002.21.10.1145.

96. Feger J, et al. Intracranial teratoma. Radiopaedia. https://radiopaedia.org/articles/intracranial-teratoma?lang=us.

97. Feldman M, Katyal S, Blackwood M. US artifacts. *RadioGraphics.* 2009;29(4):1179-1189.doi:10.1148/rg.294085199.

98. Fortin F, Goel A, et al. Pneumothorax (ultrasound). Radiopaedia. https://radiopaedia.org/articles/pneumothorax-ultrasound-1?lang=us.

99. Foster T, et al. Branchial cleft anomalies. Radiopaedia. https://radiopaedia.org/articles/branchial-cleft-anomalies?lang=us.

100. Gaca AM, Bissett GS. Diseases of the Pediatric Pancreas. *Textbook of Gastrointestinal Radiology.* 2008;2:2341-2353. doi:10.1016/b978-1-4160-2332-6.50130-5

101. Gaillard F, Desai P, et al. Choroid plexus papilloma. Radiopaedia. https://radiopaedia.org/articles/choroid-plexus-papilloma-1?lang=us.

102. Gaillard F, Ho M, et al. Porencephaly. Radiopaedia. https://radiopaedia.org/articles/porencephaly?lang=us.

103. Gaillard, F., Sharma, R. Phrygian cap. Reference article, Radiopaedia.org. https://doi.org/10.53347/rID-1870

104. Gander R, Asensio M, Royo G, Lloret J. Evaluation of the initial treatment of ureteroceles. *Urology.* 2016;89:113-117. doi:10.1016/j.urology.2015.11.025.

105. Garel, L., Dubois, J., Grignon, A., Filiatrault, D., & Van Vliet, G. (2001). US of the pediatric female pelvis: A clinical perspective. *RadioGraphics,* 21(6), 1393–1407. https://doi.org/10.1148/radiographics.21.6.g01nv041393

106. George, A. M., Roberts, M., Mackey, M., Medrano, P., Michael, K., Smith, E., Werner, E., & White, R. (2017). *Pediatric sonography.* Society of Diagnostic Medical Sonography.

107. Gaca AM, Bissett GS. Diseases of the Pediatric Pancreas. *Textbook of Gastrointestinal Radiology.* 2008;2:2341-2353. doi:10.1016/b978-1-4160-2332-6.50130-5

108. Gaillard F, Desai P, et al. Choroid plexus papilloma. Radiopaedia. https://radiopaedia.org/articles/choroid-plexus-papilloma-1?lang=us.

109. Gaillard F, Glick Y. Lymphoma. Radiopaedia.org. https://doi.org/10.53347/rID-9229.

110. Gaillard F, Ho M, et al. Porencephaly. Radiopaedia. https://radiopaedia.org/articles/porencephaly?lang=us.

111. Garel L, Dubois J, Grignon A, Filiatrault D, Van Vliet G. Ultrasound of the pediatric female pelvis: A clinical perspective. *RadioGraphics.* 2001;21(6): 1393-1407.

112. Geramizadeh B, Maghbou M, Ziyaian B. Primary hydatid cyst of the adrenal gland: a case report and review of the literature. *Iran Red Crescent Med J.* 2011;13(5):346-347.

113. Getzoff M, Goldstein B. Spontaneous Subarachnoid Hemorrhage in Children. *Pediatrics in Review.* 1999;20(12):422-422. doi:10.1542/pir.20-12-422

114. Geyik M, Alptekin M, Erkutlu I et al. Tethered cord syndrome in children: a single-center experience with 162 patients. *Childs Nerv Sys.* 2015;31(9):1559-1563. doi:10.1007/s00381-015-2748-9.

115. Ghosh T, Banerjee M, Basu S, Das R, Kumar P, De S, Ghosh MK, Ganguly S. Assessment of normal portal vein diameter in children. Trop Gastroenterol. 2014 Apr-Jun;35(2):79-84.

116. Gibson M. Renal duplex ultrasound. WikiDoc. https://www.wikidoc.org/index.php/Renal_duplex_ultrasound. Published August 20, 2012.

117. Glick RD, Pashankar FD, Pappo A, LaQuaglia MP. Management of Pancreatoblastoma in Children and Young Adults. *Journal of Pediatric Hematology/Oncology.* 2012;34(Supplement 2):47-50. doi:10.1097/mph.0b013e31824e3839

118. Gliomas. Johns Hopkins Medicine. https://www.hopkinsmedicine.org/health/conditions-and-diseases/gliomas.

119. Goel A, et al. Doppler waveforms. Radiopaedia. https://radiopaedia.org/articles/doppler-waveforms?lang=us.

120. Gokhale S. Sonography in identification of abdominal wall lesions presenting as palpable masses. *J Ultrasound Med.* 2006;25(9):1199-1209. doi:10.7863/jum.2006.25.9.1199.

121. Golriz M, Klauss M, Zeier M, Mehrabi A. Prevention and management of lymphocele formation following kidney transplantation. *Transplantation Reviews.* 2016. doi:10.1016/j.trre.2016.11.001.

122. Grimbizis G, Gordts S, Di Spiezio Sardo A et al. The ESHRE/ESGE consensus on the classification of female genital tract congenital anomalies. *Hum Reprod.* 2013;28(8):2032-2044. doi:10.1093/humrep/det098.

123. Grimbizis G, Campo R. Clinical approach for the classification of congenital uterine malformations. *Gynecol Surg.* 2012;9(2):119-129. doi:10.1007/s10397-011-0724-2.

124. Gupta, R. (2014, September). Intussusception. Retrieved from https://kidshealth.org/en/parents/intussusception.html

125. Haber H, Busch A, Ziebach R, Dette S, Ruck P, Stern M. Ultrasonographic findings correspond to clinical, endoscopic, and histologic findings in inflammatory bowel disease and other enterocolitides. *J Ultrasound Med.* 2002;21(4):375-382. doi:10.7863/jum.2002.21.4.375.

126. Jaffe S. Reye's syndrome. *CINAHL Nursing Guide.* 2016.

127. Hacking C, et al. Circle of Willis. Radiopaedia. https://radiopaedia.org/articles/circle-of-willis?lang=us.

128. Hagen-Ansert S. *Textbook of Diagnostic Ultrasonography.* 7th ed. St. Louis, Mo.: Mosby Elsevier; 2006.

129. Hagen-Ansert, SL. Biopsies and infection prevention. In Textbook of diagnostic sonography.: Vol. I & II. Elsevier - Health Science; 2022.

130. Hagen-Ansert, S. L. (2012). The gastrointestinal tract. In *Textbook of diagnostic sonography* (7th ed., pp. 337-340). St. Louis, MO: Elsevier Mosby.

131. Hayes, C. M. (2019). *Ultrasound in Global Health Radiology. Radiology in Global Health: Strategies, Implementation, and Applications* (pp. 127–140). Springer.

132. Heinonen P. Complete septate uterus with longitudinal vaginal septum. *Fertil Sterility.* 2006;85(3):700-705. doi:10.1016/j.fertnstert.2005.08.039.

133. Haldeman-Englert C, Cunningham L, Turley Jr R. Creatinine (Blood). University of Rochester Medical Center. https://www.urmc.rochester.edu/encyclopedia/content.aspx?ContentTypeID=167&ContentID=creatinine_serum.

134. Haouimi A, et al. Dysgenesis of the corpus callosum. Radiopaedia. https://radiopaedia.org/articles /dysgenesis-of-the-corpus-callosum?lang=us.

135. Haouimi A, et al. Infantile hepatic hemangioma. Radiopaedia. https://radiopaedia.org/articles /infantile-hepatic-haemangioma?lang=us.

136. Hardin et al. Age limit of pediatrics. American Academy of Pediatrics. Accessed 13 July 2020 https://pediatrics. aappublications.org/content/pediatrics/140/3/e20172151 .full.pdf

137. Harkins JM, Ahmad B. Anatomy, Abdomen and Pelvis, Portal Venous System (Hepatic Portal System) [Updated 2021 Aug 11]. In: StatPearls [Internet]. Treasure Island (FL): StatPearls Publishing; 2022 Jan-. Available from: https://www.ncbi.nlm.nih.gov /books/NBK554589/

138. Harvey J, Radswiki, et al. Nephroblastomatosis. Radiopaedia. https://radiopaedia.org/articles/ nephroblastomatosis?lang=us.

139. Hedrick W. *Technology for Diagnostic Sonography.* 1st ed. St. Louis, Mo.: Elsevier; 2013.

140. Hedrick W, Hykes D, Starchman D. *Ultrasound Physics and Instrumentation.* 4th ed. St. Louis, Mo: Elsevier Mosby; 2005.

141. Herlin MK, Petersen MB, Brännström M. Mayer-Rokitansky-Küster-Hauser (MRKH) syndrome: a comprehensive update. Orphanet J Rare Dis. 2020 Aug 20;15(1):214.

142. Hernanz-Schulman M, Ambrosino MM, Freeman PC, Quinn CB. Common bile duct in children: sonographic dimensions. Radiology. 1995 Apr;195(1):193-195.

143. Hickling, Duane R et al. "Anatomy and Physiology of the Urinary Tract: Relation to Host Defense and Microbial Infection." *Microbiology spectrum* vol. 3,4 (2015): 10.1128/microbiolspec.UTI-0016-2012. doi:10.1128 /microbiolspec.UTI-0016-2012

144. Holm, T. L., Murati, M. A., Hoggard, E., Zhang, L., & Dietz, K. R. (2018). Liver Doppler Findings in Pediatric Patients After Total Pancreatectomy and Islet Autotransplantation. *Journal of ultrasound in medicine : official journal of the American Institute of Ultrasound in Medicine*, 37(11), 2595–2601. https://doi.org/10.1002/ jum.14617

145. Hong HS, Lee JY. Intracranial hemorrhage in term neonates. *Child's Nervous System.* 2018;34(6):1135-1143. doi:10.1007/s00381-018-3788-8

146. Hosn, S., Bell, D. Twinkling artifact. Reference article, Radiopaedia.org. (accessed on 30 Mar 2022) https://doi .org/10.53347/rID-21828

147. Huang B, Castillo M. Hypoxic-ischemic brain injury: imaging findings from birth to adulthood. *RadioGraphics.* 2008;28(2):417-439. doi:10.1148/rg.282075066.

148. Intussusception in Children. Stanford Children's Health - Lucile Packard Children's Hospital Stanford. https://www.stanfordchildrens.org/en/topic/ default?id=intussusception-90-P02002.

149. Iqbal S, et al. Acute pyelonephritis. Radiopaedia. https:// radiopaedia.org/articles/acute-pyelonephritis-1?lang=us.

150. Iqbal S, et al. Fibromatosis colli. Radiopaedia. https:// radiopaedia.org/articles/fibromatosis-colli?lang=us.

151. Irani N, Goud A, Lowe L. Isolated filar cyst on lumbar spine sonography in infants: a case-control study. *Pediatr Radiol.* 2006;36(12):1283-1288. doi:10.1007 /s00247-006-0317-9.

152. Jin T, et al. Cushing syndrome. Radiopaedia. https:// radiopaedia.org/articles/cushing-syndrome?lang=us.

153. Jin T, Jones J, et al. Subependymal giant cell astrocytoma. Radiopaedia. https://radiopaedia.org/articles/ subependymal-giant-cell-astrocytoma?lang=us.

154. John Hopkins Medicine. "Anatomy of the Urinary System." *Health,* The Johns Hopkins University, The Johns Hopkins Hospital, and Johns Hopkins Health System, 2020, www. hopkinsmedicine.org/health/wellness-and-prevention/ anatomy-of-the-urinary-system. Accessed 19 Jan. 2020.

155. John J, Idell S. Pleural effusions | Hemothorax. In: Geoffrey J. Laurent GJ, Shapiro SD, eds. Encyclopedia of Respiratory Medicine. Cambridge, MA: Academic Press; 2006: 393-397.

156. Jones B, Ball W, Tomsick T. Vein of Galen aneurysmal malformation: diagnosis and treatment of 13 children with extended clinical follow-up. *Am J Neuroradiol.* 2002;23(10):1717-1724.

157. Jones J, et al. Couinaud classification of hepatic segments. Radiopaedia. https://radiopaedia.org/articles /couinaud-classification-of-hepatic-segments?lang=us.

158. Jones J, Hacking C. Inferior vena cava. Radiopaedia.org. https://doi.org/10.53347/rID-5730.

159. Kabiri H, Domingo O, Tzarnas C. Agenesis of the gallbladder. *Curr Surg.* 2006;63(2):104-106. doi:10.1016/j. cursur.2005.04.018.

160. Kaefer M, Zurakowski D, Bauer S et al. Estimating normal bladder capacity in children. *J Urol.* 1997;158(6):2261-2264. doi:10.1016/s0022-5347(01)68230-2.

161. Kang O, et al. Cervical thymus. Radiopaedia. https:// radiopaedia.org/articles/cervical-thymus?lang=us.

162. Kapoor A, Kapoor A, Mahajan G, Sidhu B, Lakhanpal V. Real-Time elastography in differentiating metastatic from nonmetastatic liver nodules. *Ultrasound Med Biol.* 2011;37(2):207-213. doi:10.1016/j. ultrasmedbio.2010.11.013.

163. Katzenstein HM, Krailo MD, Malogolowkin MH, Ortega JA, Qu W, Douglass EC, Feusner JH, Reynolds M, Quinn JJ, Newman K, Finegold MJ, Haas JE, Sensel MG, Castleberry RP, Bowman LC. Fibrolamellar hepatocellular carcinoma in children and adolescents. Cancer. 2003 Apr 15;97(8):2006-12. doi: 10.1002/cncr.11292. PMID: 12673731.

164. Kaur P, Panneerselvam D. Bicornuate uterus. [Updated 2022 May 1]. In: StatPearls [Internet]. Treasure Island (FL): StatPearls Publishing; 2022 Jan. Available from: https://www.ncbi.nlm.nih.gov/books/NBK560859/.

165. Kawamura D, Lunsford B. *Diagnostic Medical Sonography: Abdomen and Superficial Structures.* 3rd ed. Philadelphia, PA: Lippincott Williams and Wilkins; 2012.

166. Kawamura, D. M. (1992). Gastrointestinal tract. In *Abdomen* (pp. 475-488). Philadelphia, PA: Lippincott Williams & Wilkins.

167. Kazez A, Ozel S, Kocakoc E, Kiris A. Double intussusception in a child. *J Ultrasound Med.* 2004;23(12):1659-1661. doi:10.7863/jum.2004.23.12.1659.

168. Keclar-Pietrzyk A, et al. Normal kidney size in children. Radiopaedia. https://radiopaedia.org/articles/normal-kidney-size-in-children?lang=us.

169. Keeton PI, Schlindwein FS. Spectral broadening of clinical Doppler signals using FFT and autoregressive modelling. Eur J Ultrasound. 1998 Aug;7(3):209-18. doi: 10.1016/s0929-8266(98)00032-9. PMID: 9700218.

170. Khosa F, Otero HJ, Prevedello LM, Rybicki FJ, Di Salvo DN. Imaging Presentation of Venous Thrombosis in Patients With Cancer. *American Journal of Roentgenology.* 2010;194(4):1099-1108. doi:10.2214/ajr.09.2501

171. Kim, J. H. (2004, September 30). US features of transient small bowel intussusception in pediatric patients. Retrieved from https://www.ncbi.nlm.nih.gov/pmc/articles/PMC2698160/

172. Knipe H, et al. WHO grading system for diffuse astrocytomas. Radiopaedia. https://radiopaedia.org/articles/who-grading-system-for-diffuse-astrocytomas?lang=us.

173. Kraus, S. (2017, May). General pediatric radiology: abdomen pediatric fluoroscopy: tips & tricks. *2017 Annual Meeting & Categorical Course.* Symposium conducted at The Society for Pediatric Radiology (SPR), Vancouver. Retrieved from https://www.pedrad.org/LinkClick.aspx?fileticket=dqJqagdH0t8%3D&portalid=5

174. Kremkau FW. Principles of Spectral Doppler. *Journal for Vascular Ultrasound.* 2011;35(4):214-228. doi:10.1177/154431671103500405

175. Laquerre J. Intussusception: Sonographic Findings to Fluoroscopic Reduction in Pediatrics. Radiol Technol. 2020 Mar;91(4):380-384. PMID: 32102864.

176. Laquerre J. Hydronephrosis: Diagnosis, Grading, and Treatment. Radiol Technol. 2020 Nov;92(2):135-151. PMID: 33203770.

177. Lall N, Al Kabbani A. Filar cyst. Radiopaedia.org. https://doi.org/10.53347/rID-62948.

178. Lazebnik R. Neonatal cranial sonography: modern strategies and applications. *Diag Imaging: Continuing Med Educ.* 2007:1-6.

179. Lee, P.J. Glycogen storage disease type I: pathophysiology of liver adenomas. *Eur J Pediatr* 161, S46–S49 (2002). https://doi.org/10.1007/BF02679993

180. Leong L. Ultrasound of living donor liver transplantation. *Biomed Imaging Interv J.* 2006;2(2):e17. doi:10.2349/biij.2.2.e17

181. Li Y, Chetty S, Feldstein VA, Glenn OA. Bilateral Choroid Plexus Papillomas Diagnosed by Prenatal Ultrasound and MRI. *Cureus.* March 2021. doi:10.7759/cureus.13737

182. Li Y, Liu S, Xun F, Liu Z, Huang X. Use of Transcranial Doppler Ultrasound for Diagnosis of Brain Death in Patients with Severe Cerebral Injury. *Med Sci Monit.* 2016;22:1910-1915. Published 2016 Jun 6. doi:10.12659/msm.899036

183. Li Y, Pawel BR, Hill DA, Epstein JI, Argani P. Pediatric Cystic Nephroma Is Morphologically, Immunohistochemically, and Genetically Distinct From Adult Cystic Nephroma. *Am J Surg Pathol.* 2017;41(4):472-481. doi:10.1097/PAS.0000000000000816

184. Lindholm EB, Meckmongkol T, Feinberg AJ, et al. Standardization of common bile duct size using ultrasound in pediatric patients. J Pediatr Surg. 2019 Jun;54(6):1123-1126.

185. Lioubashevsky N, Hiller N, Rozovsky K, Segev L, Simanovsky N. Ileocolic versus Small-Bowel Intussusception in Children: Can US Enable Reliable Differentiation? *Radiology.* 2013;269(1):266-271. doi:10.1148/radiol.13122639

186. Lockhart ME, Sheldon HI, Robbin ML. Augmentation in lower extremity sonography for the detection of deep venous thrombosis. *Am J Roentgenol.* 2005;184:419-422. https://www.ajronline.org/doi/full/10.2214/ajr.184.2.01840419.

187. Lowe L, Isuani B, Heller R et al. Pediatric renal masses: Wilms tumor and beyond. *RadioGraphics.* 2000;20(6):1585-1603. doi:10.1148/radiographics.20.6.g00nv051585.

188. Lowe LH, Johanek AJ, Moore CW. Sonography of the neonatal spine: part 1, normal anatomy, imaging pitfalls, and variations that may simulate disorders. Am J Roentgenology 2007 188:3, 733-738.

189. Luna J. Pseudosinus tract. Radiopaedia.org. https://doi.org/10.53347/rID-94642. Lunsford B, Kawamura D. *Workbook for Diagnostic Medical Sonography.* 1st ed. Philadelphia, PA: Wolters Kluwer/Lippincott Williams & Wilkins; 2012.

190. MacKenzie MA, Hermus AR, Wollersheim HC, Pieters GF, Smals AG, Binkhorst RA, Thien T, Kloppenborg PW. Poikilothermia in man: pathophysiology and clinical implications. Medicine (Baltimore). 1991 Jul;70(4):257-68. doi: 10.1097/00005792-199107000-00003. PMID: 2067410.

191. Malav I, Kothari S. Renal artery stenosis due to neurofibromatosis. *Ann Pediatr Cardiol.* 2017;2(2):167-169. doi:10.4103/0974-2069.58323.

192. Massicot R, Rousseau V, Darwish A, Sauvat F, Jaubert F, Nihoul-Fékété C. Serous and seromucinous infantile ovarian cystadenomas—a study of 42 cases. *Eur J Obstetr Gynecol.* 2009;142(1):64-67. doi:10.1016/j.ejogrb.2008.09.007.

193. Mayo Clinic. (2018, November 6). Intussusception. Retrieved from https://www.mayoclinic.org/diseases-conditions/intussusception/diagnosis-treatment/drc-20351457

194. McCollough M, Sharieff GQ. Abdominal surgical emergencies in infants and young children. Emerg Med Clin North Am. 2003 Nov;21(4):909-35. doi: 10.1016/s0733-8627(03)00090-7. PMID: 14708813.

195. McGahan JP, Phillips HE, Cox KL. Sonography of the normal pediatric gallbladder and biliary tract. Radiology. 1982; 144(4):873-875.

196. Mendoza E, Lattimer C, Morrison N. *Duplex Ultrasound of Superficial Leg Veins.* 1st ed. New York: Springer; 2014.

197. Mercer CA, Long WN, Thompson JD. Uterine unification: indications and technique. Clin Obstet Gynecol. 1981 Dec;24(4):1199-216.

198. Mihmanli I, Kantarci F, Kulaksizoglu H, Gurses B, Ogut G, Unluer E, et al.. Testicular size and vascular resistance before and after hydrocelectomy. AJR. 2004;183:1379-1385

199. Milošević D, Trkulja V, Turudić D, Batinić D, Spajić B, Tešović G. Ultrasound bladder wall thickness measurement in diagnosis of recurrent urinary tract infections and cystitis cystica in prepubertal girls. *J Pediatr Urol.* 2013;9(6):1170-1177. doi:10.1016/j.jpurol.2013.04.019.

200. Mohseni M, Kruse BT, Graham C. Splenic torsion: a rare cause of abdominal pain. *BMJ Case Reports*. 2018. doi:10.1136/bcr-2018-224952

201. Morgan M, Carroll, D. Bladder wall thickening (differential). Radiopaedia.org. https://doi.org/10.53347/rID-32648.

202. Morgan M, et al. Autosomal recessive polycystic kidney disease. Radiopaedia. https://radiopaedia.org/articles/autosomal-recessive-polycystic-kidney-disease?lang=us.

203. Morgan M, Jha P, et al. Renal lymphoma. Radiopaedia. https://radiopaedia.org/articles/renal-lymphoma?lang=us.

204. Moriarity J, et. al. ACR Appropriateness Criteria imaging in the diagnosis of thoracic outlet syndrome. *J Am Coll Radiol*. 2006;12(5):438-443, doi: 10.1016/j.jacr.2015.01.016.

205. Muir M, Hrynkow P, Chase R, Boyce D, Mclean D. The Nature, Cause, and Extent of Occupational

206. Musculoskeletal Injuries among Sonographers: Recommendations for Treatment and Prevention. Journal of Diagnostic Medical Sonography 2004;20(5):317-325.

207. Mutaz I Sultan, MBChB, MD. Pediatric Caroli Disease. *Medscape Reference*. July 2016; http://emedicine.medscape.com/article/927248-overview.

208. Muzio B, Knipe H, et al. Adrenal cyst. Radiopaedia. https://radiopaedia.org/articles/adrenal-cyst?lang=us.

209. Nasseri F, Eftekhari F. Clinical and radiologic review of the normal and abnormal thymus: pearls and pitfalls. *RadioGraphics*. 2010;30(2):413-428. doi:10.1148/rg.302095131.

210. Neonatal cranial ultrasonography. (2016). Diagnostic Pediatric Ultrasound. https://doi.org/10.1055/b-0035-122519.

211. Nephronophthisis. MedlinePlus. https://medlineplus.gov/genetics/condition/nephronophthisis/. Published August 18, 2020. Accessed July 3, 2021.

212. Neuroblastoma. Cleveland Clinic. https://my.clevelandclinic.org/health/diseases/14390-neuroblastoma. Published December 14, 2020.

213. *Neurocutaneous syndrome*. University of Florida Department of Neurology. (n.d.). Retrieved from https://neurology.ufl.edu/divisions/neurofibromatosis-center/neurocutaneous-syndrome/

214. Neurofibromas. Johns Hopkins Medicine. https://www.hopkinsmedicine.org/health/conditions-and-diseases/neurofibromas. Published 2021.

215. Nickerson J, Richner B, Santy K et al. Neuroimaging of pediatric intracranial infection-part 1: techniques and bacterial infections. *J Neuroimaging*. 2012;22(2):e42-e51. doi:10.1111/j.1552-6569.2011.00700.x.

216. Niknejad M, Amini B, et al. Renal angiomyolipoma. Radiopaedia. https://radiopaedia.org/articles/renal-angiomyolipoma?lang=us.

217. Niknejad M, et al. Cystic fibrosis. Radiopaedia. https://radiopaedia.org/articles/cystic-fibrosis?lang=us.

218. Niknejad MT, et al. Pancreatic pseudocyst. Radiopaedia. https://radiopaedia.org/articles/pancreatic-pseudocyst-1?lang=us.

219. Obrycki, Ł., Sarnecki, J., Lichosik, M. *et al.* Kidney length normative values in children aged 0–19 years — a multicenter study. *Pediatr Nephrol* (2021). https://doi.org/10.1007/s00467-021-05303-5

220. Oh L, Fahrenhorst-Jones T. Common bile duct. *Radiopaedia.org*. https://doi.org/10.53347/rID-24814.

221. Oleszkowicz S, Chittick P, Russo V, Keller P, Sims M, Band J. Infections associated with use of ultrasound transmission gel: proposed guidelines to minimize risk. *Infect Control Hosp Epidemiol*. 2012;33(12):1235-1237. doi:10.1086/668430.

222. Onur M, Poyraz A, Ucak E, Bozgeyik Z, Özercan I, Ogur E. Semiquantitative strain elastography of liver masses. *J Ultrasound Med*. 2012;31(7):1061-1067. doi:10.7863/jum.2012.31.7.1061.

223. Pacharn P, Ying J, Linam L, Brody A, Babcock D. Sonography in the evaluation of acute appendicitis. *J Ultrasound Med*. 2010;29(12):1749-1755. doi:10.7863/jum.2010.29.12.1749.

224. Pacifico L. Pediatric nonalcoholic fatty liver disease: a clinical and laboratory challenge. *World J Hepatol*. 2010;2(7):275. doi:10.4254/wjh.v2.i7.275.

225. Papic J, Billmire D, Rescorla F, Finell S, Leys C. Management of neonatal ovarian cysts and its effect on ovarian preservation. *J Pediatr Surg*. 2014;49(6):990-994. doi:10.1016/j.jpedsurg.2014.01.040.

226. Parasuraman, S. Venous Thromboembolism in Children. Jaffray, J. Impact of Central Venous Catheters on Pediatric VTE

227. Parente F. Bowel ultrasound in assessment of Crohn's disease and detection of related small bowel strictures: a prospective comparative study versus x ray and intraoperative findings. *Gut*. 2002;50(4):490-495. doi:10.1136/gut.50.4.490.

228. Patil H, Rege S. Bilateral giant open-lip schizencephaly: a rare case report. *J Pediatr Neurosci*. 2016;11(2):128. doi:10.4103/1817-1745.187638.

229. Patino M, Munden M. Utility of the sonographic whirlpool sign in diagnosing midgut volvulus in patients with atypical clinical presentations. *J Ultrasound Med*. 2004;23(3):397-401. doi:10.7863/jum.2004.23.3.397.

230. Pediatric Follicular Thyroid Cancer. Children's Health Texas. https://www.childrens.com/specialties-services/conditions/follicular-thyroid-cancer.

231. Pediatric Radiology Normal Measurements. Oregon Health & Science University (OSHU). (2001). Retrieved from https://www.ohsu.edu/school-of-medicine/diagnostic-radiology/pediatric-radiology-normal-measurements.

232. Perlman S, Hertweck P, Fallat M. Paratubal and tubal abnormalities. *Semin Pediatr Surg*. 2005;14(2):124-134. doi:10.1053/j.sempedsurg.2005.01.009.

233. Pike I, Russo A, Berkowitz J, Baker J, Lessoway V. The Prevalence of Musculoskeletal Disorders Among Diagnostic Medical Sonographers. Journal of Diagnostic Medical Sonography 1997;13(5):219-227.

234. Pisano U, Morgan M, et al. TIPS evaluation. Radiopaedia. https://radiopaedia.org/articles/tips-evaluation?lang=us.

235. Pomajzl AJ, Leslie SW. Appendix Testes Torsion. [Updated 2022 Feb 14]. In: StatPearls [Internet]. Treasure Island (FL): StatPearls Publishing; 2022 Jan-. Available from: https://www.ncbi.nlm.nih.gov/books/NBK546994/

236. Prabhu V, Peruzzi P. Astrocytoma Tumors. American Association of Neurological Surgeons. https://www.aans.

org/en/Patients/Neurosurgical-Conditions-and-Treatments/Astrocytoma-Tumors. Published 2021.

237. Purkayastha S, Sorond F. Transcranial Doppler ultrasound: technique and application. *Semin Neurol.* 2012;32(04):411-420. doi:10.1055/s-0032-1331812.

238. Quarrie R, Stawicki SP. Portal vein thrombosis: What surgeons need to know. *Int J Crit Illn Inj Sci.* 2018;8(2):73-77. doi:10.4103/IJCIIS.IJCIIS_71_17

239. Radiopaedia. (n.d.). Radiopaedia.org, the wiki-based collaborative Radiology resource. Retrieved from https://radiopaedia.org

240. Radiological Society of North America (RSNA). (2018, February 14). Therapeutic enema for intussusception. Retrieved from https://www.radiologyinfo.org/en/info.cfm?pg=intussusception

241. Radiological Society of North America and American College of Radiology. (2020). *Thyroid ultrasound.* RadiologyInfo.org. https://www.radiologyinfo.org/en/info.cfm?pg=us-thyroid

242. Radiological Society of North America (RSNA) and American College of Radiology (ACR). (2019, March 5). *Transjugular Intrahepatic Portosystemic shunt.* RadiologyInfo.org. https://www.radiologyinfo.org/en/info.cfm?pg=tips

243. Radswiki T, Al Kabbani A. Ventriculus terminalis. Radiopaedia.org. https://doi.org/10.53347/rID-12435.

244. Rasuli B, et al. Hepatoblastoma. Radiopaedia. https://radiopaedia.org/articles/hepatoblastoma?lang=us.

245. Rasuli B, et al. Normal hepatic vein Doppler. Radiopaedia. https://radiopaedia.org/articles/normal-hepatic-vein-doppler?lang=us.

246. Rasuli B, et al. Obstructive hydrocephalus. Radiopaedia. https://radiopaedia.org/articles/obstructive-hydrocephalus?lang=us.

247. Rasuli B, St-Amant M, et al. Pulmonary sequestration (extralobar). Radiopaedia. https://radiopaedia.org/articles/pulmonary-sequestration-extralobar?lang=us.

248. Rasuli B. Pancreatoblastoma. Radiopaedia. https://radiopaedia.org/articles/pancreatoblastoma?lang=us.

249. Reddy AS, Shah RS, Kulkarni DR. Laparoscopic Ladd'S Procedure in Children: Challenges, Results, and Problems. *J Indian Assoc Pediatr Surg.* 2018;23(2):61-65. doi:10.4103/jiaps.JIAPS_126_17

250. Rescorla F. Pediatric germ cell tumors. *Semin Pediatr Surg.* 2012;21(1):51-60. doi:10.1053/j.sempedsurg.2011.10.005.

251. Reuter-Rice K. Transcranial Doppler Ultrasound Use in Pediatric Traumatic Brain Injury. J Radiol Nurs. 2017;36(1):3-9. doi:10.1016/j.jradnu.2016.11.003

252. Richter G, Friedman A. Hemangiomas and vascular malformations: current theory and management. *Int J Pediatr.* 2012;2012(645678). doi:10.1155/2012/645678.

253. Rios S, Pereira L, Santos C, Chen A, Chen J, Vogt M. Conservative treatment and follow-up of vaginal Gartner's duct cysts: a case series. *J Med Case Rep.* 2016;10(1). doi:10.1186/s13256-016-0936-1.

254. Riccabona M. Basics, principles, techniques and modern methods in paediatric ultrasonography. *Eur J Radiol.* 2014;83(9):1485-1494. doi:10.1016/j.ejrad.2014.04.032.

255. Robbins JB, Broadwell C, Chow LC, Parry JP, Sadowski EA. Müllerian duct anomalies: embryological development, classification, and MRI assessment. J Magn Reson Imaging. 2015;41: 1-12. https://doi.org/10.1002/jmri.24771.

256. Robertson WB. Uteroplacental vasculature. *Journal of Clinical Pathology.* 1976;s3-10(1):9-17. doi:10.1136/jcp.s3-10.1.9

257. Rohanachandra Y, Dahanayake D, Wijetunge S. Dandy-Walker malformation presenting with psychological manifestations. *Case Rep Psychiatry.* 2016;2016(9104306):1-4. doi:10.1155/2016/9104306.

258. Rosenbaum DM, Korngold E, Teele RL. Sonographic assessment of renal length in normal children. *American Journal of Roentgenology.* 1984;142(3):467-469. doi:10.2214/ajr.142.3.467

259. Rosenfield R. The polycystic ovary morphology-polycystic ovary syndrome spectrum. *J Pediatr Adolesc Gynecol.* 2015;28(6):412-419. doi:10.1016/j.jpag.2014.07.016.

260. Rumack C, Wilson S, Charboneau C. *Diagnostic Ultrasound.* Vol. 1. 3rd ed. St. Louis, Mo: Elsevier; 2005.

261. Rumack C, Wilson S, Charboneau J, Levine D. *Diagnostic Ultrasound.* 4th ed. Philadelphia, PA: Elsevier; 2011.

262. Saber M, D'Souza D, et al. False aneurysm. Radiopaedia. https://radiopaedia.org/articles/false-aneurysm?lang=us.

263. Saber M, et al. Mullerian duct anomaly classification. Radiopaedia. https://radiopaedia.org/articles/mullerian-duct-anomaly-classification?lang=us.

264. Saber M, Jha P, et al. Cryptorchidism. Radiopaedia. https://radiopaedia.org/articles/cryptorchidism?lang=us.

265. Saber M, Weerakkody Y, et al. Spina bifida. Radiopaedia. https://radiopaedia.org/articles/spina-bifida?lang=us.

266. Saigal G, Therrien JR, Kuo F. Ultrasound in pediatric emergencies. Appl Radiol. 2014;43(8):6-16. Available at link.gale.com/apps/doc/A381588161/AONE?u=anon~2892c6ba&sid=googleScholar&xid=2e9d5d02 (accessed March 5, 2022).

267. Saksouk F, Johnson S. Lower genitourinary tract imaging recognition of the ovaries and ovarian origin of pelvic masses with CT. *RadioGraphics.* 2004;24(1):133-146. doi:10.1148/rg.24si045507.

268. Sarwal A, Walker F, Cartwright M. Neuromuscular ultrasound for evaluation of the diaphragm. Notes: *Muscle & Nerve.* 2013;47(3):319-329. doi:10.1002/mus.23671.

269. Safak A, Simsek E, Bahcebasi T. Sonographic assessment of the normal limits and percentile curves of liver, spleen, and kidney dimensions in healthy school-aged children. *J Ultrasound Med.* 2005;24(10):1359-1364. doi:10.7863/jum.2005.24.10.1359.

270. Schneider D, Orbach D, Cecchetto G et al. Ovarian sertoli leydig cell tumours in children and adolescents: an analysis of the european cooperative study group on pediatric rare tumors (Expert). *Eur J Cancer.* 2015;51(4):543-550. doi:10.1016/j.ejca.2014.11.013.

271. Shah V, et al. Bochdalek hernia features (mnemonic). Radiopaedia. https://radiopaedia.org/articles/bochdalek-hernia-features-mnemonic?lang=us.

272. Seliga-Siwecka J, Rutkowski J, Margas W, Puskarz-Gąsowska J, Bokiniec R. Sensitivity and specificity of different imaging modalities in diagnosing necrotising enterocolitis in a Polish population of preterm infants: a diagnostic test accuracy study protocol. BMJ Open. 2020

Jul 20;10(7):e033519. doi: 10.1136/bmjopen-2019-033519. PMID: 32690727; PMCID: PMC7375631.

273. Sendic G. Pancreas histology. Kenhub. Published 2022, July 22. Retrieved from https://www.kenhub.com/en/library/anatomy/pancreas-histology.

274. Shamshirsaz A, Ravangard S, Egan J et al. Fetal hydronephrosis as a predictor of neonatal urologic outcomes. *J Ultrasound Med.* 2012;31(6):947-954. doi:10.7863/jum.2012.31.6.947.

275. Sharecare, Inc. (n.d.). What are the benefits of a child life specialist for my child? Retrieved from https://www.sharecare.com/health/kids-teens-health/what-benefits-child-life-specialist

276. Shibchurn M. Type 1 lissencephaly and multiple afebrile seizures in a 2-month-old baby. *J Pediatr Neurosci.* 2015;10(2):123. doi:10.4103/1817-1745.159198.

277. Shin, J., Jones, J. Wall-echo-shadow sign (ultrasound). Reference article, Radiopaedia.org. (accessed on 14 Apr 2022) https://doi.org/10.53347/rID-21822

278. Shorter NA, Glick RD, Klimstra DS, et al. Malignant pancreatic tumors in childhood and adolescence: The Memorial Sloan-Kettering experience, 1967 to present. J Pediatr Surg. 2002;37:887–892

279. Siegel M. *Pediatric Sonography.* 4th ed. Philadelphia: Wolters Kluwer health/Lippincott Williams & Wilkins; 2011.

280. Siegel M, Martin K, Worthington J. Normal and abnormal pancreas in children: US studies. *Radiology.* 1987;165(1):15-18. doi:10.1148/radiology.165.1.3306783.

281. Sodhi K, Gupta P, Saxena A, Khandelwal N, Singhi P. Neonatal cranial sonography: a concise review for clinicians. *J Pediatr Neurosci.* 2016;11(1):7-13. doi:10.4103/1817-1745.181261.

282. Sohn Y, Kim M, Kim E, Kwak J, Moon H, Kim S. Sonographic elastography combined with conventional sonography: how much is it helpful for diagnostic performance? *J Ultrasound Med.* 2009;28(4):413-420. doi:10.7863/jum.2009.28.4.413.

283. Sotos JF, Tokar NJ. Appraisal of testicular volumes: volumes matching ultrasound values referenced to stages of genital development [published correction appears in Int J Pediatr Endocrinol. 2017;2017:10]. *Int J Pediatr Endocrinol.* 2017;2017:7. doi:10.1186/s13633-017-0046-x

284. Souza D. Central Tendon of Diaphragm. AnatomyZone. https://anatomyzone.com/articles/central-tendon-diaphragm/. Published December 13, 2020.

285. Spada M, Riva S, Maggiore G, Cintorino D, Gridelli B. Pediatric liver transplantation. *World J Gastroenterol.* 2009;15(6):648-674. doi:10.3748/wjg.15.648.

286. Stanescu A, Hryhorczok A, Chang P, Lee E, Phillips G. Pediatric abdominal organ transplantation: current indications, techniques, and imaging finding. *Radiol Clin North Am.* 2016;54(2):281-302. doi:10.1016/j.rcl.2015.09.011.

287. Stanislavsky A, Bell D. Dot dash pattern (ovarian dermoid cyst). Radiopaedia.org. https://doi.org/10.53347/rID-19029.

288. Stenczel ND, Purcarea MR, Tribus LC, Oniga GH. The role of the intestinal ultrasound in Crohn's disease diagnosis and monitoring. J Med Life. 2021

289. Stevenson D, Benitz W, Sunshine P. *Fetal and Neonatal Brain Injury: Mechanisms, Management, and the Risks of Practice.* 3rd ed. New York: Cambridge University Press; 2003.

290. Stocksley M. *Abdominal Ultrasound.* 1st ed. New York, NY: Cambridge University Press; 2001.

291. Walsh B. Health-care facility recommendations for standard precautions. 2006. Available at: http://www.who.int/csr/resources/publications/4EPR_AM2.pdf. Accessed March 20, 2021.

292. Stringer MD, Alizai NK. Mesenchymal hamartoma of the liver: a systematic review. J Pediatr Surg. 2005 Nov;40(11):1681-1690.

293. Takuma K, Kamisawa T, Tabata T, Egawa N, Igarashi Y. Pancreatic diseases associated with pancreas divisum. *Dig Surg.* 2010;27(2):144-148. doi:10.1159/000286975.

294. The Johns Hopkins Comprehensive Neurofibromatosis Center. (n.d.). *Neurocutaneous syndromes in children.* Johns Hopkins Medicine. Retrieved from https://www.hopkinsmedicine.org/health/conditions-and-diseases/neurocutaneous-syndromes-in-children#:~:text=The%203%20most%20common%20types%20of%20neurocutaneous%20syndromes%20are%20tuberous,condition%20that%20has%20no%20cure.

295. Thibodeau G, Patto K. *Structure and Function of the Body.* 6th ed. Philadelphia: Mosby; 2006.

296. Timor-Tritsch I, Monteagudo A, Pilu G, Malinger G. *Ultrasonography of the Prenatal Brain.* 3rd ed. New York: McGraw-Hill; 2012.

297. Thurston M, et al. Pilocytic astrocytoma of the neurohypophysis. Radiopaedia. https://radiopaedia.org/articles/pilocytic-astrocytoma-of-the-neurohypophysis?lang=us.

298. Thurston M, Radswiki, et al. Testicular cyst. Radiopaedia. https://radiopaedia.org/articles/testicular-cyst?lang=us.

299. Trent M. Pelvic inflammatory disease. *Pediatri Rev.* 2013;34(4):163-172. doi:10.1542/pir.34-4-165.

300. Trenkner SW, Smid AA, Francis IR, Levatter R. Radiological detection and diagnosis of pouch of Douglas lesions. Crit Rev Diagn Imaging. 1988;28(4):367-81. PMID: 3053046.

301. Troiano R, McCarthy S. Müllerian duct anomalies: imaging and clinical issues. *Radiology.* 2004;233(1):19-34. doi:10.1148/radiol.2331020777.

302. Tubbs R, Krishnamurthy S, Verma K et al. Cavum velum interpositum, cavum septum pellucidum, and cavum vergae: a review. *Childs Nerv Sys.* 2011;27(11):1927. doi:10.1007/s00381-011-1457-2.

303. Tublin M, Squires J. Adrenal Cyst. Adrenal cyst. https://www.sciencedirect.com/topics/medicine-and-dentistry/adrenal-cyst. Published 2018.

304. Tuli G, Munarin J, Tessaris D, Buganza R, Matarazzo P, De Sanctis L. Primary hyperparathyroidism (PHPT) in children: two case reports and review of the literature. Case Rep Endocrinol. 2021 Apr 13;2021:5539349.

305. Vadera S, et al. Uretrocele. Radiopaedia. https://radiopaedia.org/articles/ureterocele-1?lang=us.

306. VanDreel A, Sutherland J, Henkle G, Wilczysnki M. Lipomyelocele in newborn. *Appl Radiol.* 2016;45(11):53-54.

May-Jun;14(3):310-315. doi: 10.25122/jml-2021-0067. PMID: 34377195; PMCID: PMC8321617.

307. Vascular Technology Professional Performance Guidelines: Transcranial Doppler in pediatric patients with sickle cell anemia (non-imaging). Lanham, MD: Society of Vascular Ultrasound; 2012

308. Vattoth S, Kim Y, Norman E, Roberson G. Spontaneous resolution of cavum veli interpositi. *Neuroradiol J.* 2008;21(6):805-809. doi:10.1177/197140090802100609.

309. Venous Malformation. Stanford Children's Health. https://www.stanfordchildrens.org/en/service/dermatology/vascular-anomalies/venous-malformation.

310. Verma A, Chauhan RS, Singh DK, Guha B, Kumar I. Multimodality imaging of vaginal rhabdomyosarcoma. *Indian Journal of Radiology and Imaging.* 2017;27(2):148-151. doi:10.4103/ijri.ijri_444_16

311. Vural F, Sanverdi I, Coskun A, Kusgoz A, Temel O. Large nabothian cyst obstructing labour passage. *J Clin Diagn Res.* 2015;9(10):QD06-QD07. doi:10.7860/jcdr/2015/15191.6630.

312. Vossen S, Goretzki PE, Goebel U, et al. Therapeutic management of rare malignant pancreatic tumors in children. World J Surg. 1998;22:879–882

313. Walsh B, Czervinske M, DiBlasi R. *Perinatal and Pediatric Respiratory Care.* 3rd ed. St. Louis, MO: Saunders; 2010.

314. Walsh B. Health-care facility recommendations for standard precautions. 2006. Available at: http://www.who.int/csr/resources/publications/4EPR_AM2.pdf. Accessed August 31, 2015.

315. Weerakkody Y, Bell D. Parathyroid adenoma. Radiopaedia.org. https://doi.org/10.53347/rID-23949.

316. Weerakkody Y, et al. Diffuse astrocytoma. Radiopaedia. https://radiopaedia.org/articles/diffuse-astrocytoma-1?lang=us.

317. Weerakkody Y, et al. Pelviureteric junction obstruction. Radiopaedia. https://radiopaedia.org/articles/pelviureteric-junction-obstruction-1?lang=us. \

318. Weerakkody, Y., Worsley, C. Necrotizing enterocolitis. Reference article, Radiopaedia.org. https://doi.org/10.53347/rID-7658

319. Weinblatt ME, Ortega JA. Treatment of children with dysgerminoma of the ovary. Cancer. 1982 Jun 15;49(12):2608-11. doi: 10.1002/1097-0142(19820615)49:12<2608::aid-cncr2820491233>3.0.co;2-0. PMID: 7074578.

320. Willeput R, Rondeux C, De Troyer A. Breathing affects venous return from legs in humans. J Appl Physiol Respir Environ Exerc Physiol. 1984 Oct;57(4):971-6. doi: 10.1152/jappl.1984.57.4.971. PMID: 6238925.

321. Wilson S, Burns P. Microbubble-enhanced US in body imaging: what role? *Radiology.* 2010;257(1):1-16. doi:10.1148/radiol.10091210.

322. Wingerd B. *The Human Body: Concepts of Anatomy and Physiology.* 3rd ed. Philadelphia, PA: Lippincott Williams and Wilkins; 2013.

323. Wood M, Romine L, Lee Y et al. Spectral doppler signature waveforms in ultrasonography. *Ultrasound Q.* 2010;26(2):83-99. doi:10.1097/ruq.0b013e3181dcbf67.

324. World Health Organization. Diagnostic imaging: ultrasound. Accessed 13 July 2020. http://www.who.int/diagnostic_imaging/imaging_modalities/dim_ultrasound/en/.

325. Xie L. Real-time elastography for diagnosis of liver fibrosis in chronic hepatitis B. *J Ultrasound Med.* 2012;31(7):1053-1067.

326. Yang N, Rasuli B. Unicornuate uterus. Reference article, Radiopaedia.org. https://doi.org/10.53347/rID-6979.

327. Yekeler E, Tambag A, Tunaci A et al. Analysis of the thymus in 151 healthy infants from 0 to 2 years of age. *J Ultrasound Med.* 2004;23(10):1321-1326. doi:10.7863/jum.2004.23.10.1321.

328. Yildiz A, Ariyurek M, Karcaaltincaba M. Splenic anomalies of shape, size, and location: pictorial essay. *The Sci World J.* 2013;2013:1-9. doi:10.1155/2013/321810.

329. Yikilmaz, A., Taylor, G.A. Sonographic findings in bacterial meningitis in neonates and young infants. *Pediatr Radiol* 38, 129–137 (2008). https://doi.org/10.1007/s00247-007-0538-6

330. Zamora C, Sams C, Cornea EA, Yuan Z, Smith JK, Gilmore JH. Subdural Hemorrhage in Asymptomatic Neonates: Neurodevelopmental Outcomes and MRI Findings at 2 Years. *Radiology.* 2020;298(1):173-179. doi:10.1148/radiol.2020201857

331. Zayek M, Benjamin J, Maertens P, Trimm R, Lal C, Eyal F. Cerebellar hemorrhage: a major morbidity in extremely preterm infants. *J Perinatol.* 2011;32(9):699-704. doi:10.1038/jp.2011.185.

332. Zivadinov, R., Chung, C. Potential involvement of the extracranial venous system in central nervous system disorders and aging. *BMC Med* 11, 260 (2013). https://doi.org/10.1186/1741-7015-11-260

Index

Note: Page locators followed by *f* and *t* indicate figures and tables, respectively.